BELLY FAT EFFECT

THE REAL SECRET ABOUT HOW YOUR DIET, INTESTINAL HEALTH, AND GUT BACTERIA HELP YOU BURN FAT

BY MIKE MUTZEL, MSC

WILSONVILLE MEDIA
OREGON

Belly Fat Effect

ISBN: 978-0-9910703-1-2

Library of Congress Control Number: 2013952470

Published by:

Wilsonville Media:
info@wilsonvillemedia.com
www.wilsonvillemedia.com

Connect with the author:
MikeMutzel.com
twitter.com/MikeMutzel
facebook.com/MikeMutzelMS

CONTENTS

BY DAVID PERLMUTTER, MD

If you were to ask people why they want to lose weight, most commonly you would hear that they just want to "look better." But excess weight, especially the type of fat that accumulates in the belly, represents a far more sinister event in human physiology than simply a cosmetic change. While body fat does indeed represent a depot of calories, it has now been shown to be a far more active player in human health than we ever imagined. Body fat itself regulates metabolism, hunger, and brain activity and even enhances the production of chemical mediators of inflammation. This likely explains why excess poundage directly relates to increasing a person's chances for just about every medical problem they don't want to have, including heart disease, cancer, diabetes, Alzheimer's disease, arthritis, and osteoporosis.

Ours is a country where being overfed while being undernourished has become the norm. Hardly a week goes by without a new diet being popularized in the media as a surefire way to drop excess pounds. And what remains a common theme—not only in the countless diet books that flood bookstores but also in the many commercial weight-loss institutions—is the notion that if we can just cut the fat and reduce our calories, we will be rewarded by aggressive and long-lasting weight loss.

But this approach to weight loss is flawed on two counts: First, this mentality is not in any way consistent with current leading-edge research. Second, the recommendation to eat low fat leads to an increased consumption of carbohydrates and a diet completely unlike what humans have ever consumed for more than 99% of the time we have existed on this planet.

In *Belly Fat Effect*, Mike Mutzel deftly presents the science that reveals how and why body fat is created and stored. He explores the fundamentals of the role of the hormone insulin in this process. Insulin signaling, by stimulating the production of life-sustaining fat, has been responsible for human survival for hundreds of thousands of years. Were it not for this adaptation, our species would have perished during times of food scarcity. The painful irony is that this very same hormonal pathway plays the leading role in the global epidemic of obesity during the current times of caloric abundance.

In the pages that follow, Mike presents the fundamentals of the compelling science related to fat—its genesis and storage. More importantly, you will be empowered by the actionable, user-friendly information that is based on this science to make substantial changes in your lifestyle choices. And these changes will pave the way for you to redirect your health destiny and ensure a longer and healthier life.

A NEW LOOK AT A GROWING PROBLEM

This book is going to change the way you look at your metabolism. Every aspect of storing, utilizing, and burning fat, protein, and sugar will be examined from the vantage point of metabolism, a perspective that has been largely unrecognized until recently. The origins of obesity-related problems are metabolic in nature and stem from imbalances in our intestinal bacteria which in turn lead to an overactive immune system. These bacteria are highly malleable.[1] Diets rich in fiber and colored fruits and vegetables foster a microbial milieu that favors fat burning.[2,3] In contrast, poor food choices initiate a cascade of events that lead to inflammation and disturbances in blood sugar and fat metabolism, precursors to obesity, insulin resistance, cardiovascular disease, and diabetes.[4,5,6]

The millions of bacteria residing in our intestines lie at the interface between two integrated bodily systems—the metabolic and the immune—that simultaneously go awry as the pounds accumulate.[7,8] You can think of the relationship between these two seemingly detached yet highly amalgamated systems as being like our government's economic and defense systems. When the bad guys threaten us, our country spends more money to bolster its defenses. If your diet leads to a proliferation of bad-guy bacteria, your body must reallocate cellular energy to combat the harmful organisms.

This defense mechanism comes at a hefty price.[9] Immune cells congregate in areas of the body that are vital to metabolism, such as the liver and fat tissue, where they pivot metabolism away from fat burning in favor of sugar burning.[10,11,12] The result is low-grade inflammation and insulin resistance, leading to obesity and eventually chronic disease.[13] Keep this national defense analogy in mind while I share with you why I've dedicated years of my life to researching and writing this book.

THE FAT PROBLEM

The obesity epidemic is hard to ignore. The media regularly features stories about some aspect of our national weight-control problem and the American Medical Association recently classified obesity as a disease. More than 35 percent of American adults and nearly 17 percent of children are obese and, therefore, at greater risk of heart disease and type 2 diabetes.[14,15] Obesity is having a body mass index (BMI) of 30 or higher. One is considered overweight when their BMI is between 25 and 30. About 68 percent of Americans aged twenty and older fall into either the overweight or obese camp because they weigh more than is ideal for optimal health.[16]

Not only do those extra pounds impact health, but they can also lead to boundless labeling and stereotyping. Obesity creates an environment where physical disease and emotional difficulties flourish.

Admittedly, I was in this camp of discriminators. Prior to working one-on-one with overweight people, many of whom also had diabetes, my view of obesity was ignorant and inaccurate. Overweight people are lazy and unmotivated, I thought. As a fully recovered victim of the "freshman fifteen," I'd ruminate with friends and family over our personal body-weight woes. The conversations always culminated with the same solution: put down the fork and go to the gym.

I made a startling discovery soon after earning my personal trainer certification during my third year in college. As a way to make some extra income, I offered my services as a fitness and weight-loss coach in online ads and at the local YMCA.

Often while sitting knee-to-knee with a person whose abdomen was nearly twice the size of mine, I realized that he or she ate far fewer calories a day than I did. True, I spent several hours strength training and doing aerobic exercise, such as bike racing on the weekends, but I ate more calories than I burned, and still I was lean.

My suspicion that there was more regulating metabolism and fat storage than calorie balance was confirmed a short time after I graduated from college and joined the integrative primary care clinic of Gerard Guillory, MD, in Aurora, Colorado. As a nutritionist and personal trainer in Dr. G's clinic, I counseled and coached clients who were either obese or had diabetes or both. I often asked clients to bring in their grocery store receipts so that we could review exactly what they were eating. Clients kept food diaries too, and if they were married, so did their spouses. In fact, spouses joined in our sessions, which helped keep both parties accountable.

Instead of diary entries loaded with sugar and carbs of the muffin, soda, and cupcake variety, my clients often described a bagel breakfast, modest sandwich lunch, and a dinner of pasta and salad. Although not ideal for many reasons, the diets of many of my clients were on par with the current diabetes prevention recommendations and USDA dietary guidelines.

I still have notes from meetings with overweight women and men who were desperately trying to shed extra pounds. They reported eating mostly cottage cheese, egg whites, apples, a little peanut butter, and some deli meats. Again, maybe not "health nut" perfect, but heck, on most days I ate more than that by 11:00 a.m. While my body fat was about 10 percent, many of these people had over 30 percent body fat. If obesity is an issue of calories in and calories out, how can a 220-pound person eat a steady diet of apples, deli meats, and cottage cheese and not lose weight, even if he or she doesn't exercise every day?

Often the people I counseled had been to weight-loss specialists and had read libraries of diet books, yet they were still overweight. They went to Jenny Craig, hospital dietitians, Weight Watchers, and anyone claiming to have an edge on weight loss. Some even worked out with personal trainers. Yet, they were fat and frustrated. But they were not giving up. They were still willing to do whatever it takes to lose their excess pounds and reign in their out-of-control blood sugar.

OBESITY-LINKED DISEASES

A major driving force behind the impetus to lose weight is prevention of heart disease, the nation's number one killer. Although some of my clients were severely obese, others were overweight and what I call "skinny but fat," meaning they were lean overall but carrying too much belly fat. Central obesity, the medical term for this condition, is as serious a risk factor for cardiovascular disease as being overweight. The majority of these people either had developed or were close to developing *metabolic syndrome*, a cluster of interrelated imbalances in both their metabolic and cardiovascular systems.[17]

Many of the overweight people I saw had at least one if not all of the other defining criteria of metabolic syndrome, which include low blood levels of heart-healthy HDL cholesterol and high levels of glucose, insulin, HgbA1c, triglycerides, and unhealthy LDL cholesterol.

Even in Colorado, one of the healthiest states in the union, poor blood-sugar control—a euphemism for prediabetes or insulin resistance—combined with obesity was rampant when I worked in Dr. G's clinic. And it still is. Not only do people with this problem live at a suboptimal level of vitality, they are also at increased risk for developing coronary artery disease, stroke, and diabetes.

Diabetes and cardiovascular disease are just the tips of the metabolic syndrome iceberg. Many of the overweight patients who I counseled at Dr. G's clinic also suffered from asthma, autoimmune conditions, sleep disturbances, low libido, hormone imbalances, depression, irritable bowel syndrome (IBS), and disabling arthritis and joint issues. Although seemingly unrelated, these conditions are different aspects of the same problem—that is, metabolic and immune dysfunction.

Unless the root cause of these malfunctions is addressed, people must rely on drugs to manage their symptoms. For example, many of the patients who found their way into Dr. G's office were taking sleeping pills for their insomnia, methotrexate for their arthritis, metformin for their blood sugar, statins for their lipids, an antihypertensive drug for their blood pressure, and a laundry list of mood-altering medications. While many of these ailments were ameliorated through Dr. G's comprehensive and integrative medical approach, including balancing thyroid and sex hormones and supplementing with vitamin D, fish oil, and more, clients he referred to me for help with lifestyle changes still had a tough time losing weight.

Despite taking blood-sugar-regulating medicines, patients' glucose levels were out of control, and they had zero energy and morbid levels of body fat. Although the majority of them had been to many medical specialists prior to seeing Dr. G, no healthcare professional or nutritionist had ever properly educated them in the basics of nutrition, exercise, and lifestyle.

When people start to feel better through simple lifestyle changes, they listen and come back to learn more. My clients were some of the most motivated, hardworking, and determined people that I've ever worked with. Their difficulties shedding excess pounds, and ultimately their successes, motivated me to set a new goal for myself: I vowed to summarize a new paradigm that is developing in metabolic research to help others break through weight-loss plateaus, release fat, and prevent chronic disease.

THE DOMINO EFFECT OF OBESITY

Recent reports suggest 145 million people now live with at least one obesity-associated disease, such as diabetes, cancer, heart disease, neurodegenerative disease, and arthritis.[18,19] Chronic conditions are responsible for 70 percent of all deaths in the United States and 75 percent of all healthcare expenditures annually.[20] In developing countries, chronic diseases represent more than half of all diseases and are expected to increase.[21]

In contrast to the infectious diseases Columbus introduced to North America, chronic diseases take years to develop, which is why their prevalence generally increases with age. But now research is revealing that diabetes, heart disease, and obesity develop in children too. Even more alarming is that since the 1980s, there has been an almost 300 percent increase in chronic conditions in children![22]

Today, 30 percent of fifty-year-olds and more than 60 percent of those over sixty-five have at least one chronic disease.[23] Twenty-five percent of Medicare beneficiaries have five or more chronic conditions.

The majority of adults between ages sixty and eighty have hypertension, a cardiovascular risk associated with obesity.[24] Shockingly, this is why life expectancy in the United States fares poorly compared to other industrialized countries.

The United States ranks 29 in the world when it comes to life expectancy at age fifty.[25] That is certainly not a statistic to be proud of! Although collectively Americans spend more than twice as much on healthcare as 19 other industrialized countries, we rank 69 out of 100 when it comes to life expectancy and preventing death.

A NEW ROAD MAP: FUNCTIONAL MEDICINE

The framework that will help us succeed in the tug-of-war over body fat is called *functional medicine*.[26] In general, this approach to health considers all possible contributing causes of disease, including suboptimal and over-nutrition, stress, poor sleep, environmental toxin overload, genetic programming, harmful *epigenetic* influences (environmental influences on genetic expression), gut microflora imbalances, and poor emotional and spiritual health. All these variables influence the "function" of the body, and when it is out of balance, the result is "dis-ease."

While I was working in a clinical setting with overweight people who had chronic diseases, I discovered a series of seemingly disparate health-related complaints that reinforce the biological imbalances that contribute to weight issues. Most metabolically challenged and overweight people have the following in common. They

- are stressed, rating their psychological stress as a 9 out of 10.
- have rampant gastrointestinal disorders. Many of these people take antacids for heartburn and suffer from constipation, diarrhea, belching, bloating, flatulence, and acid reflux.
- have thyroid disorders, especially if they are women.
- follow low-calorie diets.
- skip breakfast and eat their biggest meal at night.
- eat while watching television.

These people suffered from chronic ailments, and instead of more medications, they needed lifestyle and diet coaching to restore core imbalances.[27,28,29]

In contrast to functional medicine, the acute care model of allopathic medicine largely practiced today typically involves prescribing medication or performing surgery with little involvement or participation from the patients. While highly effective for infectious diseases and acute illness, such as lacerations, burns, and trauma, this acute care approach often fails in treating chronic diseases, such as of obesity, diabetes, and heart disease. Yet 70 percent of all deaths in the United States are caused by one of these three diseases; and when cancer is included, 75 percent of all heathcare expenditures are associated with treating them. Clearly, this reactionary—as opposed to preventive—medical approach is financially unsustainable and largely ineffective for managing chronic diseases.

GOING FOR THE GUT

While practitioners of functional and integrative medicine have long recognized that what happens in the belly doesn't stay in the belly, the hard science to support such a hypothesis is just now surfacing. I can recall sitting in continuing-medical-education events that often began with a quote from 1908 Nobel Prize winner Ilya Mechnikov, PhD: "Death begins in the colon."[30,31] This trailblazing Russian biologist proposed nearly a hundred years ago that imbalances in intestinal bacteria are linked to many different diseases.[32,33]

Researchers throughout the world have continued to unearth ways in which environmental and lifestyle factors may lead to obesity by inducing changes in intestinal bacteria, or *microflora*.[34,35,36,37,38,39,40,41,42,43,44,45,46] For instance, now we know that the trillions of bacteria in the gut constantly communicate with the body's immune and metabolic machinery.[47,48,49,50,51] Furthermore, researchers today recognize that disequilibrium between these two systems is associated with the ubiquitous metabolic problems plaguing our modern world.[52,53]

I stumbled upon these discoveries during my early years working with Dr. G.'s overweight patients. The majority of them also had tummy troubles. At the time I thought the culprit was simply the result of poor nutrition—specifically that the sugars and fats in their diets were irritating the linings of their intestines and causing intestinal symptoms. Then in 2009 one of Dr. G's severely overweight medical assistants, whom we'll call Sally, had gastric bypass surgery. Within weeks she dropped a substantial amount of weight. Six months after surgery, she was so lean I almost didn't recognize her.

While I knew bariatric surgery was effective for weight loss, I wrongly presumed that the results were due to a drop in nutrient absorption, or *malabsorption*. Malabsorption associated with bariatric surgery is not the main driver of the typical 20–40 percent weight loss following the operation.[54]

Bariatric surgery, from the Greek word *baros* meaning weight, is often dubbed "metabolic surgery" because it has benefits that go beyond weight loss.[55] Improvements in blood glucose regulation, for example, are noted within three to six days following the operation.[56] This improvement occurs even before weight loss begins.[57] And that's not all. Along with a decrease in body mass shortly after the procedure, one study found a 78 percent reduction in the incidence of type 2 diabetes a year later.

There are also beneficial changes in the gut microflora and increased hormone signaling from the intestine.[58,59] These changes appear to be the major mechanisms responsible for the operation's long-term weight-loss success.

Bariatric surgery also increases the transit time of food passing through the intestine, reducing the length of time microbial species have to ferment and extract calories from ingested foods. Ample research suggests that Roux-en-Y gastric surgery is associated with a decrease in endotoxin.[60] These are molecules originating from the outer membranes of certain intestinal bacteria such as *E. coli*. Not surprising, then, that inflammation throughout the body is diminished after the operation.

French researchers demonstrated correlations between weight loss, reduction in obesity-related hormones, such as leptin, and changes in the intestinal microflora after bariatric surgery. Other scientists reported a tenfold increase in a beneficial bacteria species of the *Bifidobacteria* in the oral mucosa and a drop in blood levels of endotoxin following bariatric surgery.[61] They also found a decrease in a proinflammatory molecule. Although dental health and the microbial composition of the mouth may seem unrelated to body weight and blood sugar regulation, oral health is intimately linked to metabolic and immune function.[62,63]

Finally, gastric bypass surgery reduces the many deleterious health effects commonly present in overweight persons. After the operation, many conditions improve including memory, mood, fertility, asthma, sleep apnea, blood pressure, blood lipid levels, and inflammation of the brain that is characteristic of Alzheimer's disease.[64,65,66] The incidence of cancer, arthritis, and fatty liver decrease as well.[67]

DANGEROUS ENDOTOXIN

The role of healthy levels of gut bacteria is underscored by the success of bariatric surgery in improving the composition of beneficial gut bacteria. Certain types of foods influence the type of bacteria inhabiting our intestines. For example, many studies confirm that the standard American diet of refined carbohydrates and processed fats creates an imbalance in intestinal bacteria, which can damage the thin intestinal barrier and increase absorption of endotoxin.[68,69,70,71,72,73,74]

Scientific evidence has also linked increased blood levels of endotoxin to obesity and diabetes.[75,76] Intestine-derived endotoxin exit the intestine and penetrate the interior of the body in one of two ways: they either pass through breaches in the damaged intestinal barrier (a condition also known as *leaky gut*) or merge among ingested fats for transport into the body. This is why excessive intake of dietary fats can inadvertently lead to increased absorption of endotoxin and all the ailments that accompany them.

In the gut, liver, and other tissues, bacterial endotoxin latch onto immune receptors, propelling the immune system into a state of inflammation.[77,78,79,80,81,82] It's this increased immune vigilance that causes aberrations in blood glucose, lipid, and fat-storing hormones, such as insulin, that are characteristics of obesity and prediabetes.[83,84,85,86]

Worse yet, overly excited immune cells begin to make their way to fat stores, where they congregate, secreting proinflammatory messengers called *cytokines*.[87,88,89,90] The end result is a vicious cycle of low-grade inflammation, metabolic imbalance, and yes, fat accumulation.[91]

This endotoxin-related inflammation is thought to skew metabolism from a fat-burning state to a sugar-burning one.[92,93,94] When inflammation becomes chronic, metabolic disturbances like insulin resistance occur, ultimately affecting energy storage and increasing the risk of obesity.

Obesity is the collateral damage of inflammation, the kind that can be caused by food-related shifts in the intestinal microflora, leading to an overabundance of harmful bacteria and their proinflammatory endotoxin.[95] The more science learns about our digestive, immune, and metabolic systems, the more clear their interconnectedness, sensitivity, and codependence become. Storing too much fat and becoming overweight is far more complicated than simply eating more calories than you burn.

BARIATRIC SURGERY AND HORMONES

The intestines release many hormones responsible for controlling appetite and processing ingested foods. For example, after you eat, the 50–70 percent rise in insulin, the pancreatic hormone that regulates blood sugar, is contingent upon the proper secretion of *incretins,* hormones released from the intestinal tract.[96] (The most widely understood incretin hormones are called GLP-1, GLP-2, CCK, and PYY.) In addition to their integral role in blood sugar and insulin regulation, incretins govern appetite, growth of intestinal tissue, and intestinal transit and emptying.[97]

Bariatric surgery and the new generation of antidiabetic medications are linked to rapid improvements in blood levels of these incretins as well as other molecules, such as *leptin*, that regulate appetite.[98,99]

AN ALTERNATIVE TO SURGERY

Bariatric surgery is often overwhelmingly effective in causing rapid and long-lasting weight loss and metabolic improvements. However, I'm not suggesting that you or any of the world's two billion overweight people and 346 million diabetics undergo the operation. Instead, I believe in using natural agents to mimic the many beneficial physiologic effects that make bariatric surgery so effective.

Research is showing that it's possible to emulate the biological responses of bariatric surgery naturally. By scheduling meals; adjusting the balance of nutrients, such as protein and colorful phytochemicals, in the diet; combining different types of fiber; and supplementing prebiotics and probiotics, you can reduce intestinal inflammation and its effects on your metabolic machinery.[100,101,102] Studies show that mindful eating and taking prebiotics, probiotics, whey and pea protein powders, and natural herbs improve many metabolic components that scientists believed were improved only by gastric bypass surgery.

YOUR BODY—A SOCIAL NETWORK

During our journey through your metabolic system in the following chapters, we will look at your body as a network of connections, like biologic Facebook friends or Twitter followers. Just as one Tweet can cost a politician his job, one small bacterial imbalance in your gut or a glitch in one biochemical pathway can instant message your fat cells to swell with fat. When you look at your organs and systems as a vast network of linked connections, you discover why obesity and its related disorders are more than just genetics, calorie overload, or too much sitting.

To unravel the core reasons behind your weight problems, you need to decipher how your environment, your mood, and the foods you eat affect the composition of the trillions of microbes in your gut, cause your metabolic engines to misfire, and put your immune system on high alert.

To achieve the lean and healthy body you've been yearning for, you need to exploit the "social network" of your body. This means taking a deeper look at how the complex systems of your body are connected and tweaking the broken-down pathways. This is how you will sustain weight loss and reverse inflammation and insulin resistance and lower your risk of heart disease, diabetes, and other chronic disorders.

The strategies you'll learn in this book may feel unnatural at first, but the information I'll share with you will help you reevaluate your lifestyle choices and achieve the body and metabolic health you desire. You will no longer see obesity and its sister disorder, diabetes, as deficiencies in willpower, but instead as conditions dominated by strong immunologic and metabolic relationships. In short, you will discover that willpower is not enough.

CHAPTER 1

BEYOND CALORIES

"Obesity is collateral damage in the battle for modernity."
—Garry Egger, PhD

Despite our mobile phones, tablets, HDTVs, and surround-sound entertainment systems, we are ancient creatures trapped in a culture that has outpaced our genetic programming. Our primitive metabolic systems are responding to modern-day nutrient excesses in the way they were designed to do in prehistoric times when nutrient supplies were scarce and starvation was a primary cause of death.[1] We're programmed to be thrifty with the nutrients we eat. When food is abundant, we store the surplus nutrients as fat to use for fuel when food is scarce.

In the simplest Darwinian sense, the cavemen and women who weren't able to save fuel in this way didn't survive long during harsh winters or famines, and so their genes were not passed on to future generations. Fortunately, our hunter-gatherer ancestors had the ability to store energy and they survived, passing this life-saving advantage to us.[2] In other words, the ability to reserve energy for later use is in our genes. Indeed, the overwhelmingly high incidence of obesity throughout the world suggests that the primitive survival programming is marvelously effective!

Today the maxim that you gain weight when the amount of calories you eat exceeds the amount you burn is generally accepted as fact. But that formula is not the whole story of obesity. It doesn't explain why antibiotics lead to an increase in body fat.[3,4,5] Nor does it explain why babies delivered by cesarean section gain more body fat later in life than those born vaginally.[6,7] Or why metabolic function improves following gastric bypass surgery.[8,9,10,11,12,13,14] It looks like the health community has some explaining to do!

Scientific studies hint that several confounding environmental factors—above and beyond excess calories—are shifting the pivot of our thrifty metabolic programming into saving mode.[15,16,17,18,19,20,21,22,23] Researchers have discovered, for instance, that when our fat stores are overfilled, our other systems, especially the immune system, go awry.[24] Eventually fat loss becomes even more difficult, which is one reason why overweight people tend to become obese and why obese people get even fatter.[25] Getting the needle to move on the scale will require some persistence to break free from this destructive cycle.

LESSONS FROM OUR ANCESTORS

While advances in agricultural practices and food processing have increased the availability of calorie-dense, refined foods to levels greater than at any other time, studies show that our prehistoric ancestors ate more calories on a daily basis than we do.[26] It's been reported that hunter-gatherers consumed about 2,800 calories per day, according to S. Boyd Eaton, MD, of Emory University in Atlanta.[27] Since our ancestors were largely hunters and foragers, they were also on the move most of their waking hours, using the saturated fat from meat and carbohydrates from fruits and vegetables for fuel.[28,29] In contrast, modern-day humans spend a great deal of their day sitting, thanks to improvements in manufacturing and transportation and a greatly diminished need for physical labor. Not surprisingly, our ancestors didn't have the chronic diseases of affluence so common today, such as obesity, diabetes, and heart disease.[30] Instead they succumbed to starvation, predators, and infection.[31,32] Hence we are apt to store fat, have a heightened stress response, and command a robust inflammatory response system, which are maladaptive in our modern environment.

Although industrialized individuals overconsume processed calories, lack regular exercise, and have a thrifty metabolism not suited for modern life, recent research indicates that there are some gaping holes in the widely accepted calorie model theory of obesity.[33,34,35,36] Although we are much heavier than we've ever been in history, we aren't putting on the pounds that quickly.

For example, while the prevalence of obesity has tripled over the last thirty years to an all-time high, calorie consumption is only up 11 percent.[37] Both the Centers for Disease Control and Prevention and the Institute of Medicine have reported that calorie consumption has increased from 1,996 calories per day in 1974 to 2,195 calories in 2012.

Despite the obesity epidemic, if eating too many calories is the main culprit behind obesity, we should actually be much fatter. University of Colorado researcher James Hill, PhD, reported in the American Heart Association's journal *Circulation* that compared to a few decades ago, modern Western men consume an extra 168 calories a day and women consume 335 more calories daily than in the past.[38] This translates into a nationwide typical weight gain of 18 pounds for men and 35 pounds for women. As a nation, we may have become fatter, but we're not that fat!

As for diminished physical activity, researchers have extensively dissected the data surrounding lack of exercise and weight gain, and the results raise doubts about the popular calories-in, calories-out equation. Hill calculated that our nation's reduced physical activity would translate into an annual weight gain of 68 pounds for women and 47 pounds for men. Combined with the increase in average calorie intake, this imbalance should translate to a thirty- to eighty-fold weight gain, he concluded, and that simply has not occurred.

Scientists have also proved that you don't have to spend hours in the gym to lose excess pounds either. For example, exercise physiologists from Denmark instructed two groups of overweight men to exercise intensely three times a week for either thirty or sixty minutes.[39] After three months, fat loss in the two groups was not significantly different. If the energy balance hypothesis was the sine qua non of overweight and obesity, the group exercising for sixty minutes should have lost twice as much weight as the group that worked out for only thirty minutes. That didn't happen.

Another aspect of exercise, however, may have an effect on weight loss. Research indicates that how long you work out isn't as important as the type and intensity of the exercise you do. In other words, as Canadian researchers demonstrated, quality of exercise appears to have a greater effect on body weight than quantity.[40] They found that combining aerobic and resistance exercise leads to greater fat loss and larger increases in lean muscle mass than aerobic exercise alone. High-intensity interval training (HIT) is surfacing as superior to steady-state aerobic training, even though it has a lower calorie-burn in comparison to traditional aerobic exercise.

Another recent study found that intense, short bursts of cycling lead to increases in a change in cellular chemistry—specifically a cellular mediator called PGC-1α—that increases both the number and function of *mitochondria*, the energy factories within each cell.[41] These increases improve insulin signaling and fat burning.[42] Just as our understanding of what a calorie is expands, the science of exercise is similarly moving forward.

Clearly there are factors other than calories contributing to our nation's weight problems. Experts have found that other modern-day phenomenon, such as excess psychological stress, prolonged sitting, and sleep deprivation, can disturb the balance between fat breakdown (*lipolysis*) and fat storage (*lipogenesis*).[43,44] Later, I'll explain how alterations in the trillions of microbes colonizing our intestines caused by mindless and quick eating, overuse of antibiotics, and exposure to environmental chemicals also contribute to this delicate fat balance.

DON'T BLAME YOUR METABOLISM

While overweight men and women often fault inherited slow metabolism on their expanding waistlines, studies involving twins are finding that genetics, like calories and exercise, may have little to do with tipping the scale. Researchers from Finland tracked obese and lean twin pairs and found that while the obese twins' activity level was low, they had higher total energy expenditure and a higher resting or basal metabolic rate (BMR) compared to the lean twins.[45]

If an overweight person burns more calories at rest than a lean person, you would expect that the heavier person would have an easier time losing weight during periods where calories burned during exercise exceeded calories eaten. Yet, once again, that assumption does not hold up under scientific scrutiny. The Finnish study showed quite the contrary: while the obese twins had a faster resting metabolic rate than the lean twins, the obese twins also had an impaired ability to burn fat. I will discuss later how inflammation can misdirect metabolism into a state of increased sugar burning at the expense of fat burning, certainly not ideal for weight loss!

Experts on the forefront of obesity research now recognize that obesity occurs as a result of several factors interacting with each other. Calories count, but they don't explain weight gain or loss entirely. A sedentary lifestyle is a player, too, but it doesn't have a starring role. Rather a myriad of influences on the body's energy system are responsible from the bacteria in the gut to endocrine-disrupting chemicals in the environment.[46,47,48,49]

CELLULAR POWER PLANTS

From high school to college and even medical school, students learn that metabolism is an aspect of a single system, the *endocrine* system, which involves how tissues respond to insulin, the blood-sugar regulating hormone. Along with fat, skeletal muscle, and the liver, the endocrine system controls energy balance. In physics, energy is the potential to do work.

Think of your body as a car: the more fuel you have in it, the longer you can drive. Through a rather sophisticated process, your body's "engine" combines oxygen with fuel from food or fat or both, and ignites the mixture via an electric spark. This "combustion" powers your cells. In other words, your body uses oxygen to break down calories, which are simply units of energy, converting them to chemical energy or *adenosine triphosphate* (ATP) that your cells can use.

Carbohydrates and proteins yield four calories (units of energy) per gram, and fat provides nine calories per gram. The endocrine system regulates the speed at which the calories in the food we eat convert into "spending money" or "savings," as in the piggy bank of fat cells on your belly, butt, and thighs. You might think of your endocrine system as a financial institution that regulates the spending and saving of your nutritional cash for moving, breathing, thinking, even sleeping.

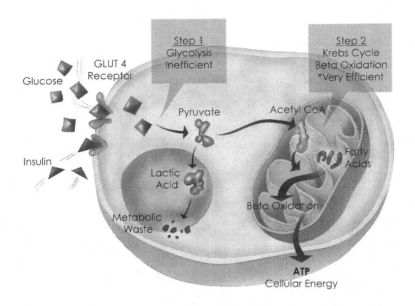

SUGAR AND FAT BURNING IN A NUTSHELL

In the first phase of cellular metabolism, insulin assists in the transport of blood glucose into the cell where it is broken down into a very small amount of ATP (two molecules per molecule of glucose) and two molecules of pyruvate. In dysfunctional metabolic states, these molecules are readily converted to lactic acid metabolic waste. In phase two, oxygen is utilized to further oxidize the pyruvate—the two molecules making roughly thirty-four molecules of ATP per molecule of glucose. Free fatty acids are also broken down inside the mitochondria and converted into usable cellular energy in the form of ATP, in a process known as beta oxidation.

Although oxygen doesn't contain calories, it serves as a critical catalyst for converting fats and carbohydrates into fuel for the activity of all your cells. This energy production occurs in these specialized cellular structures, or mitochondria. Each of them is a cellular power plant. In muscle fibers, for example, carbohydrates and fats are converted to energy to propel its fibers into high gear.

Physically fit people have increased mitochondrial functioning, while overweight and insulin-resistant folks have sluggish, poorly functioning, and fewer mitochondria.[50] The situation can become even more dysfunctional in obese people because there's a limit to how much oxygen can reach all those extra cells. *Hypoxia* occurs when the oxygen supply is deficient.[51] Instead of the fire of combustion burning brightly in those cellular powerhouses, it smolders and fat burning may come to a halt, calling in another less efficient metabolic pathway known as *glycolysis*, which doesn't require oxygen. Worse yet, the low oxygen supply that is characteristic of too much body fat triggers a molecular switch that turns on inflammation, further hampering fat burning and creating insulin resistance.[52]

Although rapid, glycolysis is inefficient and wasteful, creating only two molecules of ATP per molecule of glucose and releasing much metabolic exhaust as carbon dioxide and lactic acid.

A principle of physics is that energy cannot be destroyed; it can only be transferred to a different energy state. Translation: when the calories you consume are not needed for work and the conversion to ATP never occurs, your body will store most of those calories, or energy, as fat. At least that is how the thinking goes, and it is the basis for the common belief that if you simply match calories consumed with calories burned, you will not gain weight. The fact is, however, that your physiology is much more dynamic.

WHY DIETS FAIL

Most dieters who manage to lose weight by cutting calories regain nearly 100 percent of the weight within five years, and less than one in six dieters maintain weight loss for any extended time.[53] One reason is that cutting calories disrupts the signaling of hormones secreted in the intestine, the incretins. Incretins prompt the release of insulin when glucose levels rise and so help regulate blood sugar and appetite. When levels of incretins increase, as happens in people who have bariatric surgery, blood sugar and weight maintenance are much more likely.

Researchers are also finding that a calorie isn't just a calorie, regardless of where it comes from.[54] Rather a food may have an adverse impact on both your intestinal microflora and your metabolism when it enters your gut, depending on its composition.[55] How fast you eat, the time of day you eat, the combination of foods you consume, and the amounts of fiber, alcohol, and fructose you eat also influence how your intestinal microflora and body process calories. Furthermore, macronutrients—fats, carbohydrates, and proteins—all exert different effects on various metabolic signaling pathways, appetite centers, and gut bacteria.

THE STORY OF FRUCTOSE

To better illustrate the notion that nutrients metabolize differently, consider the metabolic effects of two sugars common to the Western diet: fructose and sucrose. Sucrose, also known as table sugar, is broken down to fructose and glucose in the body. It's been in the hot seat for decades for its purported deleterious health effects. Now corn-derived sugar additives—fructose and high fructose corn syrup (HFCS)—have taken center stage as major contributors to the obesity and diabetes epidemics.

Unlike traditional table sugar (which has a high glycemic index, meaning it is quickly absorbed and raises blood glucose levels, stimulating insulin release from the pancreas), super-concentrated forms of fructose are poorly absorbed from the intestine.[56] Fructose, therefore, has a negligible impact on blood sugar. It's for this reason that fructose still is used as a sweetener for nutrition shakes marketed to individuals with impaired glucose metabolism, prediabetes, and diabetes.

However, experts now understand that fructose's poor intestinal absorption has a major disadvantage: it is taken up by the liver where it is readily converted into glycerol, a fat. And when fat increases in the liver, insulin release is impaired, triglyceride levels rise, and there is an increase in the risks of cardiovascular disease, fatty liver disease, type 2 diabetes, and obesity.[57]

Several studies have compared drinks sweetened with either glucose or fructose and have found that fructose leads to a greater increase in unhealthy visceral belly fat, blood triglycerides, and *atherogenic*, or cardiovascular-disease promoting lipids, to a much greater extent than does glucose.[58,59] Robert Lustig, MD, of the University of California-San Francisco has been an influential voice behind the public's awareness of fructose-dangerous biology.[60]

Dr. Lustig reminds us in his web video presentations and periodicals that as humans and animals prepare for cooler winter months, a ravenous appetite and a little extra stored energy in the form of body fat is advantageous to survival. Therefore, the marked increase in consumption of fructose-rich fruits during the late summer and early autumn months would certainly have helped our ancestors in northern latitudes survive.

While scientists agree that fructose is processed differently than glucose, there is new research that exposes the differences in the two sugars' metabolic effects. For instance, fructose appears to blunt the usual satiety signals and increases levels of the hunger-stimulating hormone *ghrelin*. Another study reveals that fructose stimulates reward-seeking pathways in the brain much more readily than glucose.[61] Last but not least, scientists have discovered that fructose, but not glucose, alters intestinal bacteria.[62] Fructose also increases the porousness of the gastrointestinal tract lining, promoting absorption of bacterial endotoxin, which then prompts inflammation.[63] The effect is similar to what takes place when you drink alcohol or eat fat-laden meals.

NUTRIENTS, NOT CALORIES, COUNT

Many commercial diet programs are grounded in the belief that one must restrict calories as well as macronutrients. Typically these diets prescribe a certain percentage of calories from carbohydrates, protein, and fat. However, one reason these diets fail is that they don't take into consideration the impact each of these nutrients has on metabolism and fat storage.

A recent study spearheaded by David Ludwig, MD, PhD, of Boston Children's Hospital, found that low-calorie diets that deliver different nutrients, such as low-carb or high-fat, have different effects on metabolic signaling pathways, inflammation, fat storage, appetite, and resting metabolic rate in obese people.

Ian Spreadbury, PhD, an expert on the ancestral diets of hunter-gatherers and a researcher at Queens University in Ontario, Canada, has published extensively on the effect of grain-derived carbohydrates on metabolism.[64] Spreadbury, along with researchers S. Boyd Eaton, MD, author of *The Paleolithic Prescription*, and Loren Cordain, PhD, author of *The Paleo Diet*, propose that our ancestors were free of obesity and chronic ailments such as diabetes and cardiovascular disease because their diets were largely free of cereal grains. Indeed, Cordain is known as a "cereal killer" because he suggests that the emergence of grains into human civilization thousands of years ago is the crux of the modern-day chronic disease epidemic.

If we could turn the clock back several thousand years or study present-day hunter-gather societies in remote areas of the world, as Cordain has done, we would see that the primary foods in these primitive diets are vegetables, fruits, nuts, seeds; protein from fish and wild game; and a small amount of honey. Cordain's extensive assessment of fifty-eight contemporary hunter-gather societies that have not been influenced by modern agriculture techniques confirms that dietary fat and non-grain carbohydrates comprise the majority of the calories in these cultures, up to 58 percent and 40 percent, respectively. This flies in the face of the modern-day belief that "low-carb" diets are best for weight control.

Protein has been estimated to comprise 19–35 percent of the calories consumed by these societies. Since most of the protein comes from wild game and fish, the diet is about 20 percent fat, with oils, butter, and dairy products rarely eaten, if at all.

Eaton has quantified the calorie intake of foragers from the past one thousand years and reports that they consumed 2,800 calories a day on average.[65] In contrast, it's been reported by the Institute of Medicine that present-day Americans consume approximately 40 percent less, or 2,007 calories per day.

Despite the fact that, like our ancestors, some contemporary indigenous peoples eat significantly more calories from fat—especially saturated fat—and carbohydrates, they aren't typically obese and don't have the "diseases of affluence," such as diabetes and cardiovascular disease that threaten modern industrialized societies. Today, when hunter-gatherers leave their traditional villages and move to more populated rural and coastal regions, they undergo a "metabolic transition" that is characteristic of insulin resistance. They also experience a higher prevalence of obesity.

Studies over the last ten years of "industrialized" Pima Indians, Australian Aborigines, and native Hawaiians have found that when the amount of fat they eat is restored to levels of their traditional diets, the people lose weight and achieve a healthy metabolism.

This metabolic transition was described at the turn of the century by Westin A. Price, an Ohio-based dentist who correlated the rapid increase in the incidence of dental cavities and periodontal disease among patients in his clinical practice with their "physical degeneration." After making this observation, Price then took a ten-year sabbatical that culminated in a worldwide search for the underlying causes of the rapid increase in tooth decay that he saw in his patients.[66] He published *Nutrition and Physical Degeneration* in 1939, in which he reported that when families with children moved from an urban area to a more rural region where sugar and processed foods were less plentiful, the children born after the move had improved oral health and better bone structure than their older siblings.

Although Price didn't know it at the time, his hypotheses that a Westernized diet rich in processed carbohydrates was "transmissible" from parent to offspring and could be identified through oral health are two fundamental concepts in the new weight-loss and metabolic model presented in this book. Price's findings are important to the concept of epigenetics—that is, the study of how our environment influences our genetic programming.[67]

Experts now know that paternal and maternal malnutrition, protein restriction, environmental toxin exposure, blood-sugar imbalances, diabetes, obesity, and psychological stressors all predispose developing infants to future obesity, diabetes, and cardiovascular disease.[68,69,70,71, 72,73,74,75] Periodontal disease is linked to an imbalance in the microbes inhabiting the mucosa.[76,77] The disorder is also associated with elevated levels of absorbed bacterial endotoxin, low-grade inflammation, type 2 diabetes, and obesity.[78,79,80]

Price wasn't the only doctor to notice that parents' diets could ultimately affect the health of their offspring. Los Angeles–based physician Francis Pottenger, MD, concluded similar findings in the 1930s.[81] His famous "Milk Study" is renowned for showing how poor nutrition leads to poor health or "dis-ease" in animals' offspring. Pottenger fed cats a diet of 60 percent milk and 30 percent meat. However, the milk portion varied: one group of cats drank raw milk while the others consumed pasteurized milk. Pottenger found that the cats on raw milk thrived for generations, while those on the "cooked" or pasteurized milk had various degenerative problems, the animal equivalent of chronic diseases. Since cooking milk doesn't influence its calorie content or macronutrient profile, it was presumed that other essential components in the milk, such as micronutrients, were destroyed. It's tempting to speculate that those "essentials" were beneficial bacteria—the "forgotten organ"—which we now know to have a profound influence on metabolism and fat storage.

Researchers originally proposed that our genome hasn't programmed our digestive and metabolic machinery to digest and process carbohydrate-rich grains.[82] Our hunter-gatherer ancestors were never exposed to wheat, rice, and maize, and so they never developed the capacity to digest them. To make our metabolic and digestive lives even worse, today these cereal grains contain many anti-nutrients, including phytates, lectins, gluten, and gliadin. From obesity and insulin resistance to autoimmunity, the combination of anti-nutrients in cereal grains has been attributed to a plethora of imbalances in our microflora and digestive tract.[83]

New research suggests that cereal carbohydrates affect intestinal bacteria. Spreadbury observed that although the indigenous Kitavan Islanders and Papua New Guineans consumed a diet rich in carbohydrates and saturated fat—60 percent and 17 percent of calorie intake, respectively—obesity was quite unusual. Also, baseline levels of metabolic hormones, such as leptin, which is a marker of total fat, and fasting insulin, were far lower than those of healthy people living in modern Western societies.

Spreadbury and his colleagues suggest that the paucity of processed carbohydrates in these "ancestral diets" contributes to the people's metabolic health by promoting beneficial gastrointestinal bacteria. Spreadbury also notes that carbohydrates available to our ancestors—mainly fruits and root tubers of potato and parsnip—have a much lower carbohydrate density and higher water content compared to processed flour and cereal grains.

The present hypothesis is that the high carbohydrate content and rapid digestibility of processed carbohydrates disturbs the metabolism and composition of the trillions of microbes inhabiting our intestines. Since these microbes are inextricably linked to all body functions, especially endocrine and immune system activity, a disruption in the microflora is implicated in obesity-related diseases.

A NEW PARADIGM

Granted, people may gain weight when they consume excess calories and aren't physically active. However, suggesting that energy balance is the ultimate determination of body weight and metabolic health is an antiquated concept. Research confirms what any veteran crash dieter will tell you: restricting calories often triggers hunger and lowers your resting metabolic rate, sabotaging your attempt to lose pounds.[84] Nevertheless, calories are continually emphasized as the cause of obesity by health agencies, doctors, dietitians, and fitness experts. The Centers for Disease Control and Prevention (CDC) and the World Health Organization (WHO) continue to maintain that weight gain is solely the result of eating more calories than you burn. And these agencies obstinately continue to address obesity by recommending that people increase their physical activity, eat more fruits and vegetables, decrease their consumption of calorie-rich foods, eliminate sugar-sweetened beverages, and cut back on television time.

These recommendations may have been correct in the 1970s, but they need expanding today to reflect recent metabolic, immune, and toxicology research. Our environment is changing at a rapid pace, and experts now know that many factors contribute to obesity independent of calories eaten or burned. With seven million people transitioning from overweight to obese every year, the calorie model has clearly failed.

SUMMARY OF 2012 OBESITY AND 2020 HEALTH TARGET		
Age Group	Current Obesity Prevalence	Healthy People 2020 Target
Children (2-5 years)	10.7%	9.6%
Children (6-11 years)	17.4%	15.7%
Adolescents (12–19 years)	17.9%	16.1%
Adults (20 and above)	34%	30.6%

If we were to increase the number of states with nutrition standards for children, double the proportion of schools that do not sell sugary drinks, and triple the percentage of school districts required to offer fruits and vegetables to children, we would be making phenomenal first steps. But these are only the beginning steps. A dramatic paradigm shift is needed to make dramatic changes in the obesity epidemic. Unless we drastically change our approach, there is no indication that we'll be able to prevent obesity in the future.

KEY TAKEAWAYS

The standard weight loss theory of "burn more calories than you eat" may just be that—a theory. You can thank your ancestors for your body's strategic use of storing calories as fat in preparation for survival of the highly unlikely famine here in the United States. Our bodies haven't adapted to our modern way of living, which for the average person generally includes prolonged sitting, sleep deprivation, and psychological stress. Not only that, but other factors such as "bad" gut bacteria to endocrine-disrupting chemicals in the environment influence our body's metabolism.

Obesity can initiate a catch-22 situation as your mitochondria decrease in number and activity. With less energy, there is less motivation to exercise and thus less oxygen reaching the mitochondria, which need oxygen to function optimally and burn fat.

We now know that a calorie isn't just a calorie, especially if it's a fructose-containing calorie. Fructose is in many foods and contributes to fat storage. Increased fat in the liver impairs insulin release, raising triglyceride levels and increasing the risk of such diseases as type 2 diabetes, fatty liver disease, cardiovascular disease, and of course, obesity. Fructose also damages the lining of the gastrointestinal tract, promoting absorption of bacterial endotoxin and causing inflammation.

Our metabolic functions are many times tied in to our ancestral heritage. Studies have proven that eating foods local to your point of origin and the right combination of carbohydrates, protein, and fat will in many cases unlock the door to health and weight control.

Research has demonstrated that paternal and maternal malnutrition, protein restriction, environmental toxin exposure, blood-sugar imbalances, diabetes, obesity, and psychological stressors all predispose developing infants to future obesity, diabetes, and cardiovascular disease through genetic programming called epigenetics. What may begin as a propensity toward being overweight at birth can turn into full-fledged obesity because of easy access to high sugar and carbohydrate meals and snacks at schools. Processed carbohydrates have a negative effect on metabolism and gut bacteria. They must be eliminated or at least limited in the diet to lower the incidence of obesity. This is especially important in children.

CHAPTER 2

WHAT IS SICK FAT?

"Adipocytes in visceral fat, the favored site, in addition to storing fat, secrete adipokines and also attract and activate macrophages that release enzymes and cytokines that further drive the proinflammatory state."—Jesse Roth, MD

Fat stored on your hips, thighs, and belly is far more than a passive, energy bank.[1] It's a biologically active endocrine and immune organ and the body's primary regulator of lipid and glucose balance.[2,3,4,5,6] But too much of it is not a good thing. The body fat of overweight and obese people is out of balance, even "sick."[7] When fat cells become enlarged, their oxygen supply is inadequate.[8] The cells become inflamed and begin releasing hormones, such as leptin.[9,10,11,12] Immune cells infiltrate the fatty, or adipose, tissue and spew free fatty acids into the body.[13,14,15] A vicious cycle of inflammation and metabolic imbalances ensue.[16,17,18,19,20,21] In this section, we'll learn what assessments and blood tests to consider having in order to achieve a healthy weight.

WAIST CIRCUMFERENCE AND WHITE FAT

For nearly seventy years, scientists have known that not all fat is created equal. Actually, there are three forms of fat: white fat, protective brown fat, and beige fat, which is the intermediary between brown and white fat. White fat, particularly in the abdomen is largely responsible for many serious health problems. The French physician Jean Vague was the first to propose that the location of adipose tissue determines its metabolic effects, and as early as the 1940s he observed the diverse metabolic and immune activity of abdominal fat.[22,23]

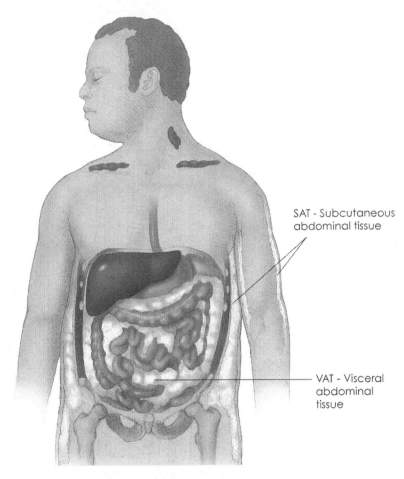

SAT - Subcutaneous abdominal tissue

VAT - Visceral abdominal tissue

THE DIFFERENT TYPES OF BODY FAT

Sick fat is the deep, intra-abdominal or visceral adipose tissue (VAT). VAT is very close to intestinal organs and is highly inflammatory. In contrast, subcutaneous adipose tissue (SAT) on the upper arms, back, legs, and buttocks has little, if any, harmful immune or metabolic effects.

Today, people with an excess of *visceral* fat, the deep belly fat around the abdominal organs, are called "apple-shaped," in contrast to the "pear shape" of those who tend to store extra fat under the skin of the arms, buttocks, and legs.[24,25] Interestingly, men tend to be more apple-shaped than women.[26] Unlike subcutaneous fat of the upper arms, visceral fat tends to attract metabolically disruptive immune cells such as macrophages and lymphocytes.[27,28,29,30,31,32,33,34] These immune cells release inflammatory messengers, or cytokines, that antagonize your metabolic machinery, disrupting your fat-loss efforts and creating a vicious cycle of more inflammation and fat accumulation.[35] Unsurprisingly, an apple shape is associated with many of the metabolic and inflammatory diseases that occur with obesity. This is why I call it "sick fat."

DO YOU HAVE "SICK FAT"?

Waist circumference and body fat percentage, not BMI, are much more reliable indicators of the "sick fat" that undermines your health. However, the vast majority of obesity facts and figures reported in the media and even some scientific journals are derived from the commonly used weight-for-height formula called body mass index, or BMI. The National Heart, Lung, and Blood Institute and the World Health Organization (WHO) classify body weight using BMI as follows:

- Underweight < 18.5
- Normal weight 18.5–24.9
- Overweight 24.9–29.9
- Obese 29.9–34.9

Some experts suggest lowering the cutoff point for obesity to a BMI of 24 for females and 28 for males. These revised BMI cutoff points are more sensitive in discerning body adiposity.[36]

WHY BODY MASS INDEX IS WRONG

Scientists have criticized this two-hundred-year-old BMI formula because it significantly underestimates adiposity and doesn't take into consideration lean muscle mass.[37,38] In contrast to body fat testing and waist circumference measures, BMI defines obesity based on a mathematical estimate, and so it tends to underestimate body fat percentage.[39]

A recent study involving nine thousand patients of an outpatient clinic found that body fat percentage analysis using an X-ray technique called *dual-energy X-ray absorptiometry* (DXA) is much more accurate than BMI measures. In fact, BMI miscalculated obesity in 48 percent of women and 26 percent of men, and the miscalculation increased with age, according to the study. These researchers reported elevated blood leptin to strongly correlate with increasing levels of body fat and suggest that physicians lower BMI cutoff points for obesity to 24 for women and 28 for men, down from 30 in both sexes.

Additionally, a recent assessment of the body fat percentage in middle-aged Indian men living in urban slums revealed that 45 percent of them had a body fat percentage greater than 25, while their BMI was only 21, which would be considered "normal."[40] The prevalence of greater than 25 percent body fat in middle-class Indian men was 84 percent, despite having a "normal" BMI under 30.

The current overweight and obesity cutoff points set by leading health organizations greatly underestimate the degree of fatness in persons with a "normal BMI." They misclassify healthy non-obese persons as obese due to increased levels of lean muscle mass and completely overlook those with "sarcopenic obesity," meaning they have a great amount of body fat and a low amount of lean muscle mass, a combination that is associated with many chronic diseases.[41]

The ever-evolving perspective is that adipose tissue of the abdomen is much more than just a collection of inactive lipid-storage deposits. Rather it becomes a metabolic organ that releases inflammatory molecules. This has been confirmed in several studies.[42,43,44,45,46] For example, in 2012, researchers at the Mayo Clinic reported that those with a normal BMI but with too much belly fat (as measured by waist-to-hip ratio) had the highest cardiovascular death risk.[47] The take-home message from this finding is that using BMI to assess weight-related health complications should be replaced with measurements of visceral abdominal fat, such as waist circumference and waist-to-hip ratio. The other message is simply that fat in general is not bad.

So take your BMI measurement with a grain of salt. Since BMI doesn't differentiate between brown and white fat or separate the subcutaneous fat from the deep abdominal or visceral fat, it's really a crude measurement. As for body fat percentage, I encourage all my female clients to be under 20 percent body fat and male clients to be under 15 percent body fat.

Since visceral, or belly fat, is the problem attributed to metabolic issues, in addition to using body fat percentage to assess "fatness," consider your waist circumference to determine your degree of "sick fat."[48,49,50,51,52,53,54] WHO defines central obesity as a waist circumference greater than 94 cm (about 37 inches) for men and 80 cm (about 31.5 inches) for women. However, more recent scientific studies feel that these values are too broad and need to be lower than 80 cm in both sexes. For example, just a slight increase in waist circumference—above 17 cm (6.7 inches) more in teen boys and 15.5 cm (5.9 inches) for teen girls—is linked with increased risk of developing diabetes, metabolic imbalances, and elevated cardiovascular risk later in life. In my opinion, the smaller your belly, the better.

ASSESSMENT	BODY MASS INDEX	WAIST CIRCUMFERENCE	BODY FAT PERCENTAGE
Target: Lean & Healthy	18	< 75 cm men < 70 cm women	< 15% men < 20% women
Overweight	22 both sexes	> 80 cm men > 75 cm women	> 25% men > 30% women
Obese	24 women 28 men	> 90 cm men > 80 cm women	> 30% men > 35% women

SKINNY FAT: LEAN BUT METABOLICALLY OBESE

Skinny people often fly under the radar despite being metabolically obese, or "skinny fat."[55] In 1981 Boston University's Neil Ruderman, MD, was the first to propose that not all lean people are metabolically healthy and subsequently coined the term metabolically obese, normal weight.[56] Ruderman noted that adult-onset obesity is associated with hyperinsulinemia and an increase in fat cell size. However, he also observed that up to 20 percent of normal-weight individuals that went on to develop type 2 diabetes presented with the same set of metabolic derangements—that is, elevated insulin and increased fat cell size—previously understood to only be a problem with obesity. His findings underscore the importance of using blood tests to assess your metabolic state.

NOT ALL FAT IS BAD

Brown fat is sometimes called baby fat since it's abundant in infants, and it was once thought to offer little benefit to adults. It plays a critical role in producing body heat, an activity called *thermogenesis*, which is why it's so important to a baby.[57] Recently though, brown fat is undergoing a resurgence of research interest. Studies now suggest that brown fat plays a critical role in regulating triglycerides, which accumulate in obesity and diabetes and increase the risk of cardiovascular problems. Since brown fat decreases as body mass—particularly belly fat—increases, researchers think brown fat may help prevent obesity.[58,59]

Brown fat is broken down to make heat by *catecholamines*, a type of adrenal hormone.[60] This reaction occurs when temperatures drop or you're plunged into cold water. Indeed, studies have shown that the stress of extreme cold prompts brown fat to increase a person's metabolic rate by up to 30 percent! [61]

Activating brown fat is known to protect against obesity, which may explain an interesting discovery by Italian researchers: they found that living in a warm home is associated with a higher incidence of obesity.[62] Unfortunately, dieting may reduce brown fat activity as the body attempts to maintain its set point body weight.[63]

METABOLIC OBESITY
AND BLOOD SUGAR

Being overweight is often connected through a kind of functional chaos with reverberations in the metabolic and immune systems.[64,65,66,67,68,69] From diabetes and heart disease to cancer and depression, obesity's contribution to what may seem to be disparate conditions can be traced back to difficulty regulating blood sugar. In fact, nearly 80 percent of obese people are insulin-resistant, which is linked to chronic inflammation.[70] While the body can normally put out the inflammatory fire, hormones released from fat impair the extinguishing process and contribute to chronic inflammation, more fat gain, and metabolic disruption.[71,72] This notion has been confirmed by recent studies suggesting that people who are overweight or who have diabetes, or both, share an inability to counter chronic inflammation.[73,74,75,76,77,78,79]

According to the 2006 National Health and Nutrition Examination Survey (NHANES), about 30 percent of adults over the age of twenty have prediabetes.[80] In this survey, diabetes was reported to afflict 13 percent of adults, suggesting that at least 40 percent of American adults have either prediabetes or type 2 diabetes.

Later in this book, I'll explain how intestinal bacterial imbalances, low-grade inflammation, and abdominal obesity create the perfect metabolic storm, leading to insulin resistance, or prediabetes, the "brewing" phase of a situation that eventually becomes type 2 diabetes. It's important to keep in mind that diabetes is a continuum with a long incubation period characterized by insulin resistance, or impaired glucose tolerance.[81]

Each year in the United States, up to 10 percent of the prediabetic population will transition to full-blown diabetes.[82] Over a lifetime, 70–90 percent of people with prediabetes will eventually develop type 2 diabetes.

Technically, one is said to have prediabetes if fasting blood glucose levels are between 100 and 125 mg/dL. Ideally, fasting glucose levels would be under 80 mg/dL. Diabetes is diagnosed when fasting blood glucose is over 125 mg/dL. However, I prefer combining waist circumference with *triglyceride* (a blood fat) levels over fasting glucose to determine who has prediabetes or diabetes.

Curiously, uncontrolled blood-sugar regulation may contribute more to cardiovascular disease development than increased blood cholesterol.[83] One study of 113 people found that impairments in fasting blood glucose—not blood cholesterol levels—indicated less elasticity of artery walls, the kind of rigidity associated with aging blood vessels, suggestive of heart disease. Considering this research, it's not surprising that in 2004 heart disease and stroke were reported on 68 percent and 16 percent, respectively, of diabetes-related death certificates.[84]

The exceedingly high rate of prediabetes at present, especially among younger adolescents and adults, may foster the burgeoning incidence of diabetes to well over 30 percent by 2050.[85] That is on the conservative side.

OBESITY'S SISTER DISEASE:
TYPE 2 DIABETES

Traditionally, type 1 diabetes occurs during childhood, but may happen at any age. In contrast, type 2 diabetes has historically been reduced to a disorder in adults brought on by a poor diet and lack of exercise.

Thirty years ago, only 2 percent of the U.S. population had diabetes. That number has skyrocketed to nearly 10 percent today and continues to climb, threatening the financial security of our healthcare system.[86,87,88,89] In fact, we have already far surpassed the direst predictions of a decade ago, when researchers estimated that 300 million people worldwide would have diabetes by 2025.[90] Instead, that number is already more than 346 million! Researchers have adjusted their projections and estimate that the rate of diabetes will increase by more than 50 percent to 552 million by 2030.[91,92] It's been reported that one in three children born in 2000 will develop type 2 diabetes in their lifetime. Although the disease historically afflicts adults between the ages of forty and sixty, the rise in childhood obesity is associated with a tenfold increase in type 2 diabetes in adolescents over the last twenty years.[93]

Additionally, this worldwide tsunami of obesity and diabetes is associated with numerous adverse health conditions, namely heart disease, cancer, and mood disorders leading to reduced life expectancy. These chronic diseases comprise the majority of our healthcare dollars and manifest as a consequence of an underlying metabolic and inflammatory-immune imbalance created as a result of many factors commonplace to our modern life.[94]

The combined direct medical costs of diabetes including amputation, kidney and retina damage, and indirect medical costs, such as for disability and loss of productivity, exceeded $245 billion in 2012 for diabetes.[95] Each year in the United States diabetes is responsible for more than 71,382 deaths.[96] Calories and sugar are the tip of the iceberg.

Preventing type 2 diabetes conditions is a lifelong feat and managing the condition medically requires an integrated approach. Excess fat is thought to contribute to 44 percent of the diabetes burden, which like obesity, is on the rise.[97] To this effect, a recent study found that obesity confers the single greatest contribution—that is, 53 percent—toward the development of type 2 diabetes in people of lower socioeconomic status.[98] Additionally, increased blood triglycerides explained about 10 percent of the diabetes burden, while alcohol and blood pressure hardly had any effect on obesity development.

EXPENSIVE RESEARCH, INEFFECTIVE SOLUTIONS

While obesity and diabetes rates flourish, preventive suggestions remain the same, even though the government-funded National Institutes of Health spends nearly $800 million dollars annually researching obesity and its related disorders.[99] The traditional model describing it suggests a long incubation period of poor diet that continually increases blood glucose levels and desensitization to the body's insulin. Conventional wisdom suggests that this dog-chasing-its-tail game can only continue for so long before the pancreas "burns out" and can no longer synthesize and release insulin from its beta cells. Or at least that is the current theory.

However, in a similar fashion to the calorie-centric view of obesity, the progression of insulin resistance to type 2 diabetes is greatly oversimplified. Many factors interfere with insulin signaling at the cellular level above and beyond too much blood glucose, or *hyperglycemia*.

The dietary and lifestyle recommendations adopted by the American Diabetes Association website suggest, for example, a whole grain bagel with orange juice for breakfast, walking more, starting dinner with a salad, and getting a good night's sleep. Similarly, the WHO and CDC websites suggest increased physical activity, eating more fruits and vegetables, and decreasing calorie-rich foods, television time, and sugar-sweetened beverages. Many of the revolutionary studies I refer to throughout this book are actually NIH-funded, yet the findings don't appear to have been disseminated.

For example, the NIH's Heart, Lung, and Blood Institute webpage contains the largely ineffectual recommendations similar to WHO's. How are tax-paying U.S. citizens benefiting from more than $800 million spent annually in NIH obesity and diabetes research? The take-home message on the NIH's site is to eat fewer calories than you burn. Thus, after millions of dollars of quality research exploring the many intricacies of obesity and diabetes, we are left with guidelines like this: eat breakfast (a bagel and orange juice, or an oatmeal breakfast bar, milk, and an English muffin), consume fewer calories in general and have a salad at dinner, exercise more, use a pedometer, and get more sleep. Is this really the best we can do for an epidemic threatening to bankrupt healthcare?

WHY GLUCOSE ISN'T THE WHOLE STORY

The main reason why I don't rely too much on fasting blood to assess metabolic health is that the body has the ability to maintain *homeostasis*, or balance, in the wake of significant post-meal surges in blood glucose. Although elevations in blood sugar and insulin are frequently observed in the insulin-resistant and prediabetic state, the body compensates by releasing insulin from the pancreas.[100] For that reason, reliance on fasting glucose and insulin levels, even in metabolically challenged persons, is inferior to more accurate challenge tests.

The Oral Glucose Tolerance Test (OGTT) has been considered the gold standard diabetes diagnostic tool. After a person drinks a sugar-laden drink, blood samples are drawn to assess how his or her blood sugar responds. This is presumed to mimic what happens after eating a meal. This same approach is now being applied to more accurately assess blood triglyceride and cholesterol handling, using the so-called lipid load test.[101,102]

AGES AND RAGES

Getting pricked with needles multiple times during a two-hour glucose tolerance test is cumbersome. This is why the World Health Organization, CDC, and American Diabetes Association have come to rely on the *glycated hemoglobin* (HbA1c) test to assess the diabetes continuum. When blood glucose is increased outside of the biological range for an extended period of time, it attaches itself to biological proteins, including the heme (iron)-containing portion of our red blood cells, through a process called glycation.[103] As such, HbA1c is widely used to quantify long-term blood-sugar control, while fasting or random glucose is more representative of short-term management.[104]

The twentieth-century chemist and physician L. C. Maillard, MD, discovered that sugars such as glucose could readily react with proteins to form a glucose-protein complex.[105] Since all proteins in the body are capable of undergoing the glycation associated with hyperglycemia, there is emerging research suggesting that glycated albumin—a protein commonly present in the blood stream—is more sensitive than HbA1c.[106] Increased glycated albumin is also an independent risk factor for coronary artery disease.

BIOMARKER	DIABETES	PREDIABETES
HbA1c	> 6.5%	> 5.7% & < 6.5%
Fasting glucose	> 125 mg/dL	> 100 mg/dL & < 125 mg/dL
75 g – Glucose tolerance test (OGTT)	>199 mg/dL (2 hours post)	> 140 mg/dL & < 199 mg/dL (2 hours post)

Glucotoxicity is an unwelcome side effect associated with increased unregulated blood-sugar levels common to insulin resistance and type 2 diabetes.[107] AGEs, or *advanced glycation end-products*, is the scientific term describing the compound created when excess sugar attaches to or mixes with proteins of the body, such as hemoglobin.[108] The immune system recognizes AGEs in a similar lock-and-key fashion that occurs when bacterial endotoxin leak through the intestine.[109] The receptors that sense these sugar-protein complexes, or AGEs, are called RAGEs, for *receptors for advanced glycation end-products*, which ignite cellular inflammation.[110]

Impaired blood-sugar control and excessive intake of fructose and D-ribose are not the only ways to unnecessarily expose your body to AGEs.[111] We are now finding that cooking methods may be as important for metabolic health as the nutrients contained within the food. For example crisp, deep-fried, broiled, grilled, and roasted foods are rich in AGEs.[112] Consumption of AGE-rich foods has recently been linked to impairments in glucose balance, satiety, and pancreatic function—that is, independent of sugar or calorie excess.[113,114,115]

Scientists at Mount Sinai School of Medicine suggest that boiling and stewing methods of cooking may be the best way to reduce the AGE content of common foods. In summary, excessive consumption of glucose, fructose, or D-ribose, and a high-AGE diet can damage bodily proteins and fuel inflammation, which is unequivocally associated with various cancers, heart disease, blood-sugar imbalances, and more.[116,117]

DIABETES + OBESITY = DIABESITY

Australian epidemiologist Paul Zimmet, MD, PhD, has sought to spread the message to the world that obesity and diabetes pandemics are not isolated conditions, but are connected.[118] As the name implies, *diabesity*, a term first reported in the medical literature during the late 1990s, describes the co-occurrence of these two overlapping conditions. It's been estimated that obesity accounts for up to 90 percent of type 2 diabetes. The diabetes risk continuum increases from about 4 fold at a BMI around 23 to over 93-fold for BMI over 35 in the extremely obese.[119]

The association between fat and diabetes in diabesity is specific to the visceral fat of the abdominal region.[120] However, diabesity fails to adequately include the associated cardiovascular risk, which is the serious consequence of both obesity and diabetes.[121] Not all obese individuals have insulin resistance or diabetes. Likewise, not all diabetics are obese. For example, a recent study of Chinese subjects reported that increased plasma leptin was more strongly associated with prediabetes and diabetes than was adiposity, or fat. Increases in leptin may indicate that the immune system is suffering from collateral immune damage and causing healthy fat to convert to sick fat.[122]

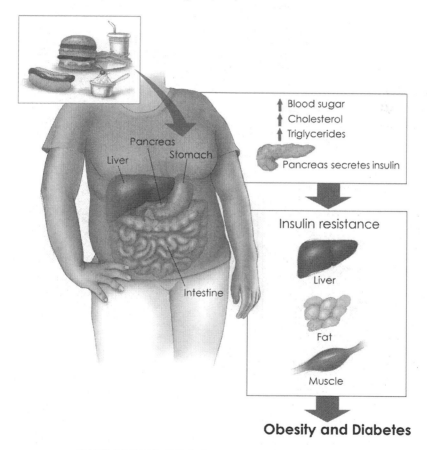

Obesity and Diabetes

THE NOW-OBSOLETE CONCEPT OF DIABETES AND OBESITY

The typical explanation of fat gain centers around calories and increased blood sugar.

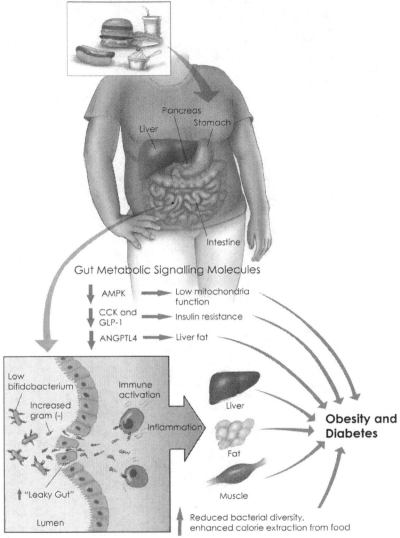

Gut Metabolic Signalling Molecules

AMPK → Low mitochondria function

CCK and GLP-1 → Insulin resistance

ANGPTL4 → Liver fat

Low bifidobacterium

Increased gram (-)

Immune activation

Inflammation

Liver

Fat

Muscle

"Leaky Gut"

Lumen

Obesity and Diabetes

Reduced bacterial diversity, enhanced calorie extraction from food

Causes of Imbalanced Gut Flora

cesarean section birthing, formula feeding, excessive hygeine, acid suppressing medications (PPIs), anti-inflammatory medications (NSAIDs), environmental toxins, mindless eating, fructose, alcohol, low fiber diet

THE CONTEMPORARY METABOLIC MODEL

The new perspective on fat gain and diabetes includes the role of gut bacteria. Western food alters the composition of trillions of intestinal bacteria, the hormones released from the intestine, and the integrity of the gastrointestinal barrier, leading to increased absorption of inflammatory bacterial particles, or endotoxin. The end result is inflammation, which impairs fat burning and leads to blood-sugar disorders.

The medical complications that have been, up to this point, exclusively a consequence of adult obesity now afflict children. It's been known for more than ten years, however, that obesity in adolescents is strongly associated with early cardiovascular disease.[123] This was first conclusively reported in the American Heart Association's journal *Circulation*, wherein autopsy studies revealed that youth obesity predicts severity of vascular damage, or *atherosclerosis*. In 2012, European researchers reported significant heart damage in overweight and obese twelve-year-olds.[124] During the last thirty years, the increase and earlier onset of obesity and diabetes have lowered life expectancy to the point where analysts are not sure whether children born today will live as long as their parents did.[125]

METABOLIC SYNDROME

Currently, the main concern about the obesity pandemic is its strong association with the increased prevalence of cardiovascular disease, type 2 diabetes and insulin resistance, and lipid disorders, or *dyslipidemia*. However, remember that not all obese people develop diabetes, not all diabetics are obese, and lean people without diabetes still develop cardiovascular disease.

Over thirty years ago, Stanford University endocrinologist Gerald Reaven, MD, proposed that people with increased abdominal fat, blood triglycerides, and blood pressure, and reduced HDL cholesterol have malfunctions in insulin signaling, despite no overt signs of insulin resistance.[126,127]

Reaven proposed that the clustering of related physiologic abnormalities comprise a "syndrome" that stemmed from one major biochemical change: resistance to insulin's ability to deposit glucose into cells.[128] Reaven and many others provided ample evidence to suggest that this insulin resistance is to blame for the diverse set of whole-body disturbances that increase the risk for diabetes, heart disease, and stroke.

According to the most current American Heart Association statistics, more than fifty million Americans are afflicted by metabolic syndrome, which is defined by three or more of the imbalances listed in the table below. It should be noted however that while there is ongoing debate about adding other criteria, such as inflammatory markers and uric acid, many studies show that increased abdominal fat proves to be one of the most reliable indicators of the disorder.[129]

AMERICAN HEART ASSOCIATION'S DEFINING CRITERIA OF METABOLIC SYNDROME	
Increased visceral adipose fat	Waist circumference in men > 40 inches in women > 35 inches
Impaired blood sugar control (insulin-resistant)	Fasting blood sugar > 100 mg/dL
Increased blood triglycerides	Blood triglycerides > 150 mg/dL
Reduced HDL-cholesterol	Low HDL in men < 40 mg/dL Low HDL in women < 50 mg/dL
Increased blood pressure (hypertension)	Blood pressure > 135/85 mm Hg

VULNERABLE AT ANY AGE

Currently more than 35 percent of the entire U.S. adult population and 23 percent of Caucasian children have metabolic syndrome.[130,131] The prevalence is much higher in overweight adults and children. Although less than 9 percent of normal-weight females meet the criteria for metabolic syndrome, 33 percent of overweight and 56 percent of obese women have three or more risk factors.[132] Only 7 percent of lean adult men have three or more risk factors, while 30 percent and 65 percent of overweight and obese men have metabolic syndrome.

Similarly 30–42.5 percent of obese children have metabolic syndrome, depending on their ethnicity, with the condition being more prevalent in non-Caucasians.[133,134] However, a recent study reported that as many as 59 percent of adolescents have one or more metabolic syndrome risk factors regardless of their ethnicity.[135]

THE COMMON SOIL THEORY

In 1995, Michael Stern, MD, proposed the "common soil" hypothesis.[136] He suggested that the origins of both cardiovascular disease and diabetes are the same. At the time, scientists perceived certain ailments to be complications of other diseases. The thinking was that diabetes occurred first and cardiovascular disease followed. The "common soil" theory was a paradigm shift. It implies that the inflammation and free-radical stress leading to insulin resistance, and eventually diabetes, simultaneously induces damage to the cardiovascular system.

Excess fat tissue, particularly around the abdomen, speeds the appearance of a myriad of age-related diseases, accelerating the aging process in general.[137] For example, a study reported in the *Lancet* suggests that the more fat you have, the more likely you are to die prematurely.[138] This study involved over 900,000 individuals and found that for each five-point increase in body mass index (BMI), there is a 30 percent higher all-cause mortality, a 40 percent increased mortality from cardiovascular disease, and 60–120 percent increase in mortality from diabetes, kidney, and liver diseases. Cardiovascular disease is the world's leading cause of mortality, responsible for nearly 30 percent of all deaths globally. Incidentally, risk of cardiovascular disease is increased in obesity.[139]

Clearly, the visceral adipose tissue around the internal organs triggers inflammation that sets the stage for cardiovascular disease.[140] Furthermore, from diabetes to cardiovascular disease to cancer and depression, obesity coexists with many inflammation-linked diseases.[141] University of California-San Francisco epidemiologists estimate that by 2035, the rates of coronary heart disease will increase from 5 percent to 16 percent, leading to an additional 100,000 cases annually.[142]

Recently, the correlation between increased body fat and cardiovascular disease risk was updated: for every BMI unit increase above baseline, there is an 8 percent increase in cardiovascular-related events and 12 percent increase in cardiovascular-related mortality.[143] Central obesity lies at the core of the fat and cardiovascular disease connection.[144]

Over the last two thousand years, humankind has experienced a slow and steady increase in life expectancy. But over the last thirty years that trend has been slowing. Today analysts are no longer sure whether a majority of children will outlive their parents.

THE DIABETES-HEART DISEASE CONNECTION

There is a high association between cardiovascular disease and the blood-sugar regulation problems characteristic of insulin resistance and diabetes. For example, people with type 2 diabetes are twice as likely to die from a heart attack or stroke, and 75 percent of them succumb to coronary heart disease.

The medical complications that have been, up to this point, exclusively a consequence of adult obesity now afflict children at increasingly younger and younger ages. There has been a ten-fold increase in type 2 diabetes in adolescents during the last twenty years.

The chronic, low-grade inflammation created by obesity throws a monkey wrench into our metabolic machinery, leading to multiple chronic diseases, and it is no longer exclusive to adults. For the first time in 2010, it was reported that chronic inflammation related to increased body weight begins as early as age three.[145]

Ten-year-olds with metabolic syndrome had an increase in biomarkers that suggested liver damage and cardiovascular disease.[146] Specifically, compared to healthy controls, children diagnosed with metabolic syndrome exhibited a 48 percent increase in liver enzymes and a 15 percent greater size of the left ventricle of the heart.

Later in this book, I will explain what scientists are learning about the origins of obesity-promoting factors, namely imbalanced gut microflora.

KEY TAKEAWAYS

The emergence of a syndrome involving imbalances in various organs and tissues stems from the same set of core imbalances—increased belly fat, inflammation, and insulin resistance. All three core physiological processes must be balanced simultaneously.

Obesity is linked to both diabetes and inflammation in children and adults, and the inflammation that results is linked to increased risk for cardiovascular disease.

Since cardiovascular disease and diabetes comprise the majority of healthcare expenditures and premature deaths, we need to focus on ways to minimize belly fat while calming inflammation and restoring balance in insulin signaling.

CHAPTER 3

METABOLISM MEETS IMMUNITY

"Immune response and metabolic regulation are highly integrated and the proper function of each is dependent on the other."—Gökhan S. Hotamisligil, MD, PhD

The energy thriftiness that was programmed into your genome many millennia ago may actually threaten your health today if you don't manage your weight.[1]

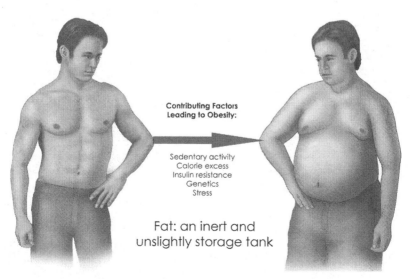

Contributing Factors
Leading to Obesity:

Sedentary activity
Calorie excess
Insulin resistance
Genetics
Stress

Fat: an inert and
unslightly storage tank

20th CENTURY MODEL OF FAT

The widely accepted, though obsolete, explanation of weight gain.

That's because fat cells are not passive storage bins, they're also hyperactive, metabolic mini-organs, secreting molecules that help your body in many ways from regulating your appetite to summoning your defenses.[2,3,4,5,6,7]

Eat enough pasta carbonara and your fat cells not only multiply, they will expand and start churning out potent chemical messengers.[8,9] Among them are interleukin-6 (IL-6) and tumor necrosis factor-alpha (TNF-alpha), which trigger inflammation. At the same time, a plethora of different inflammatory cells lock into docking stations, or receptors, on fat cell surfaces, making them receptive to incoming inflammatory messages that undermine your health.

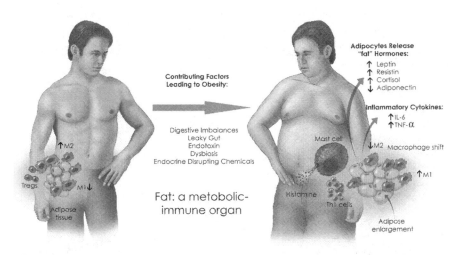

21st CENTURY MODEL OF FAT

An encompassing and scientific understanding of weight gain draws upon the close relationship between metabolism and immunity. Weight gain, particularly around the abdomen, is synonymous with an increase in proinflammatory immune cells and inflammation of fat tissue. This, in turn, antagonizes one's ability to burn fat effectively.

While nearly all tissues harbor immune cells to survey for danger and clean up tissue debris, the concentration of different inflammatory cells changes as you pile on the pounds.[10,11,12,13] This is the inherent problem with belly fat.[14] In fact, the number of inflammatory macrophages triples in abdominal fat, increasing from 4 percent of the overall fat tissue to well over 12 percent in obese people, leading to disastrous health issues.[15] An increased level of such Pac-Man-like macrophages is not exclusive to obesity but occurs in a wide range of tissues and organs contributing to cancer, brain disorders, liver disease, and cardiovascular disease, and more.[16]

Macrophages are just one of many immune cells thrown off balance as the pounds pile on, making fat loss efforts challenging.[17,18,19,20,21,22,23,24] Many immune cells can be found in common blood work received by your doctor known as a CBC (complete blood count); it's helpful to discuss what they do.

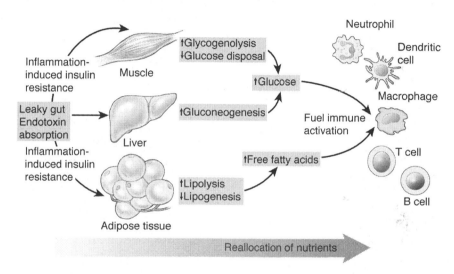

THE LINK BETWEEN POOR GUT HEALTH, INFLAMMATION, AND METABOLIC CHALLENGES

Immunological stress, such as leakage of bacterial particulate through the intestinal wall, initiates a redistribution of nutrients as the immune system attempts to fuel its defenses. Consequently, metabolic tissues, such as the liver and muscle and fat tissues, become dysfunctional and insulin resistant. Historically, this ancient protective mechanism increased human survival in the face of infectious microbes. Today the challenges to our intestinal bacteria are twenty-first-century foods. Our diets increase intestinal exposure to bacterial stimuli, igniting this ancient protective immune response at the expense of our metabolism.

When the epithelial barriers of our body, such as skin and the gastrointestinal tract, are broken, uninvited guests are greeted by our innate, or nonspecific, immune system.[25,26,27,28] These cells are constantly patrolling our body for danger signals, either damaged tissue or potential pathogens.[29,30] Using specialized antennae poised on their outer surface, they can quickly detect "uninvited guests" penetrating the body's barriers.

Generally, the sequence goes like this: hints that uninvited microbial guests have breached the barriers are messaged to other immune cells throughout the body by the surveying *toll-like receptors* (TLRs) sitting on the surfaces of the watchdog-like dendritic cells that line the gastrointestinal tract, lungs, and other mucus areas.[31,32] TLRs are found on many other immune cells, too, and even fat cells, because they have a high affinity for molecular patterns common to nearly all microbes.[33] The surface of fat cells in obese people also displays a greater concentration of docking receptors called CD40, which enable the fat cells to be hypersensitive to incoming inflammatory molecules.[34]

Neutrophils, like surveying dendritic cells, are other innate immune cells that are similar in concept to first responders.[35] They quickly migrate to the site of uninvited guests and trauma, such as a cut. TLRs also ignite the pathways of inflammation, alerting and recruiting other immune cells, killing the invader, and altering metabolism to repartition energy-rich fuels such as glucose from metabolic tissues.[36,37,38] The other immune cells recruited are monocytes and mast cells.[39] Indeed, in obesity, these "alert" signals released by immune cells (called *chemoattractant proteins* and *adhesion molecules*) are elevated in obesity.[40]

Macrophages, monocytes, and mast cells are part of the *innate immune system*, which is nonspecific, meaning it has no memory.[41] We can "restore tolerance" in these rogue immune cells by both sealing the body's protective barriers, such as the intestinal tract, and by ingesting bioactive molecules, such as vitamin D, probiotics, and plant-based phytochemicals, that relay non-danger signals.[42]

The *adaptive immune system*, which includes T and B lymphocytes, is called into action to increase production of antibodies so that the immune system can remember and better recognize invading guests, should the leak cross porous barriers again.[43] Indeed, many obesity studies have reported increases in certain types of inflammatory T lymphocytes.[44,45,46,47] It's well known in obesity investigations that groups of T lymphocytes normally congregating in and around fat tissue flip out of their chill mode and pivot into beast mode, which is incongruent with fat burning.[48,49,50]

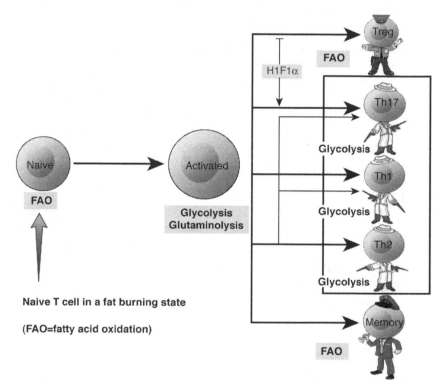

NUTRIENT METABOLISM IN
ACTIVATED T CELLS VS. TREG CELLS

The highly modifiable T lymphocytes are influenced by immune stimuli (damaged cells and microbial particles, for example) as well as local metabolism. Upon activation, inflammatory T helper cells, namely Th1 and Th17, reprogram their metabolism to favor sugar burning. In contrast, anti-inflammatory or surveying Treg cells are fueled by fat combustion.

The two packages of T lymphocytes are generally pro-inflammatory sugar burners or anti-inflammatory, fat-burning packages known as

Th1 and Th17 or Th2 and T regulatory cells (*Treg cells*). Indeed many studies hint that increased body fat is associated with the later pairing of T cells.[51,52,53,54,55,56,57,58] Treg cells normally resolve inflammation and are considered to be sentinels of the immune system, acting like security guards preventing runaway inflammation.[59,60]

So while being overweight and obese are classically thought of as metabolic disorders, with an overabundance of energy stored in fat, the condition is also characterized by inflammation and predictable shifts among various players of the immune system.[61] And these immune changes are startlingly similar to those that occur with heart disease, autoimmunity, and cancer.

Meanwhile, there are metabolic repercussions to all this immune activity. In more than 70 percent of the overweight and obese people, the inflammation that results from the expanding fat tissue ultimately changes the way those cells respond to insulin.[62,63] And since insulin is critical for controlling glucose and lipids, the levels of these nutrient metabolites in the bloodstream increase. More than twenty scientific studies over the past several decades have shown that obesity-related inflammation is linked to one disorder alone—type 2 diabetes.[64] It's not surprising that this new understanding is prompting scientists on the cutting edge of obesity research to look at new ways to help people lose weight that go beyond familiar admonitions about monitoring calories in and calories out.

PROGRAMMED TO SURVIVE

So how do the same cellular mechanisms selected over the course of humanity ultimately predispose us to chronic ailments like obesity, cardiovascular disease, and diabetes? You could blame the interdependency of the immune and metabolic systems.[65,66] That relationship is a prime biological example of too much of a good thing.

Immunity and metabolism are, as Forrest Gump would say, "like peas and carrots." One system maintains your ability to fight infection; the other enhances your ability to store energy and prevent starvation. Throughout your body what occurs in one system affects the behavior of the other, and that is especially prevalent in fat tissue, the storage bin of energy.

An expert on this topic, Gökhan S. Hotamisligil, MD, PhD, of the Harvard School of Public Health, has shown that even in the most primitive animals such as the fruit fly, both metabolic and immune response are regulated by fat tissue.[67,68] The high degree of integration of the metabolic and immune mechanisms was certainly advantageous in prehistoric times when no sanitation, immunization, animal captivity, or law and order existed. Today contagious diseases such as tuberculosis, small pox, and measles are largely under control and even infection following cuts and burns is treatable, if not preventable, but the metabolic-immune connection is as active as ever.

Here's how your immune and metabolic systems work as a team and an example of how an imbalance between them can undermine their joint efforts: when you eat something sugary or a carbohydrate that is broken down into sugar, your pancreas releases insulin, which allows your body to appropriately use the glucose or move it to various organs or store it in warehouses of fat. That's metabolism in action. When you have an infection or tissue trauma, immune cells throughout your body, including those in fat tissue, leap into action to defend against the invader, releasing cellular molecules. These include chemical messengers, such as TNF-alpha, interleukins, cytokines, leukotrienes, prostaglandins, eicosanoids, histamines, bradykinins, and eventually antibodies destroy the invaders. That's your immune system in action.

Instead of allowing glucose to be deposited into fat, liver, and muscle, the message your cells get is, "Don't take up the glucose." That's called insulin resistance. One aspect of their interaction begins when some of the inflammatory messengers released by the immune cells both kill invaders and at the same time divert energy (glucose) away from the metabolic organs back into the bloodstream for their own use.[69,70] Since about 70 percent of the fuel driving an activated immune system comes from glucose, it makes perfect sense that chemical messengers from immune cells would signal cells to resist grabbing glucose for energy and free it for use by the hungry immune system.[71] Mistakenly sensing an invader, the body is attempting to deliver glucose to cells that need it to fuel defense, such as inflammatory macrophages and infection-fighting lymphocytes.

Paralleling this cascade of events are changes in the release of more dual-acting metabolic and immune hormones from the fat cells called *adipocytokines*. *Leptin* and *adiponectin* are two well-known ones that help regulate satiety and fat storage as well as inflammation. Adiponectin is a protective, healthy *adipocytokine* released from fat tissue that helps keep inflammation in check. Leptin is more disruptive, hampering Treg cell activity, including squelching inflammation.[72] When body fat increases, leptin increases and adiponectin decreases, a pattern that is linked to inflammation and poor metabolic control.[73,74,75]

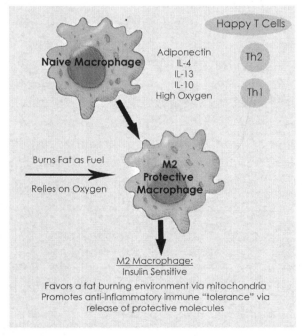

FAT BURNING
ANTI-INFLAMMATORY STATE

Regulatory and unstimulated immune cells are heavily reliant on oxygen and combustion of fats for fuel. Not so for stimulated immune cells, which thrive on glucose (sugar) in the absence of oxygen.

HOW NUTRIENTS AFFECT METABOLISM

A rich blood supply and proximity of abdominal fat to the liver enhance the inflammatory effects of fat and make fat loss especially challenging.[76] This is because when refined flours, sugar, and high-fat foods are digested, they directly trigger inflammatory switches on the surface of fat cells. The nonspecific, frontline immune cells of your innate immune system screen for and identify microbes using sensing receptors in the same way that security guards screen travelers before a flight.

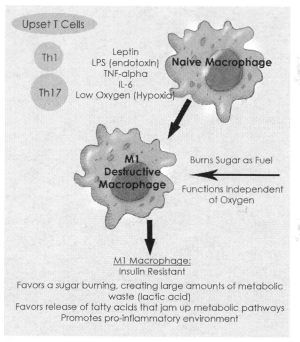

Upset T Cells

Th1

Th17

Leptin
LPS (endotoxin)
TNF-alpha
IL-6
Low Oxygen (Hypoxia)

Naive Macrophage

M1 Destructive Macrophage

Burns Sugar as Fuel

Functions Independent of Oxygen

M1 Macrophage:
Insulin Resistant
Favors a sugar burning, creating large amounts of metabolic waste (lactic acid)
Favors release of fatty acids that jam up metabolic pathways
Promotes pro-inflammatory environment

SUGAR BURNING
PROINFLAMMATORY STATE

When a person is overweight or obese, immune cells near metabolic tissues, such as fat and the liver, progress to a proinflammatory state.

These sampling receptors are called *pattern recognition receptors* (PRRs), and they seek out damaged biological molecules or DAMPs (damaged associated molecular patterns).[77] They also scan for bacterial, viral, parasitic, and fungi molecular signatures known as PAMPs (pathogen-associated molecular patterns).[78]

The sampling receptors of interest to weight loss are the TLRs (toll-like receptors), specifically one named TLR4. When it recognizes certain dietary fats and endotoxin, bacterial PAMP inflammation ensues.[79,80]

TLRs sit like watchdogs on the surfaces of macrophages and adipocytes truly bridging immunity to metabolism. With a receiving end on the outside of the cell and a transmitting end inside the cell, TLRs transmit these extracellular messages of "danger" into the cell. Common triggers of TLRs are saturated fats from the diet, lipid spillover from enlarged fat cells or damaged tissues, and endotoxin from gut bacteria.[81,82,83,84,85]

AN INFLAMMATORY MAESTRO

These triggers jump-start inflammation and shift metabolism out of the efficient (albeit slow) fat-burning state into a rapid-fire, sugar-burning state, making fat loss nearly impossible.[86,87,88,89] This is because idly sitting on the intracellular site of each TLR receiver is an inflammatory maestro, *nuclear factor kappa B* (NF-κβ). When bacterial particles such as endotoxin leak through the intestinal walls and latch onto TLR4s on fat and immune cells, NF-κβ awakes and instructs your cells to increase production of every inflammatory molecule possible, including tumor necrosis factors, interleukins, and *cyclooxygenase-2* (COX-2). When NF-κβ is activated, inflammation is in full swing.

Remember that inflammatory molecules alter how insulin communicates with your liver, fat cells, and muscles? Additionally, when excess sugars, fats, and bacterial endotoxin activate TLRs on the surfaces of these metabolic organs, NF-κβ inside these tissues directly blocks insulin's action.[90,91,92] In brief, insulin's voice is being vetoed from two angles: it's unable to assist the passage of sugar into cells and fails to prevent fatty acids from spilling out of fat cells. Blood sugar and lipid levels rise, and the cycle continues like a dog chasing its tail.[93]

PROCESSED CARBOHYDRATES: HIGH-FAT MEALS

Several studies over the last ten years have demonstrated that this complex inflammatory mechanism occurs when humans eat processed, high-glycemic carbohydrates.[94] One study found that eating pure glucose and white bread increases NF-κβ levels nearly twice as much as eating the carbohydrate-equivalent amount of low-glycemic pasta.[95] When an equal amount of calories in sugar is consumed along with polyphenolic compounds, such as those in orange juice, attenuated inflammation from NF-κβ doesn't occur.[96] (Polyphenols are the compounds that give fruits and vegetables their bright colors and are very important for fat loss, reducing inflammation, and restoring metabolism to normal.)

Sugar and processed carbohydrates are not the only nutrients known to increase inflammation. Excessive fat in the diet may be equally problematic. Endocrinologists from New York found that eating a McDonald's-type breakfast of an egg-muffin or sausage-muffin sandwich with hash browns—a 900-calorie, high-carb, high-fat meal—increased NF-κβ activity in immune cells by over 150 percent for several hours.[97] Italian researchers reported a whopping 71 percent increase in TNF-alpha and an 83 percent increase in IL-6 in the bloodstream of healthy people who ate a high-fat meal.[98]

Scientists are discovering that polyphenols and some herbs and spices block food-related inflammation. Drinking a polyphenol-rich fruit juice drink (pineapple, black currant, and plum) with a 1,300-calorie, high-fat meal blocks inflammation from NF-κβ, according to one study.[99] Scientists from Pennsylvania State University reported similar findings when adding spices such as rosemary, garlic, curcumin, and others to a 1,200-calorie, high-carbohydrate meal.[100]

One of my favorite studies conducted by Husam Ghanim, MD, at the University of Buffalo reported that when a 75 mg resveratrol capsule is combined with a 930-calorie, high-fat, high-carbohydrate meal, inflammation is attenuated.[101] This landmark study also reported two other significant findings: that the high-fat meal was associated with increases in TLR4, the antenna that drives inflammation by increasing NF-κβ, and the resveratrol supplement increased NF-κβ's anti-inflammatory opposite, *nuclear factor 2* (Nrf2, pronounced *nerf two*).

THE YIN AND YANG OF INFLAMMATION

Light and dark, fast and slow, hot and cold, inflammation and anti-inflammation: life is full of dualities. Nrf2 is the body's natural intracellular fire extinguisher. Abbot Laboratories recently paid over $400 million dollars to develop a novel Nrf2-activating drug, which would not only powerfully increase production of anti-inflammatory molecules, but also block NF-κβ, the body's main regulator of inflammatory genes. At present, plant-based phytochemicals, such as the herbs and spices used in the Penn State study, are the most potent ways to increase Nrf2-protective molecules.[102]

The three broad categories of molecules increased through Nrf2 activation are cellular detoxification molecules, antioxidants, and anti-inflammatory compounds, particularly glutathione, considered to be the body's most powerful antioxidant.[103] Specific Nrf2-activating compounds will be discussed in the treatment section. My favorites are resveratrol, curcumin, garlic, green tea, and *sulforaphane*, a compound in cruciferous vegetables.

ENDOTOXIN: THE DIET-INFLAMMATION CONNECTION

Several researchers have discovered another piece of the puzzle of how diet is related to inflammation. They found that foods high in sugar and fat increase the intestinal absorption of immune-stimulating molecules, or *antigens*.[104,105] The main inflammatory antigens linked to obesity and diabetes are substances called endotoxin, which originate from the outer membranes of certain intestinal bacteria such as *E. coli*. Endotoxin can directly bind to immune cells in the gut, or they can sneak through a leaky gut into the bloodstream, eventually clinging to immune cells, as well as fat, muscle, and liver tissue.[106] That's when NF-κβ is cranked into high gear and inflammation surges, releasing all those proinflammatory molecules like TNF-alpha and interleukin-6.

Research suggests intestinal endotoxin plays a powerful role in chronic inflammation and obesity.[107,108,109,110]

Ultimately, if you keep feeding your fat tissue excess calories, the metabolic disruption that ensues leads to a state of continuous low-grade inflammation that experts call *meta-inflammation*.[111,112] It leads to chronic diseases like diabetes and cancer. To make the situation even worse, fat cells tend to get fatter.

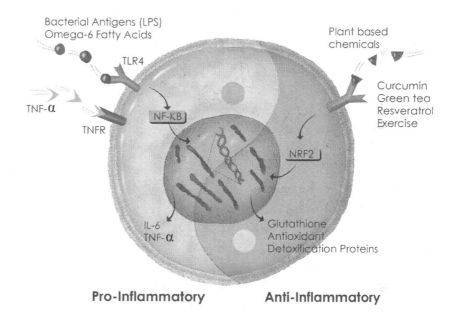

THE YIN AND YANG OF INFLAMMATION

Inflammatory triggers, such as bacterial endotoxin, dock onto cells, activating NF-kappa-B proteins and triggering inflammation. In contrast, plant-based phytochemicals stimulate a protective, anti-inflammatory pathway, Nrf2. Nrf2 activation leads to increase signaling of beneficial cellular signaling molecules with anti-inflammatory, antioxidant, and detoxification proteins.

Lean and metabolically healthy people don't get on this fat-to-fatter cycle because they have a continuous and reasonable flow of energy into fat, where it's stored as triglycerides, and out of the globules of fat as *free fatty acids* (FFAs). But in overweight people who have enlarged fat cells, triglycerides soar and free fatty acids spill out. This, if you recall, ignites cellular stress networks that derange metabolism.

IS OBESITY AN INFECTIOUS DISEASE?

The immune and metabolic responses to excess fat tissue create a biological environment that mimics what happens during an infection. But the fat tissue isn't infected. Or is it?

A recent breakthrough discovery sheds light on this question. Scientists in Texas found that overfeeding animals caused their fat cells to express a protein called *major histocompatibility complex II* (MCH II) that allows the immune system to spot an invader.[113] Normally this response should occur only when immune cells detect a bacteria or virus.

Now weight-loss experts recognize that this metabolic-immune overlap contributes significantly to obesity and that normalizing the balance between the two systems is essential for weight loss and for maintaining lifelong weight control. The role of low-grade activation of the immune system in the development of present-day obesity and diabetes epidemics is not a novel concept.[114,115] Experts, who have studied how our bodies' defense mechanisms have evolved, recognize that the original intent of insulin resistance was to protect the body.[116] If our ancestors were unable to rapidly induce a robust shift in energy allocation to the immune system, they would be very vulnerable to lethal microbes, especially those that cause infection after injury. However, what was protective when life-threatening pathogens ran amuck is no longer in our best interests. Unfortunately, this genetic heritage of molecular survival switches may be maladaptive in a world where common foodstuffs can trigger them.

MAKING ENERGY TRADE-OFFS

Just as sending troops off to battle means we have to shift federal spending from, say, building bridges to defense, the body has to shift energy from fueling day-to-day maintenance to immune defenses when bacteria in the gut leaks through gaps in its lining and enters the bloodstream. But what if there's no energy to spare? Rainer

Straub, MD, a prolific voice in the fields of neuroendocrinology and rheumatology, has written extensively on the topic of immune steering of "energy-rich fuels."[117,118] He suggests that the immune system can increase resting metabolic rate 30–100 percent.

While it's well recognized that overweight, obese, and insulin-resistant individuals have pronounced inflammation, the metabolic demands of an activated immune system have largely been under-estimated. For example, during the transition from a quiet immune state to an activated one—a phenomenon that can be evoked by eating processed foods—cells of the immune system can double in size, multiply every four hours, and synthesize many antibodies and inflammation-stimulating molecules.[119]

Just as a growing child requires more energy to synthesize new pro-teins and molecules, so does an activated immune system. And when metabolic tissues hog nutrients in the presence of a life-threatening immune threat, such as an infection, a person may die.

REINING IN THE FIGHT OR FLIGHT RESPONSE

To further confirm the modern hypothesis that obesity and diabetes are inflammatory diseases caused by eating foods that increase absorption of bacterial particles, such as endotoxin, we must look at another aspect of the inflammation response: stress. Trauma, infection, and emotional or psychological upsets create the same stress response.[120] In fact, many chronic diseases such as obesity, diabetes, and heart disease are noted to have a stress component. Since your stress response may be activated by a perceived threat, as well as actual stressors, not coping well with life's many challenges can initiate the same ancient life-saving mechanism.

Dr. Straub, in Germany, helps us to better understand how the stress response is woven into inflammation. The hormones increased upon activation of the fight or flight response, such as cortisol and catecholamine, are critical in helping the immune system thrive during life-threatening events. The stressors ramp up the hormonal signaling hub called the *hypothalamic-pituitary-adrenal* (HPA) *axis* and prompt the release of adrenal hormones, which among other things pivots the nervous system out of the rest-and-digest mode of the *parasympathetic nervous system* (PNS) into that of the "locked and loaded" fight or flight *sympathetic nervous system* (SNS) mode. This response, as Dr. Straub and others suggest, helps the body shift energy—that is, glucose and lipids—away from low-priority metabolic tissue to supply the higher-priority, activated immune system, the one required for immediate survival in a life or death situation.

OBESITY AND PSYCHONEUROIMMUNOLOGY (PNI)

Hans Selye, a mid-twentieth-century scientist, first dubbed this complex stress response as the "general adaptation syndrome." Scientists now understand that activation of the stress response doesn't just involve the *endocrine*, or hormonal, system of the body, but equally draws upon the immune system and the central nervous system in the brain. The study of these interactions is called *psychoneuroimmunology*. This complex stress response and associated increase in fat-promoting hormones like cortisol and inflammatory products can be activated by mere thoughts and perceptions of stress; it doesn't always have to involve actual physical trauma or bacterial infections.[121,122,123,124,125] For example, feelings such as loss of control, defeat, and work-related stress activate the stress response and are associated with obesity and diabetes.[126,127,128] When this primitive survival response is over-stimulated, we suffer from poor sleep, reduced energy, depression, low motivation, reduced libido, high blood pressure, plaque buildup in blood vessels, stagnant digestion, immune system changes, inflammation, and increased levels of leptin and free radicals, all of which promote fat around the abdomen and adverse metabolic changes.[129,130,131,132,133]

THE WEB OF FOOD, FAT, AND STRESS

In concert with our hypothesis that fats and processed carbohydrates alter our gut microflora, igniting our primitive inflammatory stress responses, studies show that carbohydrates, but not protein, also raise the stress hormone cortisol.[134] Additionally, scientists in Spain showed that increased cortisol following ingestion of a sugary drink is independently associated with increased blood glucose, suggesting that cortisol also raises blood sugar.[135] Like inflammatory cytokines, the stress hormone blocks insulin's action and triggers the liver to produce glucose, raising blood-sugar levels.[136,137]

Cortisol sabotages our waistline in two additional ways: first, by preferentially depositing fat in the abdominal region; and second, by stimulating appetite and creating a preference for calorie-rich foods and carbohydrates.[138,139,140,141,142,143,144] Even more troubling, as the pounds pile on, the liver and fat tissue crank up cortisol production, which normally occurs in the adrenal gland. (This effect is due to increased activity of the enzyme *11beta-hydroxysteroid dehydrogenase type 1* or 11beta-HSD1 for short.) Thankfully, losing weight and eating a low-carbohydrate diet turn down the dimmer switch on this liver and fat-tissue derived cortisol production.

Poor food choices create a viscous cycle of inflammation and release of stress hormones, creating a ravenous appetite and a desire for unhealthy food, a racing mind, and a bloodstream full of adrenaline. These choices are also a recipe for a sleepless night—which is in and of itself a stressor, appetite wrecker, and waist-line buster. In the treatment discussion, you'll learn some easy tricks to blunt the stress response, curb appetite, and squelch inflammation.

COLD VS. HOT INFLAMMATION

The classical immune survival response has been dubbed "hot" inflammation and is slightly different from those of obesity-related, metabolic-derived inflammation known as "cold" inflammation. Hot inflammation is much more complex than the cold type and involves antigen and antibody complexes and adaptive immunity, similar to that which occurs when the immune system battles a lethal pathogen, such as tuberculosis.

In contrast, cold inflammation is a new description for the kind of chronic, low-grade inflammation characteristic of persons with modern-day obesity and metabolic diseases. Cold inflammation, or meta-inflammation, can be activated both by microbes leaking through the intestinal barrier and excessive blood levels of nutrients, such as lipids dripping out of enlarged fat cells or damaged tissue. It is linked to metabolic stress, insulin resistance, and perturbations in blood glucose and fats.

Both the branches of the immune system—the *innate* system, which is the first line of defense against invaders, and the *adaptive*, the second line of defense and the one that reacts to the specific invading organism—are drawn upon, but the triggers are not generally "lethal" in the classic sense.

Today, acute immune insults have been replaced with chronic immune challenges. Food and bacterial debris may leak through your intestinal walls and enter your circulation.[145,146,147] Endotoxin from bacterial cell walls can trigger an immune response that was once protective.[148] Moreover, damaged cell components and fatty acids spilling out of fat tissue also activate the immune system, triggering inflammation and metabolic imbalances.[149] Last but not least, expanding fat tissue itself creates damage, sparking the immune system into high gear.[150,151,152] Sadly, for many people today, an immune reaction happens every time they eat, creating a scenario of chronic, low-grade inflammation.

INFECTOBESITY:
THE IMMUNE-MICROBE-METABOLIC CONNECTION

Bacterial endotoxin from the gut are not the only microbial link to obesity and diabetes. Elevated levels of circulating inflammation-stimulating immune cells have been observed in overweight and obese adults and children and in those with metabolic syndrome.[153,154,155,156,157,158,159,160] For example, one study involving more than 6,500 people found a strong correlation between total leukocyte counts and metabolic syndrome.[161] The researchers report that the increased neutrophil, monocyte, and eosinophil levels were strong and independent risk markers for obesity. (All these components are routinely measured on commercial blood tests.)

Consequences of obesity-associated skewing of the immune system include functional impairments in metabolism, namely blood sugar and fat, or lipid imbalance, which lead to insulin resistance, type 2 diabetes, metabolic syndrome, and heart disease.[162,163,164,165]

The term *infectobesity* has emerged among scientists to describe the link between being overweight and the presence of low-grade, nonpathogenic microbial manifestation.[166,167,168] With ample scientific reports confirming the presence of bacterial imbalances in the mouth, small intestine, colon, and bloodstream, and even an increase in antibodies to viruses, microbes deserve proper recognition as possible agents promoting obesity.[169,170,171,172,173,174,175] Clearly, this new understanding means a change in treatment of weight loss and metabolic disorders, with a focus on immune modulation.

The hypervigilant, proinflammatory immune state accompanying increased levels of body fat can be described as generalized immune exhaustion.[176,177] Hence, overweight persons are more susceptible to infections and related complications, periodontal disease, and autoimmunity.[178,179,180]

For the first time, in the late 1990s, scientists proved the association between viral infection and obesity in humans, confirming the findings of extensive previous animal studies.[181] A few years later, the banal human adenovirus-36 that causes the common cold and upper respiratory tract illness was also shown to increase fat mass, blood triglycerides, cholesterol, and insulin resistance in adults.[182,183] Studies also link other nonlethal viruses such as herpes simplex virus (HSV)-1, HSV-2, and enterovirus to an increase in body fat.[184]

While studies of viruses have been unable to confirm that infection causes obesity or that obesity-related changes in the immune system makes one more susceptible to viral infection, studies clearly point to an association. For example, researchers in San Diego found that 78 percent of a large group of children testing positive for adenovirus were obese. Korean researchers also found a high correlation among obesity and adenovirus infection in children, and suggested that the adenovirus may increase fat-synthesizing enzymes in the fat cells.[185]

One scientific report found that obese children and adults were at increased risk of hospitalization from the 2009 H1N1 influenza pandemic.[186] Another study found that 50 percent of Californian adults hospitalized with the 2009 H1N1 infection were obese and had an increased risk of death, and a report published in the prestigious English medical journal, *The Lancet*, concluded that obesity is a risk factor for infectious disease.[187]

Recent immune system analyses suggest that while increased fat mass is linked to inflammation, or a generalized amplification of immune defenses, there appears to be a decline in the functioning of key antiviral immune cells, such as dendritic cells (DCs) and natural killer (NK) cells, which would predispose one to infection.[188,189] This research supports the notion that metabolic and hormonal response from poor dietary choices of overweight and obese persons is inflammatory, which over time leads to a state of immune exhaustion and poor defenses. Furthermore, when overweight people start exercising, studies show they experience a significant reduction in symptoms during upper respiratory tract infections and take fewer sick days.[190]

A PEEK AT THE ROAD AHEAD

The discovery of disturbances in the cross talk between the trillions of bacteria housed in our digestive tract and our immune and metabolic systems is the most exciting breakthrough in obesity research.[191] Our intestine is lined with immune receptors whose main function is to detect pathogen-associated molecular patterns (PAMPs) common to most bacteria, fungi, viruses, and parasites.[192] The end result of microbial PAMPs and nutrients docking onto *pattern recognition receptors* (PRRs) imbedded into the intestine is a ricocheting, immunological alarm signal, tipping our metabolic physiology out of fat-burning mode and into sugar-burning mode—a physiological state that is incongruent with optimal health.

KEY TAKEAWAYS

The worlds of metabolism and immunity collide as fat tissue increases. This is evident in the number of inflammatory macrophages in abdominal fat. The surface of fat cells in those who are overweight also displays a greater concentration of docking receptors, which cause fat cells to be hypersensitive to incoming inflammatory stress molecules. Fortifying your body's protective shields, such as the intestinal tract, with vitamin D, probiotic, and plant-based phytochemicals transmits non-danger signals, thereby preventing inflammatory stress.

Misbehavior of the immune system begins when inflammatory messengers released by the immune cells destroy invaders while diverting energy (glucose) away from the metabolic organs back into the bloodstream for their own use. Bacterial particles that leak from the intestine cause a chain reaction that leads to increased production of inflammatory molecules. Research has revealed that polyphenols and some herbs and spices such as resveratrol, curcumin, garlic, green tea, and sulforaphane (a compound found in cruciferous vegetables) have the ability to block food-related inflammation.

When your body is in a state of internal stress, whether real or perceived, hormones like cortisol and inflammatory by-products increase. Although our fight or flight reaction is the same as our ancestors', it occurs in response to different circumstances. Nevertheless, it has a consequential negative effect in the form of obesity and diabetes.

Today, acute immune insults have been replaced with chronic immune challenges. The term *infectobesity* has emerged among scientists to describe the link between the conditions of being overweight and the presence of low-grade, nonpathogenic microbial manifestation. Metabolic and hormonal responses in obese people to poor dietary choices open the door to inflammation and eventual immune system exhaustion.

CHAPTER 4

TURN ON FAT BURNING

"In normal-weight individuals without the predisposition to obesity the body's ability to switch from glucose to fat oxidation is flexible, whereas pre-obese, obese and formerly obese individuals seem to be metabolically inflexible, which predisposes to weight gain and obesity during environmental challenges such as a high-fat diet and lack of high-intensity physical activity."—Arne Astrup, MD, PhD

Why are immune cells drawn to fat tissue like moths to a flame? How do they move your body from efficient fat burning to sluggish sugar burning? Are gut bacteria involved? The answers to these questions are why people can't lose weight.

Fat tissue is both an energy buffer and regulator of how much sugar (glucose) and fat (lipid) enter your bloodstream.[1] In a person who maintains a healthy weight, extra energy is stored in fat for future use, sort of like the gas in your car's tank. To use gas to turn the wheels of your car, though, the fuel can't just sit in the tank. It must flow through fuel injectors, mix with oxygen, enter the cylinders, get compressed, and finally be ignited by spark plugs. The explosion that follows drives power to the wheels.

Similarly, the nutrients in the foods you eat follow a metabolic chain of events in which they become usable cellular energy as *adenosine triphosphate* (ATP). ATP molecules drive cellular explosions, creating movement in muscles, cell synthesis and replication, and many more activities.[2]

However, unlike your car's reliance on gasoline, you can make cellular ATP in several different ways.[3,4,5] Exercise, for example, is one metabolic pathway. How long and how hard you work out will determine which pathway the sugar or fat in your body will be used.

As in cooking, metabolic pathways require certain ingredients to achieve the end goal and follow a particular recipe, often in sequence. Fats, carbohydrates, and proteins are the main nutrients required, but smaller ones, called *micronutrients*, such as alpha-lipoic acid, chromium, magnesium, selenium, and zinc are also necessary. Depending on the circumstance, B vitamins (thiamine, folate, vitamin B6, and B12) and amino acid-like compounds, such as L-leucine, creatine, carnitine, and carnosine, are needed, too.

Here is what happens when you use sugar to fuel, say, a short, intense workout. Sugar is burned by a process known as *glycolysis*, which literally translates into the splitting of sugar. In a series of steps, a molecule of glucose becomes two molecules of pyruvate and ATP (see page 6).

Glycolysis can occur with or without oxygen.[6] But when you run short of oxygen, those molecules of pyruvate are converted to lactic acid. It's what causes the burning sensation you feel in your glutes when doing a prolonged series of squats, for instance. Your breathing rate increases to buffer lactic acid buildup and to expel the CO_2 spilling off as a result of splitting glucose into pyruvate.

In contrast, when you keep the oxygen flowing, say, when working out less intensely, oxygen molecules drag the pyruvate into the cells' mitochondria. These cellular energy factories are very important for fat burning as well and comprise about 10 percent of your body weight.[7] In the presence of oxygen, the pyruvate is converted to acetyl-CoA and shuttled into the mitochondria, producing over thirty-four molecules of ATP.

Fat burning occurs in a pathway called *lipolysis*, which literally translates into lipid splitting. During exercise, *hormone-sensitive lipase* (HSL) splits stored triglycerides into free fatty acids that can be burned inside the mitochondria in the exact same way pyruvate is used after glycolysis.[8] Free fatty acids can only be shuttled into the mitochondria through a transporter molecule called L-*carnitine*, which is why some people promote L-carnitine for fat loss.[9,10] I suggest 1000-2000 mg of L-carnitine tartrate first thing in the morning before aerobic exercise.

It would seem, then, that fat loss should be pretty simple: reduce the amount of fat being deposited, while at the same time increase the amount of fatty acids exiting from fat cells to be burned in the mitochondria. But there are several things that work against this hypothesis: reduced metabolic flexibility, lipid spillover (lipotoxicity), and gut-bacteria imbalances.

USING YOUR ENERGY CURRENCY

You put coins in parking meters, carry cash at the farmer's market, and use PayPal for online shopping. The cells of metabolically healthy people have a similar ability to use energy currency in different ways. An external signal, whether it's eating a large meal or starving, will activate the most appropriate metabolic signaling network available to either store energy or burn it for fuel.[11] The scientific term for this on-demand variability in communication is known as *metabolic flexibility.*[12]

Sir Philip Randle of Oxford University coined the term in 1963, when he discovered that vascular tissue could switch back and forth between lipid and carbohydrate metabolism.[13] However, Randle also noted that insulin resistance increases cellular fatty acid production, reducing the ability of cells to use glucose.

Think about metabolic flexibility as fiscal flexibility. Let's say you wanted to take your spouse out for a nice dinner and planned to pay for it with a credit card. If you had no cash to pay the parking valet or the coat check attendant, and if the restaurant didn't take credit cards, your financial flexibility would be limited for the moment.

A similar metabolic inflexibility occurs in people who are obese or have insulin resistance or diabetes.[14] Increased levels of free fatty acids (FFAs) are characteristic of these conditions. People with these health risks also have high levels of glucose in their bloodstream, which inhibits fat burning and increases fat gain, perpetuating the metabolic syndrome. Increased free fatty acids in the bloodstream are beneficial when energy demands are high, as happens during exercise or infection.

Under normal conditions free fatty acids have two fates: (1) they can be burned inside the mitochondria to create cellular energy or ATP, and (2) they can be converted into sugar, via a process known as *gluconeogenesis*, which literally means forming sugar from anew. The later process is the body's fuel preference during sleep and exercise, while the former process is used during stages of starvation, inflammation, and stress.

In metabolically healthy persons, free fatty acids increase when *hormone-sensitive lipase* (HSL) liberates stored fats from adipose tissue, where it is burned as fuel in mitochondria-rich muscle tissue and liver. This is exactly the kind of fat release you want!

In contrast, overweight and metabolically inflexible individuals have dysfunctional fat tissue with reduced levels of *hormone-sensitive lipase* (HSL).[15] Ironically, lipids are still released from their fat cells at a very high rate. But instead of being gracefully snipped by HSL, fatty acids are pushed out of over-stuffed fat cells, raising their level in the bloodstream.[16] Trouble follows because excess lipid spillover from such dysfunctional fat tissue is not properly burned in cells' mitochondria.[17,18] Instead it accumulates in muscles and organs, such as the liver and pancreas—regions of the body where fatty acids have no business being. This state of *lipotoxicity* is linked with impaired mitochondrial function, increased inflammation, free-radical stress, and insulin resistance.[19,20,21]

In this classic model, a vicious cycle is created whereby a high-calorie, high-sugar diet creates simultaneous fat overload and insulin resistance. Much like a snowball rolling downhill, these processes feed on each other, leading to a metabolic mess.

FATTY MUSCLE

Excessive accumulation of lipids inside the muscle is a hallmark of insulin resistance.[22,23] In fact, one way that researchers create insulin resistance in the lab is to inject free fatty acids into study subjects' bloodstreams.

Think of lipid buildup inside muscles like the TV show in which people hoard things. A little storage is good, but when you don't throw anything away, it's easy to be paralyzed by your own belongings.

Hoarding of lipids inside muscle tissue is beneficial for a cyclist riding in the Tour de France, because they are actually burning the fat. However, this isn't the case for the twenty-first-century couch potato. This was recently demonstrated by researchers from the Netherlands.[24] They found that an intravenous infusion of lipids had little to no effect on insulin functioning in trained athletes, yet reduced insulin sensitivity by 63 percent in untrained people. It was noted that trained athletes had 32 percent higher mitochondrial capacity compared to sedentary study subjects.

Fatty muscle, insulin resistance, and mitochondrial dysfunction go hand in hand.[25] Research studies have reported a 30 percent reduction in mitochondrial function among insulin-resistant individuals compared to metabolically healthy counterparts.[26,27]

Researchers at the University of Colorado found that lipid deposits inside muscle tissue correlate strongly with abdominal fat and an increase in the ratio of triglyceride to heart-healthy cholesterol in adolescents prior to and during puberty.[28] This suggests that lipid accumulation in muscle tissue is an early event contributing to metabolic imbalances.

GUT BACTERIA GET INVOLVED

Nearly ten years ago, prominent microbiology researcher Fredrik Bäckhed, PhD, demonstrated that the bacteria in your intestines increases fat deposition in muscle and adipose tissue.[29]

Through a somewhat complicated mechanism, our gut microflora inhibits normal production of a protein called *fasting-induced adipose factor* (FIAF).[30,31] This protein's job is to block the transfer of fat from circulating cholesterol particles into adipocytes and muscle.[32,33] When FIAF is inhibited, more fat gets packed away in fat cells than normal. It's also been suggested that bacterial imbalances created by high-fat feeding further suppress FIAF and increase fat deposits. Even more interesting are studies showing that *berberine*, one of my favorite fat-fighting polyphenols, increases FIAF and curtails fat deposition in adipose tissue and muscle.[34] For weight loss and blood sugar improvements, I suggest 900 to 1500 mg of berberine HCl each day with a meal.[35]

CAN YOU TRICK YOUR BODY TO BURN?

Using the credit card analogy, you can see that while the overweight or insulin-resistant person has plenty of funds available, he or she may not be able to access them. A hot area of research today involves tweaking the molecular switches to make energy currency more available to mitochondria to make them more efficient fat-burners.[36] Just as NF-κβ is the molecular switch that can turn up inflammation, Nrf2 is the inflammatory dimmer switch. AMPK and PGC-1α (*peroxisome proliferator-activated receptor γ coactivator 1α*) both stimulate the mitochondria to burn fat and sugar more efficiently. When increased by fasting, exercise, cold temperatures, and certain natural compounds, the AMPK and PGC-1α pair also instruct the mitochondria to divide, a process known as *mitochondrial biogenesis*.[37,38,39] In sum, these molecular switches guide or instruct mitochondria to "burn, baby, burn," instead of "store, baby, store!"

You can think of AMPK as a fuel gauge, monitoring the energy status in your cells.[40,41] If cells are filled with fat and sugar—as in obesity and diabetes—AMPK will diminish, and the energy factories, your mitochondria, will not be able to burn fat or sugar. When AMPK is increased, mitochondria in your liver and muscles function better, so toxic fat spillover from fat cells is reduced and overall insulin sensitivity improves.[42] AMPK is so powerful that a low level may be the reason why some overweight people gain strength and stamina on an exercise program, but still don't lose weight or improve their sensitivity to insulin.[43]

One way to keep your cellular powerhouses burning fatty acids and sugar and churning out energy is regular exercise. A study of endurance athletes, for example, found that they had a 54 percent increase in energy use in their mitochondria compared to their sedentary counterparts.[44] This is the kind of fat burning that also improves insulin sensitivity. Scientists have reported that feeding animals high-fat, high-carbohydrate diets reduces the expression of AMPK and PGC-1α by up to 46 percent.[45] This suggests yet another way in which diet can influence our gut microflora. It can have a ricochet effect on our metabolism, reducing fat burning.

Metformin is the most widely prescribed diabetes drug in the world. Although it has been on the market for nearly two decades, researchers are just now beginning to understand more clearly how it improves blood-sugar control.[46]

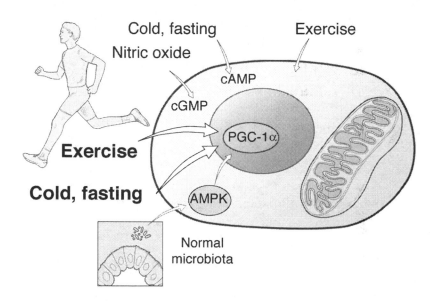

MITOCHONDRIA AND FAT BURNING

Mitochondria are critical to optimal fat burning and overall metabolic function. AMPK and PGC-1α are the master switches that ignite the flames of mitochondria. Periodic fasting, strenuous exercise, cold exposure, and healthy gut bacteria all foster healthy levels of these critical mitochondrial signaling molecules.

In 2002, a Harvard University research team found that metformin increases the signaling of AMPK to improve glucose metabolism. Prior to this discovery, researchers believed this powerful medication worked by reducing glucose production in the liver and improving glucose uptake in muscle.[47]

The health benefits of metformin extend far beyond diabetes. For instance, since it dramatically increases AMPK and improves metabolic flexibility, it helps people lose weight.[48] And diabetics who take metformin have a lower incidence of cancer compared to those who use other medications to control their blood sugar.[49] Its effects may be amplified when it is taken in the afternoon within 30 minutes after exercise. Ask your healthcare professional if metformin would be suitable for you.

As for natural products, a plethora of nutrients, herbs, and botanicals have been shown to increase AMPK signaling, optimizing mitochondrial function and fat and sugar burning.[50,51] Alpha-lipoic acid (ALA) in particular has been shown to increase AMPK signaling and fat burning signaling in humans. Italian researchers instructed 1,127 overweight subjects to take 800 mg of ALA daily for 4 months.[52] At the end of the study participants reported a 9 percent reduction in body mass, along with significant reductions in blood pressure and belly fat, compared to baseline. Korean researchers followed a similar approach, but instead they cranked up the dose to 1800 mg ALA daily for 4 months.[53] Compared with the placebo group, high-dose overweight individuals lost significantly more belly fat and body weight.

In addition to ALA, some of the best nutrients known to increase AMPK and maximize our body's fat burning capabilities include berberine, butyric acid, capsaicin (from chilly peppers), chromium, curcumin, EGCG (green tea polyphenols), genistein (soy), ginseng (*Panax quinquefolius*), quercetin, and resveratrol.[54,55,56,57,58,59,60] I suggest working with a healthcare professional to find the best sources of these nutrients so that you can add them to your program.

TOO MUCH FAT, TOO LITTLE OXYGEN

Remember that oxygen is a critical nutrient involved in the efficient burning of both sugar and fat. Yet, as the pounds pile on, the blood flow supplying oxygen to adipose tissue and the relative amount of oxygen around adipose tissue decreases. It's been proposed that as adipose tissue expands in obesity, the amount of oxygen available may decrease by as much as 70 percent.[61] This creates a low-grade lack of oxygen, or *hypoxia*, which sparks inflammation, increases leptin production, and pivots those oxygen-deprived cells from fat-burning mode into sugar-burning mode.[62,63] All this occurs simultaneously as hypoxia trips a key molecular switch known as *hypoxia-inducible factor 1 alpha* (HIF-1α).[64]

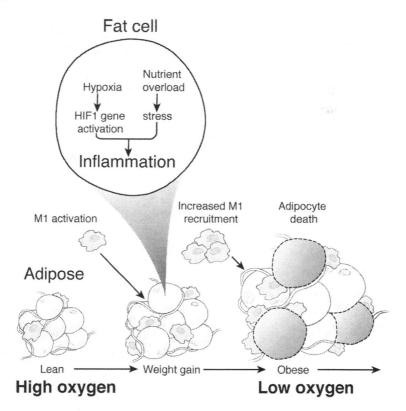

ENLARGED FAT CELLS ARE STARVED OF OXYGEN

As fat cells enlarge when a person gains weight, progressing from lean to overweight to obese, oxygen availability to cells declines. This, in combination with other cellular stress messengers, triggers a key signaling molecule called hypoxia-inducible factor 1 alpha (HIF-1α). Increased HIF-1α is linked to changes in the inflammatory predisposition of immune cells, such as increased type 1 macrophage and the Th-17 type of T lymphocytes. This "immune signature" is linked to metabolic abnormalities, such as impaired fat burning and insulin resistance.

At the start of this chapter, I asked a question: Why are immune cells drawn to adipose tissue like moths to a flame? I believe it is the combination of increased leptin and low oxygen levels in fat tissues that increase HIF-1α. That response, in combination with the surge of leptin, suppresses the immune cell guardians, the Treg cells that keep other T cells and inflammatory macrophages at bay.

By default, hypoxia is incongruent with oxygen-dependent fat burning, and so the only way immune cells can meet their increased energy demands in response to inflammation promoters like endotoxin, or HIF-1α from low oxygen, is to burn sugar as fuel.[65]

Yes. It's complicated. Here's another way to look at it: in their healthy state, working tissues, including immune cells, use oxygen to burn fat. For example, some immune cells (M2 macrophage, Th2, and Treg cells) rely heavily on fat for energy.[66,67,68] Not so for the metabolically challenged, insulin-resistant, inflamed immune cells in fat tissue, the ones that are characteristic of obesity.[69,70] These cells, which make up about 40 percent of fat tissue, shift out of fat-burning mode into sugar-burning mode.[71,72]

Inflammatory triggers such as bacterial endotoxin favor immune cells that thrive on sugar burning, including the M1-type macrophage and Th1 and Th17 types of T helper cells.[73,74,75] Unfortunately, these cells also induce inflammation, which is counterproductive to insulin sensitivity and fat burning.

In contrast, our steady-state anti-inflammatory cells, including the M2 macrophage and Treg cells, are great fat burners.[76,77] Their existence is heavily dependent on proper levels of the mitochondrial regulatory factors discussed above, including AMPK.[78]

INFLAMMATION REPROGRAMS METABOLISM

During times of immune stress, such as when leaks occur in the intestinal wall and there's increased absorption of bacterial particulate, the liver can make sugar from fats, through gluconeogenesis. At the same time, immune system stressors trigger an increase in blood-sugar levels by breaking down muscle. *Glutamine*, one of the amino acids that serves as the main building block for muscle, is used for fuel during times of inflammation. This is particularly problematic for insulin signaling because skeletal muscle is the primary professional metabolic organ that takes up glucose continually and is rich in fat-burning mitochondria. That's why the more lean muscle you have, the better suited you are to control your blood sugar. Continual muscle breakdown to fuel immune stressors is a cycle that needs to be broken for effective weight loss.

LEPTIN RESISTANCE: A NEW
LINK TO OBESITY

When it comes to understanding obesity, one of the most important hormones to consider is leptin, a hormone secreted by fat that helps you feel satisfied after you eat. The path was paved for the groundbreaking discovery of leptin partly by endocrinologists of the 1970s who made animals obese by surgically manipulating the hypo-thalamic region of their brains.[79] (As in humans, this region in the animal brain is the central hormonal processing center that regulates various aspects of metabolism.) Researchers speculated that the release of a natural chemical messenger, or *peptide*, creates a sense of satiety.

In 1994, Jeffrey Friedman, MD, PhD, and his colleagues at Rockefeller University discovered this peptide and named it appropri-ately "leptin," from the Greek word for thin, *leptos*.[80] This discovery and the awareness that one could become resistant to the chemical messenger was a major breakthrough in understanding obesity.[81]

Leptin's main role is to tell the brain how much energy is on hand and how much may be needed. Leptin is highest after a meal, when it tells the hypothalamus to reduce food intake. Because it is secreted by body fat, leptin levels generally rise in proportion to total body fat mass. Women tend to have higher leptin levels than men thanks to their higher body fat percentage.[82,83] Studies suggest leptin increases during the luteal phase of the menstrual cycle due to the effects of estradiol and progesterone.[84]

Leptin would seem to be the good guy of chemical messengers. The trouble is that when a surge of leptin is prolonged, the brain receptors designed to receive the message become desensitized or resistant to leptin and are no longer able respond to the signal. Despite an excess of leptin, the person with *leptin resistance* actually suffers from symptoms of low levels of the hormone.[85] The overweight person may be feeling hungry more often and store fat too readily. Instead of feeling satisfied, his or her brain instructs the body that it needs more energy.

Like most hormones in the body, leptin normally rises and falls with your body clock. It's highest between midnight and the early morning, allowing you to sleep without feeling hunger pangs and is at a low ebb during the afternoon.[86,87] You can use this to your advantage by eating a substantial amount of food in the morning to stimulate your resting metabolic rate.

The circadian rhythm of leptin is lost in overweight men and women, which may play a role in increased appetite and nighttime cravings.[88] In Chapter 8, we'll discuss ways to reset your circadian clock system so that the proper hormones are released at the right time.

LEPTIN AND IMMUNITY

More recent research suggests that inflammation and intestinal microbes may also increase leptin levels, and leptin is emerging as a key player not only in the regulation of fat storage but also in the regulation of immune function.[89] For instance, increased leptin release from fat cells effectively disables the security guards (Treg cells) of the immune system, setting the stage for a flood of immune cells around adipose tissue, leading to chronic inflammation, insulin resistance, and impaired fat burning.[90,91,92,93,94]

However leptin is not a kamikaze pilot set out to destroy your waistline by enabling sugar-burning immune cells to swarm the fat cells of your abdomen. Leptin actually enhanced the longevity of our cavemen ancestors by averting infection during times of famine.[95] In ancient times, starvation and infection were two driving forces of premature death. A shortage of food is a surefire way to thwart a mounting immune defense against a lethal pathogen.[96]

Leptin's dual role as an appetite suppressor and immune system stimulant circumvented immune suppression in the face of famine.[97,98] Exposure to microbes causes a leptin spike, stimulating the immune response, pushing the immune police (Treg) out of the way.[99,100] Leptin also appears to help the immune response in another way, causing insulin resistance, redirecting fuel away from muscles and liver to support the sugar-loving immune system in its quest to combat invading pathogens.[101,102,103] Indeed, after controlling for many variables, researchers have found that leptin is independently associated with insulin sensitivity in children and adults.[104,105,106]

As is often the case, a biological process that was historically protective is paradoxically problematic in the modern era. Increased leptin levels are linked to development of metabolic syndrome, cardiovascular disorders, and autoimmune diseases—including lupus, multiple sclerosis, autoimmune thyroid disease, and rheumatoid arthritis—not to mention appetite challenges in overweight persons.[107,108,109,110] One report even showed greater intestinal permeability with increasing leptin levels. In sum, leptin is a huge link to many problems with excess fat and metabolic perturbations that we've discussed up to now.

A great way to reduce leptin is to exercise more. The only caveat here is leptin promotes inflammation in the joint tissues, a condition formally known as osteoarthritis, making exercise painful and self-limiting.[111] Achy knees and painful hips were once considered to be strictly musculoskeletal; the excess pounds were stressing out the body's mainframe. Yet when studies surfaced linking a disproportionally higher prevalence of osteoarthritis in the hands of overweight persons compared to lean counterparts, that idea was explored further.[112] Low and behold, leptin emerged again as the nexus between fat tissue and joint inflammation.[113,114]

Since lowering leptin is compulsory for restoring normalcy among the immune and metabolic systems, reducing leptin is as important as loosing the pound. If you have increased belly fat, or an overall body fat percentage over 25 in women and 20 in men, it's likely that you have increased leptin above the ideal range of 15 ng/mL. To be sure, work with a healthcare professional to test your levels first thing in the morning (always retest at the same time of the day as well).

Since exercise and sleep, two significant variables influencing leptin levels, will be discussed in Chapter 7 and Chapter 8, respectively, we'll discuss the small handful of natural agents shown to modulate leptin levels and improve joint function here.

Researchers in Spain have reported that a hyaluronic acid containing product (ORALVISC) reduces symptoms of increased leptin, including pain and inflammation of the knee, while improving joint function.[115] Studies in animals link curcumin to reduced leptin release from fat cells.[116,117] Working with practitioners from Sherwood Family Medicine in Portland, OR, we observed significant reductions in serum leptin levels among six overweight patients by prescribing 350 mg curcumin, 9 grams of inulin fiber, and a symbiotic bacteria blend yielding 40 billion CFU of live organisms daily for two months.

FIGHT FAT WITH FAT

The omega-3 fatty acids docosahexaenoic acid (DHA) and eicosapentaenoic acid (EPA) common in fish, nuts, and seeds engender many fat-fighting, anti-inflammatory, and insulin-sensitizing properties.[118] They have been shown to get to the crux of the fat problem by extinguishing inflammation in fat tissue and shifting the type of immune cells to a more friendly, fat-burning pattern (M2 macrophages and Treg cells).[119,120] When endocrinologists at the University of Kentucky gave obese individuals 4 grams of fish oil concentrate a day for four months, macrophages within fat tissue declined. The protein released from monocytes that attracts macrophages to fat cells in the first place, MCP-1, dropped as well. Even more exciting, fish oil increased vascularization of the fat mass, which may help diminish inflammation-stimulating hypoxia.[121]

Curiously, this resolution of inflammation ascribed to the healthy omega-3 fatty acids EPA and DHA is actually attributed to metabolites created when these fats enter the body, not the fatty acids themselves.[122] Clearly these molecules impressed scientists, who named them resolvins and protectins after their ability to squelch inflammation, particularly in fat tissue.[123,124,125] It doesn't take much to jump-start resolvins. A daily dose of fish oil yielding 1.4 grams of

EPA and 1 gram of DHA daily is all that is required to raise blood levels of resolvins and protectins to an appreciable level, according to a recent clinical study.[126]

Research shows that omega-3 fatty acids and their metabolites are able to reduce leptin and increase adiponectin and Treg cells; short-circuiting the chronic inflammatory response.[127] Scientists in Japan noted a 60 percent increase in the anti-inflammatory cytokine adiponectin after 3 months of 1.8 grams EPA a day. When inflammation is kept at bay, the body burns fat better. For example a two-month trial of 1.8 grams of an omega-3 fatty acid supplement lead to significant reductions in blood triglycerides, belly fat, and fat cell size and an increase in adiponectin in diabetic women compared to study subjects not taking the supplement. The researchers also reported positive changes among genes in fat cells related to inflammation.

Yet another way by which omega-3 fats lend our metabolism a boost is by revving up AMPK signaling.[128] Fat making (lipogenesis) goes down and fat burning (lipolysis) and sugar burning in the mitochondria goes up. In a terminator-like fashion, omega-3 fatty acids and their metabolites reverse the buildup of toxic lipid metabolites (lipotoxicity) in muscle, the liver, and the pancreas as well. One study showed that 500 mg of DHA a day for six months improved fatty liver in children with liver disease.[129]

In a recent 12-week study, fish oil proved to be friendly to muscle and a foe to fat.[130] Researchers in Australia gave overweight people 1.9 grams of omega-3 fatty acids a day and instructed them to exercise three days a week for 45 minutes. The placebo group still exercised, but took sunflower caps instead of fish oil. Fish oil users burned more fat as a result of exercising while maintaining lean muscle mass compared to people who did not take fish oil. This muscle-sparing effect is critical, as lean muscle is the site of mitochondrial-fat burning.

Nearly all of these studies hint at the positive cardiovascular effects offered by fish oil through significant reductions in blood triglycerides and small dense LDL particles.[131,132,133,134]

An easy way to increase your EPA and DHA levels is eating three, 3-oz servings of wild-caught salmon, sardines, mackerel or herring weekly.[135] Avoid farm-raised fish altogether and when dining out, skip the Atlantic salmon, as that is farm raised too. Increasing fish intake to this level equates to roughly 400 mg EPA and DHA a day. To speed up fat loss, improve lean muscle mass, reduce blood triglycerides, and decrease inflammation, take 1,500-2,000 mg of combined EPA and DHA each day with meals.

Enteric-coated fish oil capsules make it to the small intestine, where they are better absorbed than liquids and offer greater anti-inflammatory effects.[136,137,138]

With so many brands of fish oil on the market, the easiest way to know that you are taking an ultra pure product is to ensure that it's top rated by the International Fish Oil Standards Program (IFOS)—the only third party testing company measuring purity and fish oil quality. Manufactures must submit every batch to IFOS to be tested for contaminants, heavy metals and oxidation productions. Visit www. IFOSProgram.com to learn more.

Lastly, many dietary supplement companies are promoting triglyceride (TG)- based fish oil over ethyl ester (EE) versions, claiming enhanced absorption and bioavailability. However when scientists at Stanford University compared the two versions in a 12-week study, the EE version lead to greater reductions in blood triglyceride levels and greater increases in red blood cell (RBC) omega-3 levels compared to the TG version.[133] So look for these varieties.

Blood triglycerides and the Omega-3 index are the two best used indices for assessing omega-3 fatty acid status in the body. Raising one's RBC Omega-3 Index to over 8 percent is linked to a 90 percent reduction in sudden cardiac death. So in addition to getting a metabolic boost, fish and fish oil may help you live longer! To learn more about the Omega-3 Index visit www.OmegaQuant.com or www. HDLabInc.com

KEY TAKEAWAYS

In conclusion, there are multiple links between immunity and metabolism. Excess body fat reflects this relationship. Imbalances in one system cause imbalances in another. The cellular components involved in sensing pathogens are also activated. Increased body fat elevates levels of metabolic hormones, such as leptin, which also have proinflammatory immune roles. Inflammation is so detrimental to metabolic health and weight management because it locks the body into a metabolically inflexible state, dominated by sugar burning at the expense of fat burning. This is because the body's intelligent design is such that inflammatory mediators simultaneously oppose insulin—the master metabolic hormone.

Such biological architecture was protective in historic times: it rapidly repartitioned energy nutrients to fuel robust immune and stress responses needed for infection and predation. Yet it doesn't always comport with modern industrialized life. Consumption of processed foods—particularly excess carbohydrates and fats—exploits this immune-metabolic relationship at the expense of our waistline.

Confounding the issue are trillions of bacteria residing in our intestine that can also cause inflammation as a result of poor food choices. We discussed how the bacterial appendage endotoxin can slip through a damaged intestinal barrier, igniting inflammatory sensors in metabolic organs, such as the liver and fat cells. This is not the only mode through which bacteria can make us fat. Gut microbes are capable of extracting more calories from ingested foods, altering appetite, mitochondrial function, and lipid signaling among others.

Thankfully, we can therapeutically exploit this immune-metabolic relationship by pivoting an irked immune system back into a desirable anti-inflammatory tolerant state. Anti-inflammatory immune cells thrive when the cellular switches driving fat burning are increased. When activated by exercise and intermittent fasting, AMPK and PGC-1α—the two primary cellular switches—help our metabolic organs burn fat more efficiently while simultaneously switching our immune system into an anti-inflammatory state.

CHAPTER 5

YOUR GUT AT WORK

"The gastrointestinal tract is the body's largest endocrine organ and releases more than 20 different regulatory peptide hormones that influence a number of physiological processes."
—Kevin G. Murphy, PhD

No matter the diet—low calorie, low carb, high protein—every calorie enters the body through the same orifice: the mouth. But even before food is eaten, the mere sight and smell of it triggers the release of intestinal metabolic hormones that profoundly affect how the nutrients will be processed and absorbed.[1] Furthermore, the sequential release of digestive sections—stomach acid, pepsin, secretin, and bile—influences the interaction between the food and intestinal microbes.

Poor digestion, for example, can lead to enhanced fermentation of food and synthesis of secondary compounds that promote fat synthesis.[2] That's why an awareness of the role of digestion is essential to understanding fat loss and metabolism.

The surface area of the intestinal tract that is responsible for digesting and absorbing nutrients and calories is more than 250 meters squared, about the size of a tennis court.[3] This vast biological encasement simultaneously absorbs nutrients for energy, while excluding more than four pounds of intestinal bacteria and removing fecal waste from the body.[4,5] To the average Joe, the intestine is nothing more than a food reservoir. To microbiologists, endocrinologists, and gastroenterologists, the intestinal tract and its symbiotic microbial partners comprise a "bioreactor" with a projected metabolic activity greater than the liver.[6,7] And many experts consider the liver to be the most metabolically active organ.

Long before you begin chewing food, the mind stimulates the intestine to properly handle the incoming meal by initiating the release of digestive secretions and some twenty metabolic hormones, or incretins, from the intestinal wall.[8,9] These powerful incretins improve satiety and so reduce appetite, increase intestinal barrier function, and are directly responsible for up to 40 percent of insulin's blood-sugar lowering activity.[10]

As you chew food, enzymes in your saliva mix with the food, initiating the breakdown of proteins and carbohydrates into amino acids and sugars, such as di- and monosaccharides. New research indicates that these enzymes, particularly a carbohydrate digestive enzyme called *salivary amylase*, have a fat-fighting, metabolism-promoting role. For example, a recent study revealed that people with low levels of salivary amylase don't process carbohydrate foods very well.[11] Similarly, researchers found that individuals with high levels of salivary amylase have lower glucose and insulin levels after eating compared to those with lower levels of salivary amylase.

THE GUT'S FOOD PROCESSOR

With each swallow, a bolus of chewed food enters the stomach where it's mixed and churned in a very acidic environment. The hormone *gastrin* in the stomach helps break down protein into amino acids and destroys pathogens that may have been inadvertently ingested during eating. Proper secretion of acid from the cells lining the stomach and "acidification" of ingested food may be the single most important step of the entire digestive process. The gastric contents must become acidic to facilitate the sequential digestive steps continuing in the small intestine.

Once food enters the upper portion of the stomach, it's incubated in this warm, ninety-eight-degree, acidic solution for up to seventy minutes prior to entering the small intestine where it mixes with more digestive secretions, including bile acids, as well as immunoglobulin antibodies and trillions of microbes. Many abnormalities in digestion, absorption, and metabolism can be traced to the suboptimal secretion of gastric acid in the stomach. The entire digestive process can go awry, leading to improper fermentation of ingested food and proliferation of bacteria. After churning around inside the acidic stomach, the bolus of food slowly moves through the *pyloric sphincter* into the next digestive chamber, the *duodenum*, or the first part of the small intestine.[12] This mix is now called *chyme*.

Metabolic cells called L cells in the upper small intestine sense the presence of chyme and initiate the release of a plethora of digestive metabolic hormones that are fundamental to finishing the digestive and absorptive process as well as integrating the whole-body metabolism.[13,14]

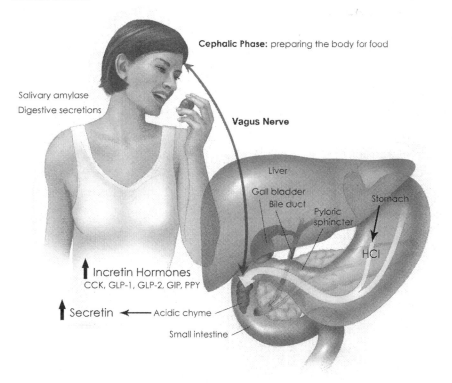

Cephalic Phase: preparing the body for food

Salivary amylase
Digestive secretions

Vagus Nerve

Liver

Gall bladder
Bile duct

Pyloric
sphincter

Stomach

HCl

↑ Incretin Hormones
CCK, GLP-1, GLP-2, GIP, PPY

↑ Secretin ◄——— Acidic chyme

Small intestine

THE METABOLIC POWER OF DIGESTION

The sequential release of various digestive hormones and secretions influence metabolism. Of particular importance are incretin hormones released from the small intestine, since they have many beneficial metabolic and immune effects.

Secretin is one example of an important intestinal signaling molecule. Acidic stomach contents trigger the small intestine to release this hormone, directing the nearby pancreas to secrete other enzymes (pancreatin, trypsin, and chymotrypsin) and pancreatic bicarbonate to digest proteins and raise the pH of the small intestine to optimize digestion.[15]

The acidic chyme also stimulates intestinal cells to release another gut hormone, *cholecystokinin* (CCK). While CCK has many metabolic functions, its major role is to instruct the gall bladder to secrete bile acids.[16] While bile is often thought of as a simple detergent-like molecule, critical for absorbing fats and fat-soluble nutrients such as coenzyme Q10 and vitamins A and D, it has metabolic and antimicrobial properties.[17]

Imagine that you take your usual dinner—a few chips, some guacamole dip, a little salad, a slice or two of beef, and a cup of pasta—and put it in a food processor. Mix in a glass of wine or some low-fat milk, maybe even a beer or two, and blend. Then heat the mixture to body temperature and take it outside during a hot summer day. Disperse the mixture evenly on a tarp lining one side of a tennis court. Pour some hydrochloric acid, pancreatic enzymes, bicarbonate, and bile salts over it and then dump a four-pound bucket of bacteria, yeast, viruses, and parasites over the mixture. Stir well, and let it heat to ninety-eight degrees. Cover the mixture by folding the other half of the doubles-tennis portion of the tarp. Seal up the edges, suck out the oxygen, and let it brew for one to eighteen hours, which is how long it would take the mix to pass through your intestine.

If putrid sights and smells are stimulating your senses already, then I've done my job. The thought of caustic gasses from microbial metabolism on digested nutrients is enough to make one gag. However, we often chew, crunch, sip, slurp, gulp, and swallow literally thousands of pounds of calorie-bearing nutrients over the course of our lifetime with no regard to what happens to them during the journey through our inner tube of life.

We are so concerned with calories that we forget about chewing. Eating while driving or watching stressful television shows is more usual than not. Bloating, belching, gas, bad breath, constipation, heartburn, and oily stools are unrelated to fat burning and body-fat synthesis, or so the thinking goes. As you'll soon see, the genesis of these post-meal intestinal discomforts suggests a communication error between gut bacteria and the intestinal wall.[18] The ensuing inflammation, leaky gut, and change in the release of metabolic hormones are how poor food choices lead to weight gain and diabetes.[19] It's no coincidence that gastrointestinal problems are present in the majority of overweight people and those with type 2 diabetes.[20,21]

A FRESH LOOK AT DIGESTION AND GUT HEALTH

Salivary and digestive enzymes, stomach acid, the antimicrobial detergent-like bile secreted by the gall bladder, and the incretins released directly from the intestine in response to a meal all play greatly underappreciated roles in maintaining metabolic balance inside and outside of the gut.

Like more than 25 percent of the population, most of the weight loss and metabolic tune-up clients I've coached over the years have bowel disorders.[22] These problems range from diarrhea, constipation, and heartburn or *gastro-esophageal reflux disease* (GERD) to more serious abdominal pain, *irritable bowel syndrome* (IBS), ulcerative colitis, and Crohn's disease.

Intestinal ailments are present in the majority of people who are overweight and have diabetes, and increase in proportion with disease severity.[23,24] For example, obese people are three times more likely to experience symptoms of heartburn and acid regurgitation.[25] Multiple studies suggest that improper movement, or motility, of the gastrointestinal tract is also much more common in obese people and those with type 2 diabetes.[26,27,28,29] Sluggish motility is linked not only to GI symptoms, such as bloating, but also to increased belly fat, because it prolongs the opportunity that intestinal bacteria have to extract excess calories from ingested food.[30]

GUTSY PARTNERS TAKE A HIT

During early embryonic development, the stomach and most of the small intestine arise from the foregut, forming the alimentary canal, our inner tube of life.[31] After about week four of fetal development, the foregut buds give rise to the liver and pancreas, two critically essential digestive and metabolic organs.[32]

The intestine is the first contact point for food, and there is a kind of cross talk between the gut, liver, and pancreas. Blood carrying recently absorbed dietary nutrients, gut bacteria, and toxins from the intestine pass through the liver before entering the systemic circulation.[33] In addition, the pancreas releases the hormone insulin after a meal, depositing nutrients into metabolic organs (muscle, liver, and adipose tissue). When food is absent, the pancreas releases glucagon to liberate stored sugar for cellular energy.

The liver is a filter as well as an immune, detoxification, antioxidant, and metabolic organ, and it is frequently stressed in a person who is overweight and has metabolic imbalances.

Diets high in fat and processed carbohydrates increase absorption of bacterial endotoxin and initiate an inflammatory reaction in the liver, stimulating inflammatory pathways and increasing fat and glucose synthesis.[34] In fact, a high percentage of obese people with intestinal bacterial imbalances also have *nonalcoholic fatty liver disease* (NAFLD).[35]

Historically, healthcare practitioners have associated fatty liver disease with alcohol excess, but the recent obesity pandemic and emerging research in toxicology have changed this view.[36] Over thirty years ago, Jurgen Ludwig, MD, was the first to report the association between the obesity-metabolic disorders with lipid overload independent of alcohol consumption, or NAFLD.[37] While there are many contributing factors leading to increased lipid accumulation in the liver, a key step lies in inflamed adipose tissue and a reduced sensitivity to insulin. This leads to lipid spillover as well as increased synthesis of lipids inside the liver. This is why monitoring the common liver function tests, *alanine amino-transferase* (ALT) and *gamma-glutamyl transpeptidase* (GGT) are important to assessing metabolism.[38,39,40,41,42]

MARKERS OF ENVIRONMENTAL TOXICITY

The enzyme GGT is intimately involved in the cellular production of a critical antioxidant and detoxification compound, glutathione (GSH).[43,44] Although the liver, as a key detoxification organ, is the primary production site of glutathione, the powerful compound is also manufactured in and used by many cells.[45,46] Ample cellular GSH levels are critical for a robust fat-burning metabolism, since the antioxidant-compound plays a critical role in keeping the mitochondria, the site of fat burning, functioning optimally.[47] The metabolic potential of these energy-making factories falters when glutathione is low and free radicals run amok.

Excessive production of free radical compounds and exposure to environmental chemicals, including dioxins, bisphenol A (BPA, phthalates, organochlorines, brominated flame retardants, and persistent organic pollutants (POPs), increase the need for glutathione. Levels of GGT rise in an effort to make more glutathione.[48,49]

Impaired glutathione signaling is implicated in many chronic diseases such as prediabetes and diabetes, cancer, cardiovascular disease, accelerated aging, and neurodegeneration.[50] Many studies have found blood levels of GGT above 26 U/L to be linked with increased risk of diabetes, metabolic syndrome, cardiovascular events, inflammation, and poor antioxidant status.[51,52,53,54,55,56] I like to see serum GGT levels under 24 U/L particularly in overweight and insulin-resistant people. Detoxification of endocrine-disturbing chemicals is imperative since they have an exceedingly long half-life.[57,58] You can minimize your exposure to them by avoiding commercially prepared foods, plastic water bottles and food-storage containers, and eating organic produce and grass-fed meat products.[59] Intravenous glutathione or oral S-acetyl glutathione and Nrf2-activating herbs such as sulforaphane, curcumin, and resveratrol can eliminate stored endocrine-disrupting compounds.

OUR TOXIC ENVIRONMENT

There's no question that consuming more calories than you expend will cause weight gain, but we cannot ignore the contribution of gut bacteria, hormones, immune messengers, and endotoxin to the rapid increase in obesity and diabetes. However, even these factors are only part of the story. The swift and unexpected worldwide rise of obesity suggests there is an environmental component that is also more powerful than calories. Study after study suggests that *obesogens* (nutritional, industrial, and pharmaceutical chemicals) alter metabolic pathways and promote fat storage and disease.[60] Obesogens include fructose, high-fructose corn syrup, certain fats, *diethylstilbestrol* (DES), *bisphenol A* (BPA), phthalates, solvents, and genetically modified foods (GMOs).[61] As an example, a recent study of 148 people in Denmark confirmed that levels of industrial pollutants are significantly higher in the blood of obese people and those with prediabetes or diabetes.[62]

LOW STOMACH ACID IS A PROBLEM

One of the most widely prescribed classes of medications is proton-pump inhibitors (PPIs), which inhibit stomach-acid production. PPIs are being criticized for being overprescribed.[63] They have long been known to cause imbalanced bacterial growth in the intestine and leaky gut syndrome.[64,65,66]

Low stomach acid is linked with intestinal tract infections and increased growth of pathogenic bacteria in the gut, such as *Yersinia*, *Clostridium*, and *Citrobacter*.[67,68] Stomach-acid suppression may also increase sensitivity to medication and foods, possibly pivoting the gut immune system into a less tolerant, more inflammatory state.[69,70,71] All of these effects make it harder to fight belly fat and rebalance blood sugar. High-fat diets may suppress stomach acid too.

Stomach acid normally declines with age. People over the age of sixty, for instance, are more likely to have hypochlorhydria, and thus imbalanced gut microflora and vitamin B12 and iron deficiencies.[72] Common symptoms of B12 deficiency include cognitive defects, poor body control, infertility, and dizziness upon standing.[73] People over the age of fifty may benefit from taking supplemental HCl with meals, particularly if they have signs and symptoms of hypochlorhydria, such as vitamin B12 deficiency, neuropathies, and mental confusion.

INCREASING YOUR STOMACH
ACID NATURALLY

For some, particularly middle-aged and elderly people, eating in a tranquil state of mind may not be enough to increase the acidity in the stomach to desirable levels. Many well-respected physicians suggest betaine hydrochloride (600 mg) with pepsin and gentian root during the middle of a meal. If you suspect you have low stomach acid, you can try one or two betaine or glutamic acid HCl (600 mg) capsules, or find a physician in your area who has a Heidelberg stomach acid test. It is the gold standard test for assessing hypochlorhydria.

If you experience upper gastrointestinal irritation, such as reflux or heartburn, you may also consider chewable zinc carnosine (75 mg). Although sold as the prescription-only product Polaprezinc in Asia, this natural product can be found in chewable tablets as a supplement. Zinc carnosine is arguably one of the most well-studied and powerful nutrient combinations known to heal the mucosa of the stomach and small intestine.[74,75] I frequently recommend it to persons suffering from digestive complaints. Results have been great.

BILE: YOUR FAT-FIGHTING PARTNER

Bile, secreted by the gall bladder, is another digestive player. It was thought to be little more than a soap-like detergent, but scientists are finding that it is involved in many aspects of metabolism and immunity beyond the intestine. From impairing bacterial growth in the intestine and improving gut-barrier and liver functioning to activating thyroid hormones and cellular signaling molecules, bile is our metabolic friend.[76,77,78]

Bile acids influence many aspects of sugar and fat metabolism as well as exert anti-inflammatory effects by activating two very important cellular receptors: *farnesoid X receptor* (FXR) and TGR5, a protein receptor.[79] When bile molecules attach to these receptors, energy expenditure and metabolic rate increase, and lipid synthesis slows. Bile acids also help to activate thyroid hormones, specifically increasing the conversion of T4 to T3. This is important since T3 is what latches on to receptors, increasing metabolism. When bile acids bind to TGR5 in muscle tissue, synthesis and mitochondria activity increase, giving cellular metabolism and fat burning a boost.[80,81]

An imbalance in gut microflora, such as increased levels of endotoxin, is linked to altered bile acid signaling, ultimately increasing fat synthesis in the liver and reducing glutathione production.[82] In contrast, supplementation with healthy probiotic bacteria reverses these changes in lipid signaling and glutathione. Bile acids are unique in that they inhibit the growth of potentially bad bacteria in the intestine.[83] Yet the majority of healthy intestinal bacterial strains are resistant to bile, which is why ingesting probiotics and fermented foods is harmless.

BILE ACID AND OBESITY

Many studies have shown impaired FXR and TGR5 signaling in people who are obese and have diabetes. Stimulating the receptors by giving a person bile-acid-like molecules improves lipid and sugar metabolism.[84] One study found that compared to lean people, obese people had a 55 percent reduction in bile flow after a meal.[85]

Improved bile acid signaling is one of the many improvements that follow bariatric surgery, leading to rapid and lasting weight loss and metabolic improvements.[86,87] Research shows that after bariatric surgery, obese people have a dramatic increase in bile flow after eating a fatty meal.[88,89]

Scientists in the United Kingdom found that the post-meal rise in bile acids was strongly linked with a healthy balance and secretion of three critical metabolic and appetite hormones: *glucagon-like peptide-1* (GLP-1), *peptide tyrosine-tyrosine* (PYY), and ghrelin.[90] And researchers in Australia who gave bile acids with a sugary drink to healthy people report that those study subjects handled the high-glycemic drink better and had an increase in the powerful GLP-1, compared to people who didn't have bile acids with the drink.

OPTIMIZING BILE OUTPUT

Since bile acid synthesis is dependent on two amino acids, taurine and glycine, it's important to consider increasing protein supplementation with them. They are hard to obtain from whole food. Additionally, release of synthesized bile is contingent upon upstream digestive processes, such as proper vagal nerve activation, chewing and proper stomach acid synthesis, and overall intestinal health, including healthy gut microflora.[91] Additionally, you can take ox bile supplements when eating fatty meals. Beets, cholagogue herbs and nutrients are also known to encourage bile production and flow.

SUPPLEMENTAL NUTRIENTS AND HERBS TO OPTIMIZE BILE FLOW		
Chamomile	Chicory root	Dandelion root
Artichoke	Greater celandine	Fringe tree
Milk thistle	Taurine (amino acid)	Glycine (amino acid)
Inositol	Methylation support	Beets

FINE-TUNING METABOLIC HORMONES

Due to the fact that the intestine is the body's largest metabolic organ, its frontline cells are able to receive anticipatory messages from the brain as well as sense food through contact as it travels through our inner tube of life. In fact, this single-cell barrier has multiple roles above and beyond absorption. As discussed previously, it acts as a metabolic liaison in bariatric surgery. Intestinal endocrine cells, or *enteroendocrine* cells, adjacent to the intestinal barrier cells in the upper portion of the small intestine release incretins.[92] While there are many incretins, the two that are most studied are GLP-1 and CCK.[93,94]

It's been suggested that these hormones travel to peripheral tissues to better prepare the body for the incoming meal. Think of them as metabolic couriers. When nutrients collide with L and K cells in the intestine, a plethora of hormones are released to alert distinct regions of the body that food is coming.

To illustrate the power of these intestinal hormones, remember that one of the main reasons why bariatric surgery is successful as a weight-loss and metabolic-restoration therapy is due to surgical sectioning of the intestine. In essence, this overloads the intestinal metabolic cells, overcoming any sluggishness that may have previously been impaired, promoting weight gain, and disrupting insulin signaling. However, since the long-term effects of bariatric surgery are not yet known, it may be best to first try to increase incretins with prebiotics, probiotics, phytochemicals, and pea protein, leaving surgery as an absolute last resort.

When incretins were first discovered more than twenty-five years ago, metabolic researchers found obese and diabetic people displayed signs of impaired metabolism as well as reduced signaling of gut peptides.[95] Over the years, scientists have found that type 2 diabetes was associated with reduced signaling of GLP-1, a major cause of blood-sugar dysregulation and eventually diabetes.[96] More recent research suggests that the normal post-meal increase in gut hormones GLP-1, gastric-inhibitory polypeptide (GIP), and CCK are out of balance in people who are obese and have diabetes.

The 30 percent or more weight regain associated with low-calorie dieting is linked to long-lasting suppression of intestinal-metabolic hormones. One study published in the *New England Journal of Medicine* found that gut hormones, namely ghrelin and CCK, remained suppressed twelve months after obese people participated in a two-month weight-loss study.[97] This underscores the notion that we shouldn't focus solely on calorie restriction, and we must include intestinal health in any approach to reducing belly fat.

GUT HORMONES AFFECT METABOLISM

Scientists suggest that GLP-1 also has anti-inflammatory properties throughout the body, including in the heart and brain.[98] One study found that a twelve-week trial of *sitagliptin*, a drug that increases intestinal GLP-1, reduces inflammatory markers in people with type 2 diabetes.[99] Endocrinologists have also reported that *exenatide*, another type of GLP-1-increasing medication, improves blood sugar and reduces cardiovascular-disease-specific inflammation.[100] And Korean scientists found GLP-1 reduces macrophage movement toward fat cells, preventing inflammation.[101] Other studies in animals using drugs designed to increase gut-satiety hormones have also revealed anti-inflammatory effects outside of the intestine.[102]

WHOLE-BODY INFLUENCE OF GLP-1	
Liver	Reduced glucose production Improved insulin sensitivity
Pancreas	Increased insulin production
Stomach	Slowed emptying
Heart	Cardio-protective effects, increased output
Muscle	Improved insulin sensitivity
Brain	Reduced appetite
Adipose tissue	Reduced adipose tissue mass

TUNE UP YOUR INTESTINAL METABOLIC HORMONES

Healthy digestive fire and increased parasympathetic tone are the main ways to activate incretins. Eating slowly is imperative. Chewing forty times before each swallow is linked to increased release of CCK and GLP-1.[103] The reduced stomach acid production that occurs with age or as a result of taking stomach-acid-suppressing drugs, such as proton-pump inhibitors, leads to an imbalance in gastrin, CCK, secretin, and other peptides involved in gastrointestinal motility.[104]

Here are some good reasons to avoid synthetic sweeteners: research shows that the synthetic sweetener saccharin suppresses GLP-1 release in animals, and that the synthetic sweetener sucralose altered post-meal changes in blood glucose and insulin in humans.[105,106]

PROBIOTICS, PREBIOTICS, PHYTOCHEMICALS, AND PEA PROTEIN

In addition to mindful eating and extensive chewing, we can also optimize our intestinal metabolic signaling hub through four simple ways: take *Bifidobacterium* probiotics, prebiotic fiber, plant-based phytochemicals, and pea and whey protein supplements.

Prebiotics are fiber-rich substances that enhance the growth of protective bacteria such as *Bifidobacteria*.[107] The inulin-rich fructans from chicory and Jerusalem artichokes are the most beneficial prebiotics. They increase the number of metabolic cells in the intestine where hormones, namely GLP-1 and GLP-2, are manufactured and released.[108]

Studies in both animals and humans have revealed the power of the prebiotic inulin to increase the intestinal release of GLP-1, improving insulin sensitivity and reducing fat mass.[109,110] A recent study demonstrated that inulin-enriched pasta reduces leaky gut, a phenomenon previously observed in animals from increased GLP-2 activity.[111]

Inulin has been found to positively change the intestinal microflora of obese women, leading to metabolic improvements. In one study the obese women who ingested 15 grams per day of inulin were found to have increased levels of the healthy *Bifidobacterium* and *Faecalibacterium prausnitzii*, which were associated with reduced endotoxin. Other studies have reported that just 10 grams per day of inulin is all that is required to increase healthy levels of *Bifidobacterium* and *Faecalibacterium prausnitzii*.[112,113]

Based on these studies, I suggest consuming 10–15 grams per day of a high-quality inulin supplement. I prefer inulin to the *fructo-oligosaccharide* (FOS) because FOS doesn't have as much data supporting increased levels of healthy *Bifidobacterium*, and FOS may also favor the growth of pathogens, while inulin does not. Lastly, prebiotic fiber is not the only protective fiber known to increase gut hormones. Soluble fiber from beta-glucan and beans has also been shown to increase levels of CCK in the intestine.[114]

PHYTOCHEMICALS AND INCRETINS

The colorful polyphenolic compounds present in our diet have multiple beneficial targets, including increasing the release of gut hormones in response to food.[115] Currently, the majority of research has been on cinnamon, berberine, resveratrol, dark chocolate, berry compounds, and ginseng. Polyphenols also exert positive effects on gut microflora balancing.[116,117,118]

Several studies conducted by neurobiologists at the University of Maryland have shown how pea and whey protein, more than other vegan and animal proteins, improves satiety and increases levels of intestinal CCK and GLP-1.[119,120,121] Prior to these studies I was actually recommending 20–30 grams of pea or whey protein in a berry smoothie as a breakfast option with great success for weight loss, and these studies validate that protocol.

KEY TAKEAWAYS

Our digestive process is sequential, and depends on proper vagus nerve activity. Enzymes in the mouth, stomach acid, bile, and incretins all influence digestion of food. Proper levels of stomach acid are needed to activate digestive functioning, including bile and key gut hormones, like secretin and CCK. Bile is a powerful antimicrobial and metabolic hormone, and it influences blood sugar. Studies show impaired bile secretion is more common in overweight people.

Proper chewing leads to the release of incretins, which help to balance blood sugar and improve metabolism. Levels of these gut hormones are often suboptimal in people who are overweight and insulin-resistant, but hormonal activity can be increased with prebiotic fibers such as inulin, pea protein, whey protein, and polyphenolic compounds. The gut-derived hormones are also anti-inflammatory.[122]

CHAPTER 6

A CHANGING VIEW OF THE GUT

"The vagus nerve regulates metabolic homeostasis by controlling heart rate, gastrointestinal motility and secretion, pancreatic endocrine and...(the vagus nerve) controls innate immune responses and inflammation during pathogen invasion and tissue injury."—Valentin A. Pavlov, PhD

With so many different types of gastrointestinal-based therapies from bariatric surgery and taking prebiotics to transplantation of microbes from lean people to obese ones, scientists now recognize that the cornerstone of our fat-burning and metabolic machinery lies within our digestive tract.[1,2,3,4,5,6,7,8,9] In fact, cutting-edge science suggests that the origins of obesity-related metabolic problems stem from imbalances in our intestinal bacteria.[10,11,12,13] These imbalances can disrupt the release of protective metabolic signaling hormones from the gut, change gut motility, and create secondary toxic compounds, all of which disrupt the integrity of the intestinal barrier and activate a massive immune response in the intestine.[14,15,16]

This twenty-first-century understanding of metabolic functioning is much more intricate than the obsolete and discernibly ineffective fat-loss models that focus on calorie counting and/or the glycemic index of meals. I suspect that the intestine has been largely underappreciated as a metabolic organ because experts thought of the internal portion of the intestine containing the microbes and the food passing through; it was perceived as technically outside of the body. Similarly, the lungs were thought to be outside the body. For instance, immunology texts often discuss the lungs and intestinal tract together since both are lined with mucosal epithelial tissue.

Either way, our gastrointestinal tract performs seemingly contradictory roles: absorption of nutrients and exclusion of foreign material. For example, the epithelial barrier in the lungs is thin enough to allow oxygen to pass into the bloodstream and eliminate carbon dioxide, while at the same time keeping dust and other noxious substances out. Similarly, along the intestinal tract, the lining is so thin that nutrients can be absorbed through it, yet thick enough to prevent harmful compounds and microbes from passing into the rest of the body.[17]

Imbalances in intestinal bacteria, along with stress, medications, alcohol, and processed foods, increase gut permeability (*leaky gut*) and allow immunologically stimulating particles, such as endotoxin, to be absorbed.[18,19,20,21,22,23] These inflammatory molecules stimulate components of the immune system, which as you know by now, is synonymous with belly fat and metabolic aberrations.[24,25,26] Indeed, many studies have found leaky gut to coexist alongside obesity and metabolic syndrome.[27,28,29,30]

In sum, the intestinal tract is far more than just a laundry shoot for food: it's a dynamic, metabolic-immune-microbial orchestration. Food and bacteria interact to influence our metabolism, energy storage, and response to invaders.[31]

SLOW DOWN AND CHEW

Your personal trainer may encourage you to "Eat more protein!" Your doctor is likely to advise, "Watch those saturated fats and reduce your calories." But your grandma, who told you to "Chew your food," probably knows best. Granny intuitively sensed that the only way her home-cooked meals would be able to fuel our scrawny childhood bodies would be through slow and proper digestion. Now experts recognize that chewing is one of the major contributors of nutrient absorption in the bloodstream.

Recently scientists revealed how fast eaters were at increased risk for being overweight and having metabolic syndrome and multiple cardiovascular-disease risk factors.[32,33,34] Rapid eaters don't fully chew their food and may not activate the neurological pathways needed to light the digestive fire. Two studies have found that chewing forty times before swallowing led to decreased levels of the hunger hormone ghrelin and increased levels of two critically important gut peptides, *cholecystokinin* (CCK) and *glucagon-like peptide-1* (GLP-1).[35,36]

Overall, mindful eating and chewing at least forty times per swallow is linked to reduced food intake.[37] Thorough chewing may activate the vagus nerve that communicates with the digestive tract, optimizing digestion and the release of gut hormones, which help us to balance blood sugar and burn more fat.[38,39]

TIMING MEALS FOR FAT LOSS

Despite widely accepted admonitions against skipping breakfast, the majority of clients I've worked with either don't eat breakfast or eat a very small one. It's long been known among professionals in the fitness community that eating a large breakfast is key to maintaining a lean, muscular physique. Science has confirmed that people who eat late in the day have a harder time losing weight compared to those who eat early.[40,41,42] In one study, late eaters had less calorie-dense breakfasts or skipped breakfast altogether compared to early eaters, and the late eaters lost less weight at the end of the twenty-week weight-loss study.[43] Another study of healthy males compared the differences in blood glucose, insulin, and two gut hormones (GLP-1 and PYY) after the men either drank a high-calorie, high-carbohydrate shake two and a half hours after breakfast or ate no breakfast at all.[44] Those who had the breakfast shake had significantly lower post-meal blood glucose and insulin. Compared to those who didn't eat, the men who drank the shake had a greater sense of fullness and less hunger, which is no surprise, but they also ate 17 percent fewer calories during their next meal.

Other similarly designed studies have been conducted in women, comparing the metabolic responses of test meals in breakfast eaters versus non-breakfast eaters.[45] The non-breakfast eaters ate more calories later in the day and had impaired blood lipids and insulin levels compared to the breakfast eaters.

In sum, skipping breakfast clearly leads to altered insulin signaling and increased calorie intake later in the day.[46] Multiple studies suggest that eating a hearty breakfast of ample protein and complex carbohydrates decreases cravings later in the day and improves insulin signaling. I suggest eating lean protein, a root vegetable and fruits, as well as healthy fats from nuts and coconut oil for breakfast.

GIVING DIGESTION A BOOST FROM THE HEART

One of my most effective tips for weight loss is helping clients to practice meditative breathing prior to a meal. Eating in a rushed, stressed physiological state leads to poor chewing, improper digestion, and imbalanced gut microflora. In contrast, mindful strategies such as deep breathing will increase the "rest and digest" or parasympathetic nervous system including the vagus nerve, which activates digestive juices and gut hormones such as CCK and GLP-1.[47] Vagus nerve activation is key to optimal digestive health.

There are two divisions of your nervous system running on autopilot in the background: the parasympathetic nervous system, or the rest and digest system, and the sympathetic nervous system, the "fight or flight" response. We are hardwired to survive as if we lived in prehistoric times when life expectancy was contingent upon surviving predators, starvation, and infection. When prehistoric man was fighting or fleeing from a life-threatening altercation, our nervous system pivoted out of rest and digest status (parasympathetic dominance) into fight or flight mode (sympathetic dominance).

Such a shift in nervous system signaling drives the adrenals to release more stress hormones, which increases blood sugar, constricts blood vessels, raises blood pressure, and speeds heart rate. The shift also reallocates nutrients and blood to the lungs, heart, muscle tissue, and brain. Digestion, muscle building, production of growth and sex hormones—all of which are activated by the vagus nerve of the parasympathetic nervous system—come to a screeching halt, since these activities aren't critical to survival during life-or-death situations. However, that's not true in the long term.

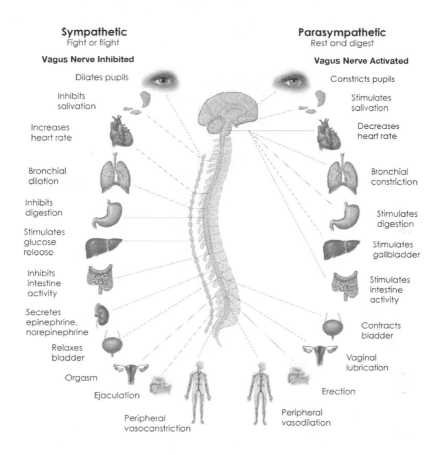

OVERVIEW OF THE AUTONOMIC NERVOUS SYSTEM

The autonomic nervous system governs many body functions. The key to fat loss and blood sugar balance is to tip the balance of this system in direction of the parasympathetic nervous system.

The modern-day challenge is that your body interprets present-day life stressors—traffic, work overload, sleep disturbances—as though they are life threats. The morning and evening rush-hour commute, work deadlines, financial uncertainties, and even the Western diet, lock our nervous system thermostat on stress and inflammation mode. Intestinal bacterial imbalances and associated leaky gut lead to increased absorption of endotoxin, driving the stressful, inflammatory branch of our nervous system.[48]

Since inflammation disrupts metabolism and normal hormone functioning, this leads to insulin resistance, prediabetes, and other obesity-related abnormalities. Furthermore, impaired blood-sugar regulation, as in prediabetes and insulin resistance, sets up a state in which activating the vagus nerve and parasympathetic nervous system becomes increasingly challenging.[49] This sets up a cycle of poor digestive and hormonal function and inflammation and metabolic imbalances that are incongruent with fat burning.

Scientists have found that fat tissue from obese subjects has reduced levels of the receptor (*nicotinic acetylcholine*) through which the vagus nerve and parasympathetic nervous system operate. This discovery confirms what we already know: fat tissue is unable to suppress an over-activated immune system, and that inability is at the crux of the belly fat problem. However a three-month lifestyle therapy program, involving a phytochemical-rich diet program, significantly increases the expression of the acetylcholine receptor in obese people.[50] This suggests that simple lifestyle modifications can reduce our inflammatory load and restore metabolism quite effectively.

THE BRAIN IN YOUR BELLY

In addition to directly suppressing inflammation, the parasympathetic nervous system, specifically the vagus nerve, activates a network of six hundred million neurons—the brain of our gut—which is called the *enteric nervous system*.[51] Since this neuronal extension of the parasympathetic nervous system contains as many neurons as the spinal cord, it's often referred to as our "second brain."[52]

Your central nervous system is much like the Federal Reserve, and the enteric nervous system is like a local bank. Just as constant communication between the Fed and local banks is vital to fiscal health, ongoing cross talk between the "gut-brain axis" is vital to the overall health of the body.

The balance of intestinal bacteria in our gut and the integrity of our gut barrier, along with proper vagus nerve activation from outside the intestine, are essential for optimal metabolic health because the nerve fibers stimulate the brain in our gut and liver.[53] Balance of this two-way communication system inside and outside of the gut maintains proper GI motility and levels of hormones that help to process nutrients and communicate sensations such as hunger, satiety, food cravings, and feelings of anxiety, depression, and "butterfly" sensations.[54,55,56]

Many studies in both obese and diabetic individuals suggest that gut-brain signaling may lead to gastrointestinal symptoms, including heartburn, impaired motility, and intestinal pain. Moreover, gut-brain signaling is implicated as a major culprit of the glucose-insulin imbalances leading to obesity.[57] Altered inputs from the brain to the gut, as in psychological stress, negatively alter intestinal immune response to ingested foods, leading to gut inflammation, a major contributing factor to gastrointestinal disorders and obesity.[58]

ACTIVATE YOUR VAGUS NERVE

Mindful lifestyle practices, such as meditative breathing, yoga, and other centering activities are able to activate our vagus nerve, and thus our parasympathetic nervous system, to suppress inflammation and alleviate metabolic imbalances.[59,60] Scientists have demonstrated through many human studies that increased parasympathetic nervous system tone is essential for preventing inflammation and metabolic health.[61,62] Moreover, healthy PNS tone has been shown to block endotoxin-mediated inflammation, which is linked to obesity, insulin resistance, and heart disease.[63] It helps to fight fat and metabolic disease through multiple mechanisms ranging from improved insulin sensitivity, increased digestive capacity, and sending anti-inflammatory messages throughout the body.

One of the easiest ways to assess your level of inflammation, metabolic control, and overall stress balance is through heart rate variability (HRV) assessment.[64] Multiple studies have shown increased parasympathetic activity to be strongly linked with increased variability, or frequency, in the beating of the heart. In contrast, reduced heart rate variability is linked with inflammation (elevated c-reactive protein and white blood cells), metabolic dysfunction, cardiovascular disease, and an overall stress response.[65,66,67]

Portuguese physicians tracked over 160 healthy patients for three years and found reduced heart rate variably (HRV) to strongly correlate with metabolic syndrome and inflammation.[68] In contrast, improved physical activity was positively correlated with increased heart rate variability and reduced levels of inflammation.

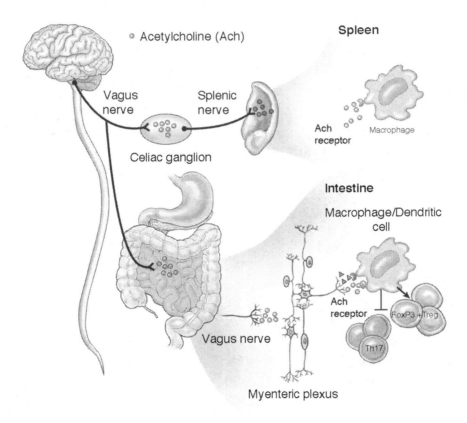

THE MIND-BODY CONTROL
OF DIGESTION AND INFLAMMATION

Mind-body therapies such as HeartMath, yoga, and meditation ignite a powerful anti-inflammatory pathway in the body via the vagus nerve. Vagus nerve activation is also required to properly turn on digestive secretions as well as prompt movement of the gastrointestinal tract.

My favorite tool for increasing activity of the vagus nerve, and thus HRV, is HeartMath. This small handheld biofeedback tool measures the subtle rate and rhythms of the heart. States of appreciation and goodwill are associated with increased HRV, while stress, frustration, and anger are associated with reduced HRV. Increased HRV is synonymous with increased parasympathetic nervous system tone and feelings of gratitude and calm.

Through the use of the HeartMath device, you can practice generating positive thoughts and taking deep meditative breaths for five to ten minutes to improve your parasympathetic tone. I ask all of my clients to use HeartMath five minutes prior to eating meals, up to three times a day. Ideally, one would be able to work up to 10–20 minutes of HeartMath activity one to three times a day. This will both prime the digestive tract for the incoming meal and help to offset inflammation associated with it. To learn more, go to www.BellyFatEffect.com/heart-math.

KEY TAKEAWAYS

Food interacts with trillions of gut microflora and digestive secretions before it enters our body for utilization and storage. The quality of this interaction is proving to be an important facet of our health. Digestive imbalances are more common in overweight persons, and may be a core dysfunction contributing to metabolic aberrations. Meal timing profoundly influences how the body processes and desires foods. The digestive tract and its associated secretions are regulated by the vagus nerve, which can be activated by relaxing behavior and deep breathing. Studies show overweight and inflamed subjects have poor heart rate variability, which is directly associated with reduced vagus nerve functioning.

I suggest eating a high-carbohydrate and high-protein breakfast daily and incorporating stress reduction techniques into daily life, particularly prior to eating. HeartMath is arguably the best and most effective therapy for learning how to achieve this physiologic state of relaxation and increase vagus nerve stimulation, for maximum digestive fire.

CHAPTER 7

EXERCISE TO LOSE BELLY FAT

"Even short periods of physical inactivity are associated with metabolic changes, including decreased insulin sensitivity, attenuation of postprandial lipid metabolism, loss of muscle mass and accumulation of visceral adipose tissue."
—Bente Klarlund Pedersen, MD, DMSc

Remember how those ten billion energy factories in your cells, the mitochondria, convert lipids and carbohydrates into cellular energy? They are not self-sufficient, but are dependent upon a few important cellular signaling molecules, such as AMPK (*adenosine monophosphate-activated protein kinase*).[1] One way you can keep your AMPK levels up is with exercise. Now researchers are learning just what kind of exercise will do the job.[2,3]

AMPK: THE BODY'S FUEL GAUGE

After you eat a meal, your energy fuel levels are high and your AMPK level is low. The AMPK circulating increases as you use that energy fuel, say for example, when doing intense exercise, during cold stress, and if you restrict how many calories you eat at the next meal. As AMPK increases, cells get the message to make more mitochondria, which enhances your ability to burn fat instead of sugar as fuel.[4,5] AMPK and other enzymes in the intestine are known to coordinate mitochondrial function by up to 46 percent.[6]

AMPK also plays a key role in regulating the appetite center in your brain and improves your sensitivity to insulin.[7] That's why AMPK is often regarded as the body's master energy regulator.[8]

Lastly, AMPK inhibits lipid signaling in pathways involved in making cholesterol and triglycerides, offering protection against heart problems and metabolic diseases.[9]

Exercise and intermittent fasting are not the only ways to increase cellular AMPK.[10,11,12] Cells in the intestinal tract and gut microflora also help regulate AMPK and mitochondrial activity. The gut is both the first point of contact for ingested nutrients as well as the main converter of whole food into energy that cells can use. Studies have found that consumption of processed carbohydrates and high-fat meals decrease AMPK.

A recent study reported that a high-fat diet reduces AMPK in fat tissue and in the liver, preceding elevations in blood sugar and markers of inflammation.[13] This suggests that diet-induced changes of AMPK directly affect nutrient and inflammatory signaling in the rest of the body.

SUMMARY OF AMPK'S EFFECTS	
TISSUE	ROLE IN METABOLISM
Liver	Decreases production of glucose, cholesterol, triglycerides Increases oxidation (breakdown) of fatty acids
Muscle	Increases glucose uptake and fat oxidation (breakdown)
Adipose (Fat)	Prevents fat storage Increases oxidation (breakdown) of fat

Since AMPK plays such important roles in fat burning, blood-sugar regulation, and appetite control, it's no surprise that AMPK is reduced in overweight, insulin-resistant people. In fact, research reveals that increased body fat, particularly abdominal fat, a primary source of inflammation, is associated with a 45 percent reduction in AMPK. Scientists have also found that a proinflammatory cytokine, TNF-alpha, alters AMPK's ability to burn fat.[14]

Hormones involved in the stress response may also perturb AMPK signaling. According to one study, increased levels of the stress hormone cortisol, which rises during both stress and inflammation, decreases AMPK in fat tissue.[15]

In contrast, increased cellular AMPK levels are linked with reduced inflammation.[16] More specifically, researchers suggest that healthy cellular AMPK levels block a major inflammatory signaling molecule (NF-κβ).[17,18,19] Recent studies have revealed a novel finding: AMPK is linked to both improved fat combustion and anti-inflammatory signaling pathways. Scientists associate increased AMPK with simultaneous improvements in metabolism, enhancing fat burning and suppression of inflammation.[20]

HORMESIS: YOUR INTERNAL METABOLIC SWITCHES

Thankfully, we have many ways to increase our AMPK levels as well as other protective metabolic signaling molecules. Mild stressors, such as exercising intensely, restricting calories for a short period, and eating a plant-rich diet place healthy stress on our metabolic networks.[21,22,23,24,25,26,27] These positive stressors increase AMPK in our muscles and liver tissue, optimizing our fat-burning and anti-inflammatory capabilities.[28]

Edward Calabrese, PhD, of the University of Massachusetts at Amherst, has characterized many examples of *hormesis*—that is, the concept that intermittent exposure to mild stressors leads to adaptations in metabolism.[29,30] Think of hormesis as school or work stress that causes you to burn the midnight oil to get a project completed. If you had no pressure or deadline to meet, you might not push yourself to learn new information or develop a particular skill, and so you wouldn't improve academically or professionally. Similarly, intermittent, short-term stress through high-intensity interval training, modified calorie restriction, and plant polyphenols are key to tuning your metabolism and maintaining an anti-inflammatory state. In contrast, sedentary activity, overeating, and consumption of colorless (white, processed) foods lead to metabolic imbalances and inflammation.

EXERCISE, AMPK, AND LONGEVITY

Exercise is a transient stressor, lowering body fat and maintaining a healthy blood-sugar balance by tweaking cellular energy gauges, such as AMPK.[31] Short duration, high-intensity exercise offers many metabolic benefits above and beyond simply burning calories and fat: intense activity improves metabolic efficiency and flips on longevity genes called *sirtuins*, producing anti-aging effects.[32,33]

AMPK and sirtuins work together to improve your fat-burning potential while simultaneously pivoting your cells into an anti-inflammatory state and protecting DNA from damage.[34] This is important because poor dietary choices (for example, eating refined sugar and fat) and increased belly fat are associated with shorter DNA strands, a marker of cellular aging.[35,36]

Sirtuins are enzymes that offer protection to the more than six feet of double-stranded DNA in every cell of your body.[37] DNA is subjected to many insults, including free-radical stressors from inflammation, radiation from excessive sun exposure or X rays, and consuming heavy metals, such as lead and arsenic, in water and food.[38,39,40] Damaged DNA is analogous to a computer virus that misguides your computer's hardware into doing things it shouldn't. In the body, DNA damage leads to aberrant protein synthesis, unregulated cell growth, premature cell death, and cancer.

Sirtuins protect our cellular instruction manual, or DNA, by increasing the tautness of its binding around DNA compactors called *histones*.[41,42,43] Histones are like a garden hose that compresses and compacts the six-foot-long DNA strands into cells so small that they can only be viewed under a microscope.[44] In essence, they "silence" the information of DNA through the removal of biochemical groups called acetyl groups and the addition of methyl groups.[45] Methylation is a critically important aspect of DNA protection as well as immune function, detoxification, hormone and neurotransmitter synthesis, and glutathione protection.[46,47,48,49] For more information on methylation, please visit the website of Benjamin Lynch, ND, at www.MTHFR.net.

The most well studied of the sirtuins is SIRT1.[50,51,52] It extends the life of yeast, fruit flies, and mice when upregulated during calorie restriction and administration of the polyphenol, resveratrol.[53] Sirtuins help link our metabolism with the pacemaker in our brain, ensuring that the proper hormones are released at the right time of the day.[54] We'll learn more about the importance of optimal sleep and our internal clock system in Chapter 8. Maintaining the integrity of our genes so that we can live longer is just one of many roles that sirtuins, specifically SIRT1, play in the body.

EXCESS BODY FAT AND CELLULAR AGING

Telomeres are protective caps on the ends of DNA strands that protect our genetic material from damage.[55] The sirtuins described above augment telomere length, combating cellular ageing. The enzyme that acts like a handyman, protecting our chromosomes from unwiring and shortening, is called *telomerase*.[56] Low telomere length—shortened DNA— is linked with obesity, diabetes, cardio-vascular disease, cancers, and depression. Elizabeth Blackburn, PhD, won the 2009 Nobel Prize in Physiology or Medicine for her work with telomeres.[57,58,59,60,61,62]

Many studies have since demonstrated a strong correlation among excess body fat, accelerated cellular aging, and shortened telomeres.[63,64,65] For example, one study found that the telomeres of obese children were over 23 percent shorter than their non-obese counterparts.

Obesity, insulin resistance, inflammation, and inflammatory disease are associated with reduced telomere length in adults too.[66,67,68,69] Shortened telomere length isn't linked to fat of all types, but researchers do believe it's linked to the "sick fat" of the abdomen.[70] For instance, people with type 2 diabetes also have shortened telomeres.[71]

Regular exercise; taking multivitamins, vitamin D, and essential fatty acid (EFA) supplements; and eating color-rich fruits and vegetables or following a Mediterranean diet are all associated with longer telomeres.[72,73,74]

In sum, diet, exercise, and our metabolic machinery elegantly converge with cellular housekeeping features to protect the single entity that makes us human: our DNA. This critically important cellular instruction manual is highly sensitive to free radical and toxin damage. Telomeres serve as umbrella-like caps, preventing damage to DNA from the rain of cellular and environmental toxins. Fine-tuning our metabolic machinery not only helps us shed fat and balance blood sugar, but also improves sirtuin activity and protects telomere length, combating cellular aging. The answer to long-lasting health is simple: stress reduction, high-intensity exercise, intermittent calorie restriction, and a microbial-friendly diet rich in polyphenolic compounds from vegetables, fruits, herbs, and spices.

MODIFIED CALORIE RESTRICTION

Scientists suggest that a 25 percent calorie reduction is needed to increase AMPK and sirtuin activity leading to improved mitochondria function. However, cutting back that much on calories is too challenging for most people. Another option is to occasionally fast for a day. Here is a healthy way to do it: pick one day a week and simply don't eat for twenty-four hours. If you're the type that gets jittery with no food, you can drink a pea-protein shake in the morning and evening. (The protein also prevents loss of lean muscle mass.) Try to fast on days when you are relatively inactive.

Alternatively, you can try night fasting, my personal favorite. Pick three nonconsecutive nights out of the week and fast for twelve or more hours. For example, on Monday, Wednesday, and Friday eat dinner before 6:00 p.m. and then don't eat anything else for the rest of the evening. By the time you awake at 6:00 or 7:00 a.m., you've gone twelve or more hours without food.

Layering regular and intense exercise over this modified calorie restriction program will super-charge mitochondrial activity, boosting fat burning and blood-sugar metabolism and protecting your DNA.[75,76]

EXERCISE FOR FAT LOSS AND OPTIMAL CELLULAR HEALTH

Humans are meant to move. Research shows time after time that exercise is a not an option for reducing sick belly fat, it's a requirement.[77,78] In my own experience of vigorous weight lifting five days a week for the last fifteen years and as a personal trainer for others for eight years, I've noticed that people who push the envelope at the gym, inducing mild cellular stress, achieve the best results. Those that cruise in their comfort zone or follow the same exercise program and don't push through the "burn," hardly ever improve. Their ability to burn fat never changes.

The best workout for losing belly fat is short-duration, moderate-to-high intensity exercise that combines both aerobic (cardiovascular training) and anaerobic movements (resistance training).[79,80] Blending these two types of exercise is key to losing belly fat, improving metabolism, and preventing age-related chronic disease.[81,82,83,84]

Resistance training builds lean muscle, which improves insulin sensitivity, while aerobic exercise burns fat most effectively.[85,86,87,88,89,90] More specifically, researchers suggest that thirty minutes of moderate to vigorous exercise five days a week is optimal for reducing belly fat and improving cardiovascular risk factors. And this occurs with no change in diet.[91,92]

However, dietary changes and exercise are more powerful together than either is alone. For example, according to one study, leptin decreased more than 50 percent with forty minutes a day of vigorous activity, five days a week, combined with a moderately low-calorie diet.[93] (Remember, leptin increases with fat and is involved in driving inflammation that often makes fat burning impossible.)

HIT THE BELLY FAT

High-intensity interval training, or HIT, is a method that includes bursts of very intense exercise followed by a brief period of rest during the course of a workout.[94] HIT will give you the most benefit from your aerobic exercise, since it efficiently exploits your cellular metabolic machinery.

An example of HIT is four thirty-second spurts of all-out effort on an exercise bike, followed by four minutes of low-to-moderate recovery cycling during the course of a bout of cycling. Intervals can be performed indoors on the stair-climber, treadmill, or elliptical machine or outdoors on inclined roads, stairs, and trails. These short bursts of intense effort offer the best of both worlds: maximizing results from exercise, while preventing injury and maintaining the enjoyment of exercise.

HIT training is so powerful that in as little as six sessions over the course of two weeks, you will experience dramatic improvements in metabolic control and an enhanced ability to burn fat.[95] Compared to longer-duration aerobic training, HIT leads to dramatic improvements in muscle cell AMPK and another cellular signaling molecule called PGC-1α.[96]

Most importantly, studies report that when overweight people do HIT, abdominal fat decreases by up to 48 percent and insulin sensitivity improves up to 58 percent in just eight weeks.[97] A more recent study reported that after just three months of HIT for twenty minutes three days a week, visceral fat was reduced by over 17 percent in untrained, overweight men.[98] One study found that just two weeks of HIT every other day, consisting of ten four-minute bouts of vigorous efforts on an exercise bike followed by a two-minute rest, increased fat burning by 36 percent.[99]

HOW TO START HIT

The easiest way to start HIT is to add "bursts" of intense effort to a twenty-minute steady pace of cycling, stair climbing, or uphill treadmill walking. (I like to begin with four twenty-second all-out bursts for every fifteen minutes of exercise.) Two recent studies found that just four seconds of an all-out burst every two minutes during a twenty-minute cycling session was more effective than twenty minutes of solid-state cycling.[100,101]

There are a few ways to track intensity. You can use the heart rate or power output. I prefer the latter. At your workout facility, find an exercise bike that has watts as a metric to gauge workout intensity. *Watts*, a measurement of power over time, is a much better barometer to assess exercise efforts than heart rate monitoring because it's not affected by stress, hydration, or sleep as is heart rate. To assess your target "interval power," do a warm-up spin for five minutes and then increase the resistance to an effort that is very difficult yet manageable for 45–60 seconds. You'll know you're doing this right if your legs and lungs are burning and you're really out of breath.

Record the average number from this test effort. My average one-minute power output is 450 watts. So when I do longer ninety-second bursts at 80 percent intensity, and I'm peddling or stepping on the stair mill, I'm stepping at 360 watts. For more details, visit www.BellyFatEffect.com/exercise.

Now that you have a general idea of what 100 percent intensity feels like, you can gauge your bursts of intense exercise. The burst periods should vary for 45–90 seconds, followed by two minutes of active recovery, three days a week. For example, on Monday, try four, ninety-second bursts at 80 percent intensity followed by a four-minute rest. Then on Wednesday, do six forty-five-second bursts at 100 percent intensity followed by a four-minute rest. Then Friday, do five sixty-second bursts at 85 percent intensity. As you progress into month three of training and beyond, I suggest increasing the number of burst periods to four to six per aerobic workout.

THE DOWNSIDE OF ENDURANCE

In college, I raced road bikes competitively and quickly moved to the elite level while living in Boulder, CO. Some weeks I would train twenty-five hours or more, riding around the beautiful hills of Boulder and beyond. Six-hour group training rides on the weekends were the norm. Although I would wake up feeling utterly exhausted and with a ravenous appetite, I continued the torturous workouts for years, hoping to advance from the category 2 level to the pros. Thankfully, three major bicycle wrecks in successive weekends motivated me to move on from competitive sports.

I share this story because I witnessed what endurance training does to you: I was emaciated, hormonally imbalanced, stressed, and constantly tired. Excessive endurance training is very *catabolic*, meaning it breaks down cellular material. It is the antithesis of anabolic, which means to build.[102] In other words, long-duration, steady-state exercise causes a hormonal milieu fostering both muscle tissue and fat breakdown. Due to the pro-metabolic effects of muscle tissue, this is obviously undesirable. So while hiking and biking is healthy, making a habit of intense, long-duration exercise is counterproductive.

Curiously, my body fat percentage when I was cycling, as well as that of many others I trained with, was high, considering the amount of calories I burned every day. Prolonged endurance training is similar to the body's response to stress. Muscle-wasting cortisol increases and anabolic hormones, growth hormone, and testosterone decrease. Worse yet, after a long duration of aerobic training, it's common to have a ravenous appetite. The perception among many is, "I earned it. . . so I can eat whatever I want." Such a spike in appetite doesn't occur during short-duration HIT.

THE IMPORTANCE OF MUSCLE

Some people are so focused on fat loss that they forget about muscle. The health potential of lean muscle mass is largely underestimated. Metabolically, it is very active and rich in mitochondria, making it a powerful fat-fighting factory.[103] Muscle is actually a critically important metabolic organ, releasing a plethora of metabolic and immune-signaling molecules, including AMPK, which has many health benefits.[104]

LEAN MUSCLE AND FAT-SHEDDING EXERCISE PROGRAM		
DAY OF THE WEEK	BODY PARTS INCORPORATED	DETAILS
Monday	Shoulders and triceps: 20 minutes of stair climbing with 4 x 60-second bursts at 80% on stair stepper.	I'm a huge fan of standing military presses for both men and women.
Tuesday	Back and calf strengthening followed by bursts on exercise bike. Keep intensity very high, 95% max. Do 6 x 40-second bursts.	Dead lifts are fantastic to begin a back workout. Follow them with bent-over rows, dumbbell rows, and pull-ups.
Wednesday	Alternate between yoga and cross fit and core work every week. Walking uphill on treadmill for 25 minutes is great too.	This is a modified rest day. Stay active but at low intensity.
Thursday	Legs and biceps strengthening: 20 minutes walking uphill on treadmill. Do 4 x 90-second bursts on steep incline of 10% or more. Keep intensity at 80% of max during bursts.	It's important to do compound movements for legs, such as squats and leg presses.
Friday	Chest and core strengthening: 20 minutes cardio on exercise bike. Do 5 x 60-second intervals at 75% of max.	I really like incline dumbbells and push-ups with feet elevated.
Saturday and Sunday	Get outside for some uphill hiking during the summer or snowshoeing during the winter. Keep the intensity low and a 45-second burst every 20 minutes. Try to keep duration under 90 minutes.	The goal is to reduce stress, get some sun with family and friends.

Not surprisingly exercise, particularly resistance exercise, may one day be a primary modality for countering inflammation in chronic inflammatory diseases, such as autoimmunity and cancer.[105,106] Lean muscle is also linked with improved insulin sensitivity and reduced inflammation. Just as fat tissue can become inflamed during insulin resistance and obesity, muscle tissue can be affected too.[107]

In addition to HIT, I recommend that both men and women also participate in high-intensity resistance training at least three days a week. The goal is to train each body part at least once a week. Researchers have concluded that high-intensity weight lifting for 6–12 reps, or to failure, engenders the most muscle hypertrophy.[108] (Muscle hypertrophy is when cells increase in size, giving muscles definition.) Such intense resistance training also positively affects various hormones of the body, facilitating fat burning and improving blood-sugar control.

Many people wrongly believe that such training will make one overly muscular like a bodybuilder. The reality is that most male and female bodybuilders who look like that have too much muscle because of anabolic steroid use. Only the most genetically gifted and those who eat an uncomfortable amount of food could become so overly muscular.

As such, it's in your best interest to really push your muscles to failure, while maintaining correct form. For full details and descriptions of these exercises, please visit www.BellyFatEffect.com/exercise to learn more.

TOOLS TO HELP BUILD MUSCLE, BURN FAT

There are a few tricks to help maximize your workouts. I like to ingest coffee or tea in the hours leading up to my workout. This will enable you to burn more fat and be able to sustain a harder workout.[109] Also pre-workout, I like to take the following:

- Niacin: nicotinic acid, not *inositol hexanicotinate* (1,000 mg)
- *L-arginine alpha ketoglutarate* (4,000 mg)

- *Beta-alanine* (1 gram)
- *Creatine*: Creatine MagnaPower®(2.5 grams)
- Branched-chain amino acids, or BCAAs (5 grams)
- Taurine (750 mg)
- L-carnitine tartrate (1000-2000 mg)

The niacin and arginine increase peripheral blood flow while the beta-alanine, L-carnitine, creatine, and BCAAs support exercise performance and recovery.[110,111,112,113,114,115,116,117,118,119]

Immediately following my workout, if I've exercised very intensely, I make a smoothie that includes polyphenol-rich berries, a banana, honey, and the following:[120,121,122,123]

- *Creatine*: Creatine MagnaPower® (2.5 grams)
- Whey protein concentrate from New Zealand grass-fed cows (25 grams)
- L-glutamine (5 grams)
- Branched-chain amino acids, or BCAAs (2.5 grams)
- Immunoglobulin concentrate (2.5 grams)

The post-workout shake is critically important to maintaining lean muscle mass after exercise and for aiding in fat burning. Those who prefer to drink a Starbucks latte after a workout won't achieve the same benefits as those who consume a protein shake in the thirty-minute post-workout window.

Optimal adaptations to muscle building and fat burning can occur when exercise is done in the afternoon because cortisol, the body's primary catabolic hormone, is lowest at this time.[124] If morning is the only time that you can exercise, then make sure to have a whey or pea protein shake during exercise or else you'll catabolize your metabolically protective muscle.

SITTING IS DEADLY

Just because you exercise, doesn't mean you can sit all day. In fact, despite recreational exercise, prolonged sitting is associated with inflammation.[125,126] Science is showing that low "non-exercise physical activity," such as little activity at work, is linked to a higher incidence of death from cardiovascular disease.[127] However, breaking up prolonged sitting time with a walk every ninety minutes or so offsets that danger.[128] Some studies suggest getting up for five minutes or so every half hour may offer similar benefits.[129] Researchers recently reported that five minutes of exercise at intervals throughout the day, for forty minutes total was more effective at burning fat than forty-five consecutive minutes.[130]

You should move every 45–90 minutes for a few minutes of working out. Run the stairs, do push-ups, sit-ups, something to get your blood pumping. This will lead to beneficial changes in your skeletal muscle physiology and the genetic expression of your mitochondrial regulatory proteins.

KEY TAKEAWAYS

Shedding fat, especially belly fat, can seem like a monumental task, but addressing key components of fat metabolism will have you sporting a slimmer waistline in no time! First, your body's high-octane fuel of choice is AMPK, which is essential in regulating appetite, energy, and cholesterol. Studies have found reduced levels of AMPK in overweight and insulin-resistant people; increased abdominal fat is linked to reduction in AMPK levels. The good news is that the right diet and exercise can effectively increase AMPK.

Intermittent fasting also increases AMPK. So does high-intensity interval training or short bursts of intense exercise supported by healthy intestinal flora. Increased AMPK levels promote healthy metabolism and anti-inflammatory pathways. AMPK has another partner in health called sirtuins, which are responsible in part for longevity by protecting DNA from damage. Without sirtuins, we would have runaway aging!

DNA preservation comes from preventing the shortening of telomere protective caps on the ends of DNA strands. Long telomeres have been associated with health and longevity. Incorporating foods such as fruits and vegetables that are high in vitamins C, D, and E, and protein, such as fish, will enable your body to whittle away that sick fat!

The companion of diet is exercise, and stubborn belly fat requires both high-intensity interval aerobic and resistance training. For fat loss, the goal in exercise is not time duration or endurance, but intense sequences of exercise that will change your cellular chemistry.

CHAPTER 8

SLEEP MORE, WEIGH LESS

"Among the well-known consequences of a disrupted circadian function are altered metabolism and even life span, which may be all adversely affected when the circadian time-keeping system is altered."—Marta Garaulet Aza, PhD

The recent spike in overweight and obesity prevalence is associated with a simultaneous decline in sleep time. According to the Centers for Disease Control and Prevention and the National Sleep Foundation polls, Americans are sleeping less than seven hours per night, down from the more than eight hours reported just 50 years ago.[1] The number of adults sleeping less than six hours per night is between 30 percent and 40 percent, according to several recent reports.[2,3]

Since sleep is one of the body's ways of conserving energy, curbing that resting time is linked to many metabolic derangements and fat gain.[4] Endocrinologists now recognize that poor sleep habits and sleep loss are risk factors for obesity and diabetes.[5,6] People who sleep five or less hours per night have a 46 percent increased risk of developing diabetes compared to those who sleep seven to eight hours a night. Other biological consequences of burning the midnight oil are insulin resistance, increased blood triglycerides, altered levels of sex and adrenal hormones, disruption of the vagus nerve, increased susceptibility to inflammation, and increased hunger, particularly for after-dinner snacks.[7,8,9]

Poor sleep hygiene and altered meal timing desynchronize our delicate internal clocks and thus affect our metabolism.[10] Worse yet, disruption of our circadian clock system also throws a monkey wrench into the critically important anti-inflammatory mechanism controlled by the vagus nerve. Up to 20 percent of our genes adhere to some degree of daily oscillation.[11] Circumventing proper sleep and wake cycles leads to imbalanced circadian rhythms.[12] This partially explains why most heart attacks occur in the morning, why shift workers have a higher incidence of cancer, and why poor sleepers tend to be more overweight.[13,14,15] Altered circadian rhythms are skewed in persons with depression, anxiety, schizophrenia, neurodegenerative disorders, gastrointestinal (GI) problems, and cancer.[16,17,18,19]

Abnormal rhythm of secretion of the hormone cortisol, for example, has been linked to poor survival in patients with breast and colon cancer.[20,21]

CIRCADIAN CLOCK SYSTEM 101

Many crucial aspects of our metabolic and hormonal functions operate in a rhythmical fashion corresponding to the rise and fall of the sun. In fact, the word *circadian* is derived from the Latin words *circa* and *dies* for "around" and "day."[22] From primitive unicellular bacteria to complex organisms like humans, the so-called clock gene networks in these life forms align the daily rhythms of the body's functions with the light and dark cycles of each day.[23,24,25]

Many aspects of our bodies—from hormone levels and cognitive performance to body temperature—operate under the direction of the hypothalamus's attempt to coordinate our physiology with the 24-hour cycle of the earth.[26] As such, many hormones discussed up to now exhibit some degree of circadian rhythm, including hormones released from fat tissue, such as leptin and adiponectin; the hunger-inducing hormone ghrelin; metabolic hormones insulin and glucagon; inflammatory cytokines, such as TNF-alpha; the adrenal stress hormones; and melatonin.[27,28,29] Loss of circadian rhythm of the core clock genes, or chronodisruption, is associated with obesity and diabetes.[30,31,32]

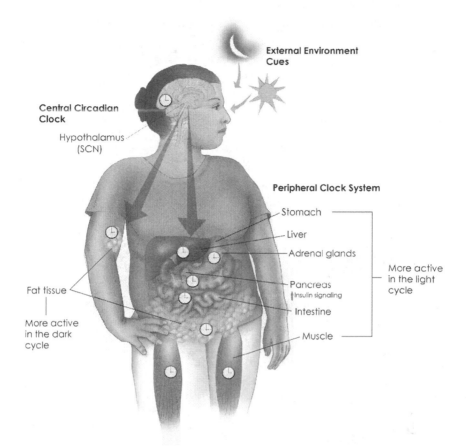

External Environment Cues

Central Circadian Clock

Hypothalamus (SCN)

Peripheral Clock System

Stomach

Liver

Adrenal glands

Pancreas
Insulin signaling

Intestine

Muscle

More active in the light cycle

Fat tissue

More active in the dark cycle

THE CIRCADIAN CLOCK SYSTEM

The master pacemaker in the brain translates external light and dark cues and relays them to internal clock systems in the digestive tract and various tissues throughout the body, including fat and muscle. Getting adequate sleep and eating early in the day keeps these clocks, and thus metabolism, in alignment.

In humans, the master pacemaker, called the suprachiasmatic nucleus (SCN), is strategically positioned in the hypothalamus region of the brain. The SCN, also known as your central clock, keenly detects light and dark and relays this information to peripheral tissues.[33] Located within these peripheral tissues are networks of core circadian clock genes found in many peripheral metabolic, cardiovascular, and immune tissues.[34] This aligns the 24-hour cycle of the earth to many of our organs, including the stomach, small and large intestines, pancreas, liver, heart, adrenal glands, endometrium, ovaries, prostate, spleen, and muscles as well as fat tissue (adipocyte), and many immune cells (CD4+ and CD8+ T cells, neutrophils, monocytes, and macrophages).[35,36,37,38,39]

The chain of communication goes something like this: The master pacemaker, the SCN, detects morning light cues and evening dark cues through nerves in the eye and transmits messages by way of the nervous system to peripheral tissues. Muscle, fat, liver, and cardiovascular tissues respond by activating or deactivating core clock genes in an oscillatory manner. This maximizes our ability to adapt to our environment. The core clock genes, which are tightly aligned with many metabolic signaling hubs, are turned on or off depending on the time of day.

It's therefore critical to a healthy metabolism to align your biological clock with the rise and fall of the sun.[40,41] Stress reduction, exercise, diet, and optimal GI health are only complete when one's circadian clock is rhythmically aligned to the external environment. Sleep and a properly tuned circadian system are paramount to shedding belly fat and attaining an optimal metabolism.

PUT YOUR BODY CLOCKS TO WORK

In the field of oncology, it's well known that the timing of the administration of cancer drugs is very important to the medication's effectiveness. The goal of many of these agents is to interrupt the cell replication cycle, which is on hyperdrive in rapidly replicating tumor cells. Since so many functions at the cellular level display a peak and nadir at different times of the day, aligning chemotherapy drugs with the "cellular clock" improves response to the drugs and minimizes the side effects of chemotherapy. If taking into account the influence of the body's rhythms on cancer therapy is successful, why shouldn't chronotherapy be used to maximize fat-loss efforts?

During the day, or wake phase, the pacemaker-like SCN sends messages from the brain to the periphery of the body to optimize metabolic activities with daytime functions, which include eating and movement. In circadian-aligned healthy persons, light stimulates the release of the adrenal stress hormones cortisol and catecholamine most during the morning, and this stimulation lessens as the day progresses.[42] Exposure to light also stimulates the sympathetic or "fight or flight" branch of the nervous system. The absence of light at night stimulates the parasympathetic or "rest and digest" branch of the nervous system.[43]

Several studies have demonstrated how curtailment of this daily spike and dip in cortisol levels is linked with insulin resistance and type 2 diabetes. Researchers at Johns Hopkins University, for example, found that people with diabetes have a significantly lower rise in cortisol in the morning compared to healthy controls.[44]

Chemical messengers that signal hunger and prompt eating shift according to this light-darkness cycle. Leptin, the hormone released from fat cells signaling satiety, is highest in the night and declines upon waking.[45] A high leptin level during sleep is beneficial, since it signals to the brain that there is plenty of fuel available and that there is no need to hit the fridge for a midnight snack. Ghrelin levels, in contrast, spike in the morning and trigger hunger. Cut back on your sleep, though, and those leptin and ghrelin levels become skewed, exaggerating daytime appetite and cravings for high-calorie foods.[46,47]

Blood sugar and insulin have long been known to display diurnal rhythm, at least in metabolically healthy people.[48] Not so for those with insulin resistance or type 2 diabetes. Normally, blood glucose is highest in the morning and diminishes as the day progresses while insulin's rhythm is the reverse—it is lowest in the morning and peaks in the afternoon.[49] Since insulin is involved in storing glucose, amino acids, and lipids after eating, it's programmed to peak during the day when eating takes place. However, sensitivity to insulin progressively diminishes as the day advances, so it's best to eat carbohydrates (sweet potatoes, black rice, or fruit) in the morning.[50]

Timing exercise around the peak surges of the anabolic hormone insulin and valleys of the catabolic hormone cortisol is important. Since insulin peaks in the afternoon and the muscle-wasting hormone cortisol is at its nadir in the afternoon, early to mid-afternoon is the best time to do resistance training.[51] Also, muscle power peaks between 4 and 6 p.m.[52] By weight training in the afternoon, you'll not only work out harder, but you'll take advantage of the extra anabolic potential of insulin to develop more metabolically healthy muscle mass.

LEAKY GUT AND CIRCADIAN RHYTHMS

The gut is a major processor and repository for the food you eat, and it's highly regulated by circadian clock genes. GI tract motility, gastric emptying, and food absorption are much more active during the day than at night.[53] This is why it's important to keep your body on a regular sleep schedule and eat your largest meal early in the day when the gut is best able to process the food and absorb nutrients.

Levels of gut-hormones such as GLP-1 and CCK, are highest during the earlier part of the day, which may be why insulin sensitivity is also highest in the morning and diminishes as the day goes on.[54]

The ability to digest and process fats is best in the morning as well. Post-meal fat processing, cholesterol synthesis, and levels of bile—the detergent-like molecules involved in fat digestion—are largely under the control of core clock genes. Lipases, enzymes involved in cleavage of fats, are highest in the morning compared to the evening.[55]

The fact that our bodies naturally lose metabolic flexibility—the ability to efficiently utilize different fuels, such as fats and sugars—as the day progresses means that eating fat at night is very problematic for our waistlines and metabolic health. That's because lipids not stored in fat or in the liver are placed in non-storage tissues, such as muscle tissue.[56] This can lead to a state of lipotoxicity, which is associated with insulin resistance and metabolic disease. Likewise, intestinal absorption of dietary fats and proper packaging into chylomicrons, the form in which fat is transported into the bloodstream, is most efficient in the earlier part of the day.[57]

An impaired ability to process dietary fats in the evening may explain why the body is more susceptible to the deleterious effects of intestinal-derived endotoxin in the evening.[58] Increased endotoxin burden may also be the result of leaky gut formed from disturbances in the circadian rhythm, as some animal studies have shown. A recent study reported increased endotoxin burden and poor barrier function in the intestines of animals that had been exposed to changes in light/dark cycles, which shifted their circadian clock out of sync.[59]

Moreover, the circadian clock system influences many aspects of metabolism, and vice versa. Research shows that ingestion of excessive fats can derail the rhythm of the clock.[60] By feeding mice high-fat meals near their sleep cycle, mimicking a late-night standard American meal, researchers were able to pivot the cellular clocks of these animals right out of their rhythm and increase fat storage. So, if late-night snacks are a must, it is recommended to keep the carbohydrates and fats to a minimum and limit the meal to vegetables, lean protein, and easily digested fats from coconut oil.

Due to the high degree of coordination in human metabolism and the circadian clock system, fluctuations in cellular energy and nutrient levels known to influence metabolic signaling, such as AMPK, also affect circadian clock genes. For example, both calorie restriction and calorie excess can skew one's circadian clock.[61] That is why it's not just what you eat that affects weight gain, but when you eat it.

METABOLISM IS CYCLICAL: FAT BURNING OCCURS AT NIGHT

Enzyme activity and levels of proteins involved in detoxification and lipid synthesis increase during the dark phase of the circadian rhythm.[62] Just like nutrients can affect our internal circadian clock, environmental toxins and xenobiotic compounds in the environment can similarly skew this pacemaker system.[63]

During the night cycle, the liver also increases levels of many enzymes involved in mitochondria function and lipid and cholesterol synthesis. A recent study revealed that fat burning in the mitochondria is most active during the sleep phase, peaking just before waking.[64,65] At night, our master pacemaker (SCN) helps to increase fat burning (lipolysis), which has the effect of reducing hunger so that we can stay asleep. As the master pacemaker in the brain detects light, the body shifts out of a lipid-burning mode and into a more sugar-burning state.[66]

Shiftwork increases the risk of developing fatty liver, a disease often associated with perturbed fat metabolism, increased belly fat, and metabolic syndrome. Researchers report that people with fatty livers have mitochondrial dysfunction, which impairs fat burning.[67] Now we know that this may be a result of a skewed circadian clock.

Very lean fitness competitors plan their aerobic sessions first thing in the morning, so they can ride on the coattails of their natural circadian system and exploit its fat-burning potential.

For maximal belly fat burning, perform interval-based aerobic training first thing in the morning on an empty stomach. Drink one to two cups of coffee or green tea prior to exercise, as caffeine helps to increase fat lipolysis burning.

Before we learn more about how to optimize our circadian clocks, let's first see how disruption of this critical biological rhythm can cause the pounds to stack up and increase fat storage.

CYCLES OF IMMUNITY

The immune system is also affected by the cyclical patterns of nature.[68] Although both the metabolic and immune systems beat to the same drum, which is the hypothalamus, one peaks as the other reaches its lowest point. That is, many metabolic hormones are highest in the morning and lowest at night.[69] The inverse is true for the immune system. Studies have shown that levels of inflammatory cytokines such as TNF-alpha, neutrophils, and macrophages are most active during the night in healthy people.[70] In contrast, people with rheumatoid arthritis display perturbed circadian patterns of inflammatory signaling, with levels peaking at 6 a.m.[71] Many studies have also shown increased cardiovascular-related events in the early morning as well, when inflammation is highest.[72]

DISRUPTED SLEEP CAN MAKE YOU FAT

From narcolepsy to sleep apnea to shiftwork, disturbing your sleep takes a toll on your waistline. As with the liver and gut, more than 21% of the genes expressed in fat tissue exhibit circadian rhythm.[73] Misguided environmental cues, such as sleep loss or late-night eating, disrupt these networks and disturb your metabolism. Studies confirm that overweight people have imbalanced circadian rhythms in their fat tissue.[74]

Sleep lab studies have quantified how sleep curtailment bulges your belly. Just five consecutive nights of five hours of sleep led to a 42 percent increase in post-dinner snacks and smaller breakfast, which translated to a 1.7 pound weight gain on average.[75] A similar small study sought to examine the effects of five consecutive days of just four hours of night sleep in 14 men. This team reported a 15.5 percent increase in evening cortisol and an 11.4 percent increase in blood glucose, particularly after breakfast. Additionally, marked changes in sex hormones, including reductions in testosterone and sex hormone binding globulin, were observed. This is a hormone pattern that's linked to increased belly fat and poor glucose control. Another research study reported that 40 percent of type 2 diabetic subjects slept less than six hours per night, had increased levels of ghrelin, and experienced hunger cravings.

While chronic sleep deprivation will surely have a negative effect on metabolism, just two consecutive nights of only four hours of sleep are enough to throw a monkey wrench into the system. Researchers from the University of Chicago and Belgium demonstrated how quickly a few days of sleep restriction can increase the hunger hormone ghrelin by 28 percent, leading to a 24 percent increase in hunger ratings, particularly for high-calorie and carbohydrate-rich foods. Overall, sleep deprivation demonstrably alters blood sugar balance and sensitivity to inulin.

Larger research studies involving over 13,000 participants have revealed similar findings to smaller studies mentioned up to now. The findings show that less than seven hours of sleep per night is linked to increased belly fat.[77] But that's not all. Compared to those who sleep seven to nine hours per night, people who sleep six or less hours per night have a higher incidence of cardiovascular disease, diabetes, lung disorders, arthritis, and depression.

Researchers at Rush University Medical Center in Chicago recently described the deleterious metabolic effects of a "late chronotype" in diabetic patients. (A late chronotype is defined as a person who goes to bed late and wakes late in morning.) These people are more likely to eat larger dinners and skip breakfast and so have poorer glucose control compared to those who go to bed early.[78]

In addition to eating up to 50 percent more calories after 8 p.m., late sleepers eat more fast food, drink more soda, and eat fewer fruits and vegetables than do their countertypes.[79]

Sleep duration and fat loss may be more connected than previously thought. Scientists have revealed how short sleepers have a harder time burning fat compared to long sleepers, despite losing similar amounts of overall weight. Another weight-loss study reported how weight loss increased sleep duration in short sleepers prior to weight loss interventions.[80] However, weight loss had no effect on lengthening sleep duration in long duration sleepers prior to the study.

In sum, many recent clinical studies have revealed that sleep loss, and thus alteration of the circadian rhythm, increases fat gain, snacking, and nighttime appetite. Sleep disruption also reduces physical activity.[81]

SLEEP LOSS INCREASES RISK OF HEART DISEASE, DIABETES, AND METABOLIC SYNDROME

Circadian clock genes are not confined to fat and liver cells, but are also found in many other cells, including those of the cardiovascular system.[82] Not surprisingly, perturbations in the circadian clock system increase cardiovascular disease risk.[83] Moreover, studies suggest that the majority of heart attacks, strokes, arrhythmias, and sudden cardiac death events occur between 6 a.m. and noon.[84,85] This may be due to the fact that blood pressure begins to rise during the transition between the sleep and wake cycle, peaking first thing in the morning and dipping at night. Persons with elevated blood pressure that do not dip—so-called "non-dippers"—have increased cardiovascular risk.[86]

Even more fascinating, the frequency of cardiovascular events, including strokes, is highest in the winter when temperatures are lowest. Blood pressure and stress hormones increase to raise body temperature. These increases may be problematic to persons with damaged or inflamed cardiovascular conditions.

About a third of Americans suffer from metabolic syndrome, which, along with increased belly fat and poor blood sugar control, raises the risk of cardiovascular disease. Poor sleepers are at an increased risk of developing metabolic syndrome.[87] Several large studies reveal how sleeping less than six hours per night is linked to significant increases in metabolic syndrome and is independently linked to metabolic syndrome risk factors such as increased belly fat and triglycerides.[88]

Sleep is intended for the body to restore and conserve energy. Poor sleep hygiene or altered sleep-wake cycles, including shift work, desynchronize our internal circadian clocks and throw our metabolism into disarray.[89] Worse yet, since our metabolic machinery and our clock gene network are intimately connected, mistiming meals and eating too much alters our internal circadian clocks. The good news is that you can easily restore your own circadian rhythm, reset your clock, shrink your waistline, and minimize your chronic disease risk.

RESETTING YOUR CIRCADIAN CLOCK: SLEEP HYGIENE

As night approaches, the circadian clock system releases a powerful hormone from the pineal gland called melatonin. Conversely, exposure to lights at night stimulates the sympathetic nervous system and is a sure-fire way to suppress natural melatonin release and pivot one's circadian clock system right out of gear.[90,91] Although it may be challenging at first, it's critically important to turn down the lights, computers, tablets, smart phones, and television after 8 p.m. Instead, choose light reading, socializing with family, yoga, stretching, or mindfulness-based deep breathing techniques in the evening. Aim to be in bed by 9 or 9:30 p.m.

Ensure that there is absolutely no light in your bedroom, nor any television or alarm clocks that produce light. If you need to get new blinds to block outdoor light, get them. When traveling, you may wish to bring duct tape to keep light from beaming through your blinds as hotel rooms are notorious for having excessive light pouring through the shades. It's also a good practice to turn off your cell phone and cover the television screen in your room with a towel.

Avoid strenuous exercise and alcohol two hours prior to sleeping. Other agents known to negatively alter our circadian rhythm network are caffeinated beverages, sugar, excessive sodium, thiamin, and endotoxin. When possible, minimize exposure to these agents.

When you awaken in the morning, hopefully eight hours after falling asleep, it's best to go outside for exposure to natural light. This will entrain your circadian clock system. During the wintertime in higher latitude regions, it is wise to purchase a full-spectrum light system that can function in place of the sun, again stimulating the light cycle of your circadian system upon awakening.

SOCIAL JET LAG AND MELATONIN

It's best to go to sleep at the same time every night, but work, school, travel, and social schedules often contribute to "social jet lag" because the body gets disconnected from its biological rhythms.[92] Falling asleep at irregular times, even if you sleep seven to eight hours, is still disruptive. Sleeping in on the weekends doesn't counteract social jet lag; your sleep centers and circadian system will still be misaligned. And, when you awake late, you're likely to be exposed to lights, food, and other forms of stimulation which are out of sync with the night cycle of your circadian rhythm.

So, while catching up on sleep is beneficial, when your lifestyle repeatedly clashes with the rise and fall of the sun, your clock genes in your gut, liver, heart, and fat cells will still be out of sync.[93] For this reason, social jet lag is linked to poor heart health, depression, and obesity. Just like you'll need to plan out healthy meals ahead of time, you'll also need to work diligently to correct an irregular sleep schedule. Short 20-minute power naps in the early to mid-afternoon are a fine start, but the real magic happens with a regular sleep pattern and sleep supporting supplements, including melatonin.

MELATONIN: THE KEY TO RESTORING YOUR CIRCADIAN CLOCK GENES

Melatonin is an over-the-counter supplement with no known side effects and can be used in the late afternoon or early evening to help kick-start your circadian clock system back into a regular pattern. Doses of melatonin ranging from 0.5 mg to 10 mg taken in the evening have been shown to restore normal circadian rhythms and sleep in blind patients who have zero perception of light.[94,95] Melatonin use also reduced the number and duration of naps needed by blind people.[96] Melatonin and dark glasses have also been shown to be effective in realigning the circadian rhythm in people working night shifts.[97,98] For shift workers, world travelers, and late-night partiers alike, it's best to take melatonin during the time that you should be sleeping. If you're on a new time zone, for example, you should take 1-5 mg of melatonin in the afternoon; likewise shift workers should take melatonin near the end of their shift and avoid direct sun exposure in the morning.

ADDED HEALTH BENEFITS OF MELATONIN

With melatonin being so central to aligning the cogs of our circadian clocks, it makes sense then that the health benefits ascribed to melatonin reach far beyond sleep promotion.[99] Receptors for melatonin are abundant in the central nervous system (CNS), cardio-metabolic system, and the immune system.[100] Polish scientists revealed the power of melatonin in metabolic syndrome.[101] Two months of nightly melatonin use—5 mg, two hours before bed—led to a 12-point drop in blood pressure, as well as significant reductions in LDL-cholesterol and increases in antioxidant scores. Several months of 10 mg of melatonin per day in subjects with fatty liver, a common metabolic problem linked to increased belly fat, led to significant improvements in liver enzyme levels.[102] The same research group reported a 60 percent improvement in glucose and insulin sensitivity measures in patients with fatty liver disease during just one month of a daily dose of 10 mg melatonin.[103]

Melatonin has been studied extensively in people with cardio-vascular disease.[104,105] While also shifting biological rhythms into healthy patterns, melatonin has been shown to increase the protective HDL-cholesterol and to decrease atherogenic markers, including triglycerides and LDL-cholesterol.

In addition to many positive cardiovascular and metabolic effects, melatonin also has powerful anti-inflammatory effects and has been shown to ameliorate free radical stress and DNA damage-associated with extreme exercise.[106] In football players, 6 mg of melatonin reduced exercise-related immune dysfunction and oxidative stress.[107] Long-term melatonin therapy of 8 mg per day in women with irritable bowel syndrome has been shown to reduce pain, bloating, and constipation by over 50 percent.[108]

In sum, many human clinical studies as well as test tube and animal studies demonstrate the power of melatonin in restoring sleep and circadian rhythms and in improving cellular metabolism and reducing inflammation.

KEY TAKEAWAYS

It's essential to get to sleep at the same time every night and to minimize both chemical and social stressors as well as light at night. Our metabolism operates in a circadian fashion and is largely under the influence of melatonin. Light cycles correspond with taking in nutrition, so eat early in the day and expose your body to light upon awakening. Avoid eating rich meals at night for the reason that your metabolism grows increasingly inflexible as the day progresses.

When trying to restore your natural sleep cycle, or when obligated to stay up late or travel to different time zones, take 5 mg of melatonin before bed to keep your biological clock in rhythm.

CHAPTER 9

ARE GUT BACTERIA MAKING YOU FAT?

"The recent discovery that metabolic diseases are associated with a change in intestinal and tissue microbiota opens a new era of putative therapeutic and preventive strategies to reduce the economic and social burden of diabetes and obesity."
— Rémy Burcelin, PhD

Microbiology changed the fate of the world in 1493. Christopher Columbus brought malaria, typhoid fever, tuberculosis, cholera, meningitis, diphtheria, small pox, and influenza to the New World, landing a devastating blow to the health of indigenous people that reduced the population of the northern hemisphere by more than 75 percent.[1] Fast-forward more than five hundred years later to the Western world where people live in an ultra-sterile environment and are now immunized against the same infectious microbes that once plagued our ancestors.

Today microorganisms are poised to change the fate of our species once again. However, instead of swiftly killing people, today's microbes are surreptitiously promoting an explosion of waistlines and terrorizing our ability to regulate blood sugar, leading to chronic type 2 diabetes.[2,3,4,5,6,7]

UNDERCOVER MICROORGANISMS

Although sloth and gluttony garner most of the blame for the obesity epidemic, recent research suggests that microorganisms, namely bacteria, but viruses as well, are key contributors to obesity.[8,9,10,11,12,13,14] But unlike the pathogenic microorganisms that Christopher Columbus experienced hundreds of years ago, microorganisms today often operate in a more insidious fashion. Low-grade, prolonged exposure to noninfectious microbes stimulate the immune system and redirect stored nutrients—glucose, proteins, triglycerides, and free fatty acids—to engender even greater immune system activity.[15,16,17,18,19]

Indeed, obesity and associated chronic conditions of insulin resistance, diabetes, metabolic syndrome, and heart disease are not only linked to changes in metabolism and nutrient availability but also chronic inflammation.[20,21,22,23,24,25,26] The trillions of microbes living in your gut are significant players.[27] In fact, the gut *microbiota*, as scientists refer to these organisms, dramatically influence metabolism and inflammation, which can lead to obesity and type 2 diabetes: two of the most prevalent conditions threatening our nation's health today.[28,29,30]

As many new studies can attest, the importance of intestinal flora as a factor in obesity cannot be underestimated.[31,32] The stage for a healthy balance of bacteria is set in the first few months of life.[33] It begins with the way in which you were born and whether you were breast-fed or given antibiotics as an infant.[34,35,36] Later, what you eat—your choice of carbohydrates, for instance—and how you eat—whether you chew your food mindfully or swallow hard-to-digest-chunks—affect your gut and metabolism.[37,38,39,40,41] The amount of fat you eat and the alcohol you drink and the medications you take, such as acid suppressants to alter your intestinal secretions and digestion transit time, have an influence on your gut bacteria.[42,43,44,45,46,47] Which microorganisms thrive in your intestines, and in what proportion, affects your metabolism and how readily you store excess calories as fat.[48,49]

Considering this new knowledge, it's clear that the calorie-is-a-calorie model of weight loss, which counts a calorie of sugar in the same way as a calorie of fat, totally ignores our intestinal bioreactor, the four pounds of one hundred trillion single-cell organisms living in the gut.[50,51] We need to start appreciating the notion that prior to nutrient absorption, ingested foods collide with our inner fermentation tank and influence how our bodies regulate energy, with regard to storing or burning fat, as well as affect our mood and appetite. Our intestinal microflora is as impressionable as a child on a schoolyard playground. And food can change that playground.[52]

Evaluating foods for how they influence the type and behavior of our gut microorganisms will prove to be more important than counting calories. Food is a source of nutrients, and most importantly, information for our microbes and our genes.[53,54] For instance, the type of fat is as important as the amount of fat.[55] The eloquence of cellular biology can be appreciated with a closer look at trans fats, which are distinguished from other fats because of a small geometrical difference in their molecular structure. However, this small difference enables a change in signaling pathways that over time predisposes a person who eats a large amount of trans fats to an increased risk of obesity and heart disease.[56] In understanding how a subtle molecular change in the structure of one fatty acid can cause disease, we can also then conceptualize how an intentional administration of molecules, which at one time offered plants protection, can favor the growth of beneficial microorganisms.[57,58] (These molecular patterns affect the color of plants, too, creating colorful polyphenols in herbs and spices, such as rosemary, cocoa, curcumin, resveratrol, and green tea.)

GUT BACTERIA: THE FORGOTTEN METABOLIC ORGAN

Gut health has been the focal point of traditional Asian medicine for centuries. For example, the Japanese have coined such phrases as "honored middle" and "center of the spiritual strength" to describe the human intestinal system.[59] Although Russian scientist Ilya Mechnikov, PhD, won the Nobel Prize in 1908 for works done in the field of gut microbiology and bowel health, it wasn't until the early twenty-first century that Western science began to rapidly clarify the various components of gut microflora and their relationship to modern-day immune malfunctions and metabolic diseases.[60] In recent years, scientists from around the world have linked imbalances in gut microbes with a range of modern health epidemics, including autoimmunity, asthma, allergies, depression, mood disorders, acne, heart disease, diabetes, and obesity.[61,62,63,64,65,66,67]

Living throughout your intestine are more than one hundred trillion bacteria from some forty thousand species that collectively have a level of metabolic activity that exceeds that of the liver![68,69] These intestinal microflora also contain their own genes, 3.3 million of them, which is nearly 140 times those in our own genome. These genes direct 6,313 unique metabolic functions.[70,71]

This massive microbial genome, or *microbiome*, engenders humans with many physiological functions that would otherwise be unavailable. From assisting in the release of intestinal hormones that regulate appetite, augmenting digestion, and extracting energy from ingested foods to synthesizing essential vitamins and protecting us from ingested pathogens, this three-pound "microbial organ" is essential to our survival.[72]

For instance, gut microbe fermentation of intestinal nutrients creates short-chain fatty acids such as *butyrate*, which in and of itself exerts systemic metabolic effects.[73,74] Even more intestinal microbes influence the intestinal release of the critical metabolic-signaling molecule AMPK, sparking our cellular powerhouses, or mitochondria, into high gear and improving fat and sugar burning.[75]

The trillions of bugs in our gut live side by side with 80 percent of our body's immune system cells, which, together with digestive tract organs such as the pancreas and liver, make up a huge metabolic-immune regulatory organ system. Imbalances in gut microbes may lead to metabolic disturbances.[76,77,78] Indeed, a recent analysis of several human studies suggests that obese people tend to have a lower level of bacterial diversity, a higher level of *Staphylococcus aureus*, more intestinal bacterial overgrowth, and a lower level of *Bifidobacteria* compared to lean people.[79] *Bifidobacteria* are well known to be more "friendly" strains, while *Staphylococcus aureus* are known to be more immune stimulating.

One need not harbor pathogenic strains of microbes to gain weight. Researchers at Cedar-Sinai Medical Center in Los Angeles found that obese people have greater levels of intestinal methane-producing bacteria known as *Methanobrevibacter smithii*.[80] These bacteria slow down intestinal transit time by up to 60 percent, prolonging the period during which intestinal bacteria are exposed to food. As a result, more calories are absorbed from that food, and there is more weight gain.[81,82] That's one reason why even if you were to eat fewer calories than you actually burn, imbalances in your gut microflora might cause you to gain weight.

The scientific community has confirmed the notion that gut microflora play an important role in the onset and development of obesity, diabetes, and cardiovascular disease.[83,84,85,86] Moreover, research suggests that just one day of eating a Western diet that is high in fat and simple carbohydrates leads to changes in both the structure of the intestinal microbiota and metabolic pathways governing fat storage, and is consistent with fat gain.[87] This makes sense, given the fact that our gut microflora participate in various aspects of metabolism, including energy extraction from food, fat storage, glucose and insulin regulation, as well as appetite, satiety, liver function, and immunity.[88]

Gut microbes are able to do this because of their intimate contact with our intestinal cells, which constantly relay messages to the brain about what's happening inside the intestine, including what hormones are being secreted, what foods are coming in, what kind of bacteria are present, and how many are thriving.[89,90] The brain then responds with its own messages along a nerve network that's like a neurological freeway from your brain to your tummy. This vagus nerve pathway is bidirectional, going from the gut to the brain and back, and is constantly relaying messages back and forth.[91]

We've learned from people who have had bariatric surgery, which reduces the size of the stomach and/or small intestine, that this gut-metabolic axis can be made to function better.[92,93,94] For example, supplementation with certain *probiotics*, healthy bacteria strains; prebiotics, fibers on which healthy microbes can feed; and certain proteins, such as whey and pea protein, encourage the release of gut hormones that improve our metabolism.[95,96,97,98,99,100]

THE GUT BUG-OBESITY LINK

Many of the initial breakthroughs in the understanding about how the gut and its associated microflora contribute to obesity and metabolism emerged from the lab of biologist Jeffrey Gordon, MD, at the Washington University School of Medicine in St. Louis, MO.[101,102,103] In 2004, Gordon's team discovered that when eight-week-old germ-free mice are inoculated with the fecal contents of ordinary mice, their fat content increased by 57 percent, even though they ate 29 percent less food.

Gordon's group found that adding intestinal microbes into germ-free mice was associated with increased transport of carbohydrates from the intestine to the liver. This interfered with signals from a gut hormone that inhibits a particular enzyme—in this case an enzyme that normally delivers fat from the liver to the fat cells. The end result of these and other physiologic changes led to more fat accumulation in the liver and abdomen.

This emerging "super organism" paradigm is changing our perspectives about immunity and nutrient digestion, absorption, and metabolism. Diet, stress, genetic programming, hygiene, allergen exposure, antibiotic use, and intestinal immune responses all affect our gut bacteria. The earliest and most profound influence is how we are born—that is, literally, the way in which a newborn exits the sterile maternal womb and enters the microbial-rich world.

THE BEST START IN LIFE

Being born vaginally, as opposed to delivery by Cesarean section, and breast-fed point your metabolism in the right direction by establishing a stable, metabolically healthy gut microflora environment.[104,105] Researchers have found, for example, that babies delivered vaginally are immediately inoculated with their mother's vaginal flora, which is dominated by healthy *Lactobacillus* and *Prevotella* strains.[106] And scientists know that infant inoculation with maternal microflora is among the earliest and most powerful environmental variables molding our gut and hence our metabolism.[107]

In contrast, babies born by C-section are inoculated by the more pathogenic bacteria, common to the skin and hospital air, such as *Staphylococcus aureus* and *Clostridium difficile*.[108] Incidentally, studies link child and adult microflora profiles rich in these bacteria to obesity and possibly diabetes.[109,110,111] Moreover, a recent study of 1,255 children found that the prevalence of obesity in children born via Cesarean section by age three is twice that of children born vaginally.[112]

Evidence linking harmful intestine microflora in early life with metabolic dysfunction and obesity is continually emerging.[113,114,115,116] For example, researchers in Finland reported that obese seven-year-olds have a twofold increased level of *S. aureus* in their stool when compared to lean children of the same age. Scientists in Sweden found that obese four-year-olds have significant increases in *Enterobacteriaceae* bacteria associated with obesity, compared to their lean peers.[117]

In 2011, the Centers for Disease Control and Prevention (CDC) reported that 32.8 percent of babies were delivered by C-section, up from 20 percent just ten years earlier, and today a full 20 percent of children under the age of five are overweight.[118] Is this a coincidence? I don't think so. Rather, I agree with many researchers who believe that birthing methods create a predisposition to obesity and underscore the importance of proper bacterial colonization early in life. Weight-loss studies in adults and children show that potentially harmful intestinal bacteria correlate with both early life events, such as breast-feeding, and the degree of weight loss or gain later in life, independent of calories.

In the last decade, many studies have found that specific components in breast milk—namely certain prebiotics (soluble fiber, for example)—act as "fertilizers" that encourage the proliferation of beneficial intestinal microflora, namely *Bifidobacteria*, and offer some protection against obesity.[119,120] Breast-fed infants also have increased levels of *Bifidobacteria* and *Lactobacillus* strains in their intestinal tract while formula-fed infants have lower amounts of these strains but greater numbers of endotoxin of *Clostridium* and *Enterobacteria* strains as well as *Bacteroides*. Research indicates that most *Bifidobacteria* and some *Lactobacillus* strains offer protection against obesity, diabetes, and inflammation.[121,122,123]

A study of teenagers found that those who were breast-fed for at least six months weighed less and had less belly fat than their peers who were bottle-fed formula as infants.[124,125] In contrast, infant formula, which has been pasteurized and lacks the obesity-fighting bacteria common to breast milk, and infants' early introduction to solid foods appear to negatively influence the development of protective *Bifidobacteria* strains of intestinal microflora.[126]

In fact, more than ten years ago, a German research team tracked 1,314 children for five years and found that infants who were exclusively breast-fed for six months had significantly lower body fat than their bottle-fed counterparts.[127]

In 2011, the CDC endorsed breast-feeding as a prevention against obesity, suggesting that nine months of nursing can reduce the odds by 30 percent that the child will become an obese adult.[128] Nevertheless, in the United States, of the 75 percent of new mothers who begin nursing their babies, 35 percent stop after three months. Less than 15 percent are still nursing at six months. This is unfortunate since research shows that lack of breast-feeding appears to play a role in the fact that one in three American children are overweight or obese.

Breast-feeding may also transfer immunity to the baby and provide hormones—leptin, adiponectin, and ghrelin—that assist in energy balance and storage. Research suggests that the presence of these hormones in early life regulates growth and programs energy balance later in life. Pasteurized infant formula obtained from grain-fed cows probably doesn't contain the same quantities of metabolic hormones.[129]

ANTIBIOTICS AND OBESITY

Another salient event that alters gut microflora early in life and leads to obesity later is antibiotic use.[130,131] The prolific researcher Martin Blaser, MD, of the New York University Langone Medical Center showed that the incidence of obesity among toddlers who received antibiotics during their first six months of life is twice that of infants who were not given the drugs.[132] The association between exposure to antibiotics and obesity is not exclusive to children. French scientists reported significant increases in body weight in a large group of adults receiving intravenous antibiotics for treatment of infective endocarditis.[133] A third of the adults in this study had more than a 10 percent increase in their BMI, while only 2 percent of the non-treated controls had a similar increase in body mass.

These reports are not surprising for two reasons. First, more than sixty-six years ago, scientists discovered that the antibiotics *streptothricin* and *sulfasuxidine* increased growth of baby chickens.[134] During the 1950s, the antibiotic tetracycline was given to premature infants of U.S. Navy doctors to fatten them up.[135,136] Today, farmers commonly give their animals low doses to increase their growth rate. The livestock industry uses more than 29.8 million pounds of antibiotics annually, and much of that is spent to spur animals to grow bigger, faster.[137]

Second, Blaser's group recently confirmed the mechanisms by which antibiotic therapy increases fat mass. In this seven-week study, weaning mice were administered various common antibiotics in doses approved by the FDA for agricultural use.[138] This group reported that compared to nonantibiotic-treated mice, the treated ones had a demonstrable change in their gut microflora, increased concentrations of bacterial fermentation products (short-chain fatty acids), and increased activity in genes of the liver involved in fatty acid metabolism and cholesterol synthesis.

WHAT'S GOING ON IN YOUR BELLY?

The most compelling study confirming the gut bacteria–obesity link in adults was done in China and reported in 2012.[139] Liping Zhao, PhD, a microbiologist and prolific researcher in the field of gut microflora, metabolism, and obesity, lost over forty pounds by regulating his own gut microflora with a diet rich in prebiotic foods.[140] When Zhao prescribed a prebiotic-rich diet of whole foods, an exercise program, and traditional Chinese herbs, including berberine, to an overweight man, the fellow lost over one hundred pounds in less than six months. His blood sugar returned to normal, and there was a 35 percent reduction in the endotoxin-producing *Enterobacteriaceae* in his gut.

Then, in order to further confirm the association between the gram-negative bacteria and obesity, Zhao's research team extracted the *Enterobacteriaceae* from the man's intestine and placed it in the intestinal tract of lean, germ-free mice. The mice became obese and exhibited signs of increased inflammation.

Other research using DNA stool analysis found increased levels of *Bacteroides*, *Clostridium*, and *Escherichia coli* in the stool of people with type 2 diabetes, but not in healthy control subjects.[141] Researchers from Spain have also found significant alterations in the intestinal bacteria of obese pregnant women, but not in their lean counterparts. Using DNA-based stool analysis, the obese mothers-to-be had fewer *Bifidobacteria* and an increase in *Staphylococcus*, *Enterobacteriaceae*, and *Escherichia coli*.

A French research team also confirmed the link between microbes and obesity in adults. They were the first to show that an increase in the concentration of bacterial genetic material (DNA) in the blood predicted the amount of abdominal fat present and the onset of diabetes.[142] Moreover, a recent groundbreaking study found a correlation between the levels of antibodies against intestinal microbes in the blood and the degree of insulin resistance and obesity.[143]

INTESTINAL ENDOTOXIN

Shortly after French microbiologist Louis Pasteur's discovery that germs cause disease in the mid-1800s, Robert Koch discovered that specific microorganisms are responsible for causing tuberculosis and cholera.[144] In 1884, Koch identified cholera (*Vibrio cholerae*) and postulated that a toxic substance was responsible for the disease. His coworker Richard Pfeiffer later discovered that even after he killed the bacteria with heat, it was still toxic to animals when it was injected. Pfeiffer determined that a component of *V. cholera's* bacterial cell wall was responsible for its toxic effects. He subsequently conceived the concept of the *endotoxin*, or the "toxin within."

Professor Patrice D. Cani, PhD, a researcher at the Fund for Scientific Research at the Louvain Drug Research Institute in Brussels, Belgium, was one of the first to demonstrate in animals that an imbalance in gut flora and a condition called "leaky gut" increase endotoxin, a part of the cell wall of bacteria.[145] In humans, endotoxin is now being linked to obesity, insulin resistance, diabetes, high blood pressure, high cholesterol, high triglycerides, and increased risk of heart disease.[146,147,148,149,150,151,152]

Thanks to the trailblazing researcher Cani, we now have ample scientific validation linking the same bacterial endotoxin *lipopolysaccharide*, found by Koch, with modern-day obesity and the diabetes epidemics. Cani's work motivated me to write this book. I feel that everyone should know how eating the Western diet of high-fat and high-carbohydrate foods acts like a Trojan horse, piggybacking endotoxin through the walls of our intestine and into the bloodstream.[153,154] The ensuing inflammation and deranged metabolism has been coined *metabolic endotoxemia*, which is different from the often-fatal *endotoxemia* of septic shock.

If you recall from a previous chapter, our immune, liver, and fat cells have antennae-like structures called *toll-like receptors* (TLRs). Endotoxin as pathogen-associated molecular patterns (PAMPs) latch like a key into the TLR lock, driving cells to increase inflammation-perturbing metabolism.[155] For example, a diet rich in processed foods and high in calories, fat, and sugar, such as high-fructose corn syrup, shifts our gut ecology and increases the absorption of endotoxin, which cranks up inflammation in the gut, liver, and fat tissues.[156]

It's been suggested that food-related inflammation in the intestine is an early event that precedes obesity.[157,158,159] Scientific articles have documented intestinal inflammation in obese children and have linked weight loss with reduced levels of inflammatory markers.[160,161]

Researchers reported in 2009 that infusing endotoxin into the bloodstream of healthy adults led to rapid increases in the inflammatory signaling among fat cells, recruiting more metabolically disruptive immune cells, which in turn led to elevations in proinflammatory molecules and insulin resistance.[162]

More recently, scientists found that high endotoxin levels are associated with early-onset diabetes and many components of insulin resistance, including increased blood pressure, vascular abnormalities, and a rise in blood lipids. Studies also show elevated endotoxin and inflammatory signaling molecules in pregnant, obese women.

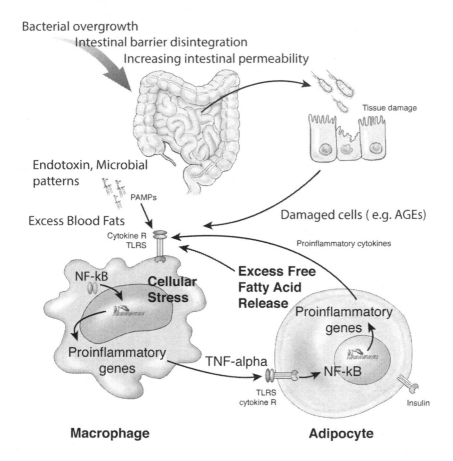

THE WEB OF LEAKY GUT, INFLAMMATION, AND FAT GAIN

Dysbiosis of the intestine created by eating processed foods, poor chewing and digestion, antibiotics, and antacid medications leads to a double whammy of leaky gut and increased endotoxin absorption. The end result is whole-body inflammation, insulin resistance, fat gain, and increased risk for cardiovascular disease.

Research published in the American Dietetic Association (ADA) publication *Diabetes Care* suggested that the increased blood levels of intestinal-derived endotoxin are associated with increased risk of diabetes and the kind of inflammation that is characteristic of obesity. These associations between endotoxin and increased diabetes risk were independent of other known risk factors. *Diabetes Care* has published several articles suggesting that diet-related changes in our gut microflora activate inflammation and metabolic disorders. The ADA has also reported that environmental toxins are associated with diabetes.[163] Another groundbreaking National Institutes of Health-funded study found a correlation between serum levels of antibodies against endotoxin-containing intestinal microbes, which indicate a bacterial infection, and the degree of insulin resistance and obesity.

HIGH-CALORIE, HIGH-FAT DIET DANGERS

Studies suggest that excessive calories and fat overload increase the absorption of endotoxin in both healthy and morbidly obese people and those with type 2 diabetes. The degree of a post-meal rise in triglycerides coincided with the amount of endotoxin absorbed. Collectively, these recent scientific studies confirm Cani's earlier finding in animals: unhealthy foods lead to inflammation, blood-sugar disturbances, and increased energy storage as fat by changing the ecology in our gut to favor unhealthy bacteria.

PUTTING THE BRAKES ON ENDOTOXIN

Harvard scientists recently found that by supplementing the diets of mice with an enzyme that inhibits absorption of endotoxin blocked diet-induced fat gain and metabolic disorders.[164] This enzyme, *alkaline phosphatase*, is normally found on the surface of our intestinal wall and may be a critical component in keeping gut microbes in check.[165,166,167] Alkaline phosphatase may preserve favorable microbes while excluding the growth of more problematic microbes like *E. coli* and *Salmonella typhimurium*. Some researchers suggest that this enzyme is depleted when a person continually eats a high-fat diet.[168]

This protective enzyme is sensitive to the acid-base balance, and functions better in a more alkaline environment. Acid-suppressing medications, artificial sweeteners, and acidic foods, such as hard cheeses and refined carbohydrates, may reduce alkaline phosphatase's protective ability. In contrast, green leafy vegetables, fruits, fish, butter, fibers, fish, and seeds appear to increase intestinal alkaline phosphatase and detoxify endotoxin.[169]

HOW STRONG IS YOUR GUT?

While most of the more than one hundred trillion microbes residing in our gut are friendly, there are some rough characters (like endotoxin) in the mix that must be kept in check by our intestinal barrier and our gut immune system. However, research suggests that increased permeability of the intestinal barrier is independently associated with abdominal fat.[170,171] Along with absorbing nutrients, the intestinal lining also acts as a protective barrier, keeping the trillions of bacteria from entering our bloodstream. Or at least that's what it's supposed to do.

An abundance of research has connected a compromised intestinal barrier with many of the same ubiquitous, modern-day health conditions also associated with imbalanced gut microflora, including autoimmune disorders, cancer, mood disorders, and fat storage and blood-sugar imbalances.[172,173,174] This is due in part to the fact that a leaky gut activates a variety of immune messengers, which alter how insulin, a critical hormone involved in controlling excess energy from fat and blood-sugar through storage, functions.[175,176,177] The end result is insulin resistance (prediabetes) and increased belly fat.[178,179]

In 2011, research published in the journal *Obesity* revealed for the first time that the permeability of the intestinal wall is associated with abdominal and liver fat.[180] Nearly a year later, scientists from three different parts of the world linked gut permeability with obesity, insulin resistance, and metabolic syndrome.[181,182,183] It seems that the strength or integrity of the intestinal wall can be compromised, leading to leaky gut syndrome. When bacteria (or bacterial fragments like endotoxin) are able to slip between the cells lining the intestinal wall and enter the sterile environment of your bloodstream, your immune system reacts, causing inflammation and predisposing you to metabolic imbalances and chronic health problems.

If the intestinal epithelial cells are bricks, then "tight junction" proteins are the mortar holding them together.[184] These mortar-like proteins hold adjacent intestinal cells together, favoring absorption of nutrients while preventing the bad microbial characters from entering.[185,186] Spanish endocrinologists confirmed a relationship between leaky gut and belly fat: they found that increased blood levels of a protein called *zonulin*, which opens the junctions between cells of the intestinal wall (essentially making the gut permeable), is associated with obesity and insulin resistance.

Since 2001, Alessio Fasano, MD, a pediatric endocrinologist who founded the University of Maryland Center for Celiac Research, has been one of the most vocal researchers about the connection between zonulin deregulation, leaky gut, and the development of autoimmune diseases, such as irritable bowel syndrome and celiac disease.[187] Other researchers have linked a compromised intestinal barrier and gut bacteria imbalance with inflammation, increased fat storage, and blood-sugar-regulating problems. This appears to occur because a leaky gut activates a variety of immune messengers, altering insulin function and predisposing the body to obesity and insulin resistance, leading to prediabetes and type 2 diabetes.

KEY TAKEAWAYS

Modern scientists have confirmed what John Pickup, MD, proposed over fifteen years ago: type 2 diabetes is as much a disorder of the immune system as the metabolic system.[188,189] Dr. Pickup noticed that people with insulin resistance—low HDL cholesterol, increased abdominal fat, high blood pressure, high cholesterol, high blood sugar, and reduced sensitivity to insulin—also exhibit characteristics of the acute phase of an immune response. Several years later, researchers confirmed Pickup's findings: elevated blood levels of two inflammatory compounds—C reactive protein (CRP) and interleukin-6 (IL-6)—are strongly correlated with the development of adult-onset type 2 diabetes.[190] We now know that gut microbes, such as endotoxin, are linked to inflammation as well as diabetes and obesity.[191,192,193]

It is this chronic, albeit low-grade, activation of the immune system that leads to the kind of inflammation linked to obesity and diabetes.[194,195] The immune response throws a monkey wrench into our metabolic machinery, leading to prediabetes, diabetes, autoimmunity, and cancer. For the first time, in 2010, scientists reported that chronic inflammation related to increased body weight starts as early as age three.[196]

Certainly, one of the many consequences associated with ingesting processed foods—namely refined sugars, carbohydrates, excessive fats, and alcohol—is obesity and insulin resistance.[197] However we now know that these foods don't cause weight gain because they are inherently fattening. Rather, they disturb the delicate cross talk between gut microflora and the intestinal barrier, leading to a cascade of immune system disruptions. These events promote fat gain around the middle, insulin resistance, and eventually diabetes.

The overwhelmingly high incidence of overweight and obese adults and children throughout the world suggests that primitive survival features of our past are indeed working as they should. In particular, the rapid increase in the prevalence of obesity in both adults and children over the last few decades hints that other confounding environmental factors are shifting our thrifty metabolic programming toward saving mode.

A low-calorie diet and exercise are not enough. An effective fat-loss program must also support the immune system, gut microflora, and intestinal barrier. Adjusting for early life events that negatively shape your inner microbial organ—including birthing method, breast feeding, and antibiotic exposure—will help achieve these goals. Individuals born by cesarean section, given antibiotics in the first 6 months of life and/or fed formula will require extra gastrointestinal support in the form of prebiotics, probiotics, and herbal compounds like berberine, garlic, oregano, and peppermint oil.

CHAPTER 10

HOW TO KEEP
YOUR GUT HEALTHY

"The gut microbiota is situated on the intersection between the diet and host genome and thus has important implications for food processing and making nutrients available to the host."
— Fredrik Bäckhed, PhD

One way that poor food choices and digestive dysfunction contribute to obesity is by promoting bacterial imbalances in your intestine, a condition called *dysbiosis* or *small intestinal bacterial overgrowth* (SIBO).[1] Many studies have demonstrated this imbalance in metabolically challenged people.[2,3,4,5]

SIBO occurs in 20–41 percent of obese people, according to one survey. It is also associated with many other disorders, including fatty liver disease, diabetes, autoimmunity, and depression.[6]

IS YOUR GUT MICROFLORA
OUT OF BALANCE?

The quick questionnaire below will give you an insight into whether you have *dysbiosis* and, if so, the degree of imbalance among your gut microbes.

1. Were you born vaginally?
   (a) Yes.
   (b) No. I was delivered by Cesarean section.

2. Were you breast-fed exclusively for the first six months of your life?
   (a) Yes.
   (b) No. I was fed formula partially or entirely.

3. Have you been fortunate enough not to need antibiotics?
   (a) Yes. I've taken few, if any, antibiotics.
   (b) No. I've taken multiple rounds of antibiotics.

4. Have you been able to avoid taking an acid-suppressing medication, such as Nexium, or a proton-pump inhibitor (PPI), such as Prilosec?
   (a) Yes. I have not taken acid-suppressing drugs.
   (b) No. I have taken an acid-suppressing drug for stomach irritation and symptoms of acid reflux.

5. Did you spend most of your childhood on a farm?
   (a) Yes.
   (b) No.

6. Did you have large pets as a child?
   (a) Yes.
   (b) No.

7. Growing up, did you play outside in the dirt?
   (a) Yes.
   (b) No. I played mostly indoors.

8. Do you have three or more siblings?
   (a) Yes.
   (b) No.

9. Is gas or GI distress after eating rarely a problem for you?
   (a) Yes. I rarely have intestinal distress.
   (b) No. I frequently have intestinal distress.

10. Do you eat slowly, taking your time to chew thoroughly?

    (a) Yes.

    (b) No, I eat quickly.

11. Is it true you rarely have more than one or two alcoholic drinks a week or sweetened soda and tea and/or fruit juice?

    (a) Yes. I rarely drink these beverages.

    (b) No. I drink more than two alcoholic drinks a week and/or enjoy sweetened soda and tea and/or fruit juice.

KEY

Although crude, if you have five or more "no" responses, it's likely you have imbalanced gut microflora. Vaginal birthing, breast-feeding, being raised on a farm, being from a large family, having pets, playing in the dirt, and avoiding the use of antibiotics, alcohol, and sugar-sweetened beverages favor healthy gut microbes.

Another noninvasive and simple test is to see if you get bloated after drinking 12–16 ounces of sugary fruit juice, such as apple or pomegranate juice. If you get bloated or gassy within the hour, you probably have imbalanced gut microflora or dysbiosis. Imbalanced gut microbes thrive on sugar, which creates gas and distension of the abdomen.

Stool testing is the gold standard assessment to see if the bugs in your gut are making you fat. Metametrix Clinical Laboratory offers a state-of-the-art test known as GI Effects that uses a DNA-based probe to identify intestinal bacteria. You can find clinicians that offer the test at www.metametrix.com.

OBESITY AND BACTERIAL IMBALANCES

The main consequences of perturbations in the balance of the one hundred trillion single-celled organisms in your intestine are an inflammatory state throughout your body and increased gut permeability, which promotes absorption of endotoxin.[7] Many recent studies strongly link high-fat and high-carbohydrate diets with increased gut inflammation, leaky gut, a big belly, and altered metabolism due to increased absorption of endotoxin-containing bacteria.[8,9,10,11,12,13] Increased levels of bacteria endotoxin in the intestine create a vicious cycle of inflammation and metabolic challenges. The more endotoxin present, the greater the expression of receptors—such as toll-like receptor 4 (TLR4)—that detect endotoxin and stimulate inflammatory reactions.[14]

Gram-negative, endotoxin-containing bacteria are not the only bugs that make you fat. Although one recent study found that metabolically challenged, overweight women have higher levels of gram-negative bacteria compared to lean women, the researchers also found increased levels of the endotoxin-free bacteria *Eubacterium rectale* and *Clostridium coccoides*.[15] Also, scientists have established that overweight and obese adults and children tend to have an increase in bacteria belonging to the *Firmicutes* phyla, including species of the *Lactobacillus* genera, and reduced bacteria belonging to the *Bacteroidetes* phyla.[16,17] (A phyla is a higher order to genus and species.) In one study, bacteria of the *Firmicutes* phyla were 10 percent more numerous in obese subjects compared to lean ones.[18] These overweight adults also had threefold fewer *Bacteroidetes* bacteria compared to lean people. Many studies suggest that an increased ratio of *Firmicutes* to *Bacteroidetes* is strongly linked to increased body fat and possibly a reflection of increased calorie intake.[19] However, not all studies consistently show that this happens in obesity.

For example, consider this study done in Amsterdam in which scientists transferred intestinal microbiota from healthy lean donors to obese individuals with metabolic syndrome.[20] Prior to the transplant, the obese people had elevated *Bacteroidetes* phyla and reduced bacterial diversity compared to their lean counterparts. (The finding of reduced bacterial diversity is consistent with many studies of obesity.) Following the microbial transplant from lean donors, the metabolically challenged people had an increase in bacterial diversity and improved insulin sensitivity. More specifically, the recipients of the lean microbiota were found to have significant increases in butyrate, a beneficial short-chain fatty acid (SCFA) produced by bacteria.[21,22,23]

Bacteria affect insulin signaling. For example, French researchers extracted bacterial DNA and RNA from the appendix of overweight people and found that certain bacterial gene signatures clustered strongly with insulin resistance.[24] Researchers suggest that over-weight people have reduced bacterial diversity in their intestines. Additionally, many other studies suggest that the reduced concentration of *Bifidobacterium* species may foster increased body fat mass and metabolic aberrations, since *Bifidobacterium* is thought to help exclude absorption of endotoxin from the intestine.[25,26,27,28] I can say with certainty that strains of the *Bifidobacterium* genera and bacterial diversity protect against obesity.

BARIATRIC SURGERY BENEFITS

The microbial shifts associated with bariatric surgery have been well-documented. One study found that the reduced ratio of *Bacteroides* to *Prevotella* in obese people increased following bariatric surgery and weight loss.[29]

Another study found *Escherichia* and *Akkermansia* populations to increase substantially after *Roux-en-Y gastric bypass* (RYGB) surgery, suggesting that these two bacteria strains are deeply involved in controlling fat deposition.[30] *Akkermansia muciniphila* has been shown to prevent absorption of endotoxin and is increased by eating prebiotic fiber, such as inulin.[31]

BACTERIA THAT MAY MAKE YOU FAT

There are many human clinical studies comparing fecal levels of bacteria in overweight and lean people. Here are a few examples of the bacterial increases they identified in the overweight group:[32,33,34,35]

- *Staphylococcus* species, *S. aureus* in particular
- *Prevotella*
- *Methanobrevibacter smithii*
- *Enterobacter*
- *Escherichia coli*
- *Archaea*
- *Klebsiella pneumoniae*
- *Vibrio*
- *Yersinia eubacteria*

- *Clostridium bifermentans*
- *Firmicutes phylum*
- *Lactobacillus*

The intestinal bacteria that diminish in overweight people are:[36,37,38,39,40,41,42]

- *Akkermansia muciniphila*
- *Bifidobacterium* species, specifically *B. longum* and *B. adolescentis*
- *Allistipes et rel.*
- *Lactobacillus paracasei, L. plantarum*
- *Bacteroides fragilis* group
- *Parabacteroides* group
- *Clostridium perfringens, Clostridium leptum*
- *Ruminococcus flavefaciens*
- *Faecalibacterium prausnitzii*
- *Verrucomicrobia* group
- *Lachnospira* family
- *Gammaproteobacteria*
- *Fusobacteriaceae*
- *Methanobrevibacter*

GUT MICROBES BREACH THE BARRIER

Imbalances in the intestinal bacteria are a primary cause of increased gut permeability, or leaky gut, but not the only cause. Anti-inflammatory medications, physical and psychological stress, acid-suppressing medications, alcohol, and high-fat and high-carbohydrate meals open the door for the absorption of immunity-stimulating particles, which can lead to belly fat and metabolic challenges.[43] Indeed many studies have found leaky gut to coexist alongside obesity and metabolic syndrome.[44,45]

Leaky gut opens the door for inflammation to strike.[46] That's because interspersed among and just beneath the single-cell-thick intestinal barrier is the largest immune organ in the body—that is, the *gut-associated lymphoid tissue* (GALT).[47,48] This immune-cell-rich connective tissue comprises more than 80 percent of the body's immunologically active cells.[49] So when the cellular shoelaces, or tight junction proteins, that link epithelial cells together become altered, the largest mucosal immune system in the body is challenged.[50,51]

Many things loosen these laces, from intestinal bacterial imbalances to inflammatory components of poor lifestyle choices, endotoxin, food-derived components (casein and gluten), and damaged molecules from cooking (AGEs).[52,53,54,55] You can now see why Dr. Alession Fasano of Johns Hopkins University referred to these tightly interlocked proteins as the biological door to various inflammatory diseases.[56,57]

TUNING GUTSY DEFENSES TO LOSE WEIGHT

Gut microflora help to shape the intestinal barrier as well as immune reactions of the gut, and thus the rest of the body, underscoring the importance of a proper balance of intestinal microbes.[58,59,60] Researchers see this in the lab when they raise mice in a sterile environment.[61,62] They have no intestinal microflora, their immune systems are impaired, and they have many other intestinal alterations.

A high incidence of inflammatory disease in humans is a testimony to microbes' ability to mold the immune response in response to Cesarean section delivery, formula feeding, antibiotic use, small family size, and poor diets. All of these factors lead to imbalanced gut microflora.[63,64,65,66,67] It's known, for instance, that children raised on a farm have a lower incidence of inflammatory diseases, such as asthma. Farm living, like vaginal birthing and breast-feeding, exposes the developing gut and immune system to a diverse collection of microbes, nudging immunity to subsist in a less inflammatory, more tolerant state.

Intestinal immunity is relevant to maintaining a narrow waistline and finely tuned metabolism because many of the immune actors cross talking with intestinal microbes also directly communicate with belly fat and metabolic tissues.[68] You may remember from earlier chapters that when the immune system is under fire, it redirects nutrient traffic away from metabolic tissues, causing insulin resistance.[69,70]

It shouldn't be surprising that children and adults with asthma have metabolic abnormalities.[71] Likewise, leaky gut and translocation of intestinal microbes that activate the intestinal immune system are similarly linked to increased body fat and metabolic disorders.[72] This process is exacerbated by a Western diet of high-fat foods and processed carbohydrates.[73] It is linked to reduced microbial diversity, leaky gut, and increased absorption of inflammatory bacterial particles, or endotoxin.[74,75]

RESTORING TOLERANCE

Even though the majority of our immune system is just an earshot away from trillions of nonhuman bacterial cells that it normally would attack, the healthy gut immune system exists in a quiescent or tolerant state. You can think of immune tolerance as a very patient parent. On a good day, you may tolerate misbehavior from your child. However, after a stressful day at the office, you will have little tolerance for the same behavior.

The intestinal immune system is continually probing our inner tube of life, looking for strange and dangerous molecules.[76] Tolerance occurs when the cross talk between gut immune cells and microflora is cordial.[77] For this reason, our gut microflora is both an asset and a liability.

It's an asset because it shapes our whole-body immune response, pivoting the immune system into an anti-inflammatory state of tolerance.[78] A tolerant immune system is less reactive to potential immune stimuli, such as microbes and foods. Remember the patient parent? Such a state of immune suppression, or tolerance, is similar to tolerating noisy children.[79] Physiologically, this is achieved with help from the actors discussed earlier, including the immune sentinels, or T regulatory cells.[80,81,82] Remember that elevated leptin from excess body fat suppresses Treg cells, so fat loss is necessary.[83,84]

INTESTINAL HISTAMINE AND LEAKY GUT

Intestinal histamine can instigate intestinal inflammation, leaky gut, and reduced immune tolerance, especially to foods.[85] Histamine is a well-known signaling molecule recognized for its ability to increase the porosity of epithelial barriers, including that of the intestine, lung, and even vascular system, in an attempt to draw more immune cells to the inflammatory site.[86,87]

What's troubling is that we are getting bombarded by histamine in two ways: externally—ingestion of histamine-containing foods and beverages—and internally—by triggering histamine release from mast cells.[88,89] Even more, bacterial endotoxin stimulate mast cells in the gut to puke out more histamine, prompting more intestinal permeability.[90] No matter the source trigger, histamine helps drive the inflammatory response inside and out of the intestine.

Classically, histamine and mast cells have been pigeonholed as the factors driving environmental allergy, hay fever, and the like. However, environmental histamine and the associated mast cells that store and release the molecule are now understood to be critically involved in the smoldering inflammatory state present in many overweight and metabolically challenged individuals in the twenty-first century.

Thankfully, our intestine is equipped with a natural histamine fire extinguisher—an enzyme called diamine oxidase, or DAO for short.[91] Like water on fire, DAO smothers histamine. Healthy levels of this enzyme are needed to prevent some of the deleterious inflammatory effects of histamine on the intestine.[92] Scientists attribute many of the detrimental health effects ascribed to the consumption of processed Western foods to a combination of excessive histamine release in the intestine and poor levels of DAO.[93] Furthermore, persons with irritable bowel syndrome (gut inflammation) and histamine intolerance have low levels of the DAO enzyme.[94]

The list of organs and tissues that display symptoms of excess histamine doesn't stop at the gut. Histamine overload can affect the whole body. Other common symptoms include skin irritations and flushing, brain fog, cardiovascular complications, nausea, menstrual issues, circadian rhythm imbalances, and nasal congestion.

Histamine-intolerant persons commonly react to nuts and seasonings, food additives (like sulfites and benzoates), fermented beverages, seafood, preserved meats, cheeses, breads, and cereals. Scientists in a European study reported the prevalence of histamine intolerance to be

22 percent.[95] Adverse reactions to wine were most common, followed by nuts, apples, and dairy. Alcohol is a known inhibitor of DAO.

SUBSTANCES THAT INCREASE HISTAMINE	
Nuts and spices	All nuts, sunflower seeds, cinnamon, nutmeg, cloves, anise, and curry powder
Fruits	Oranges, grapefruits, lemons, limes, apricots, plums, cherries, cranberries prunes, dates, raisins, currants, dried cranberries, bananas, pineapples, papayas, mangos, strawberries, raspberries, and loganberries
Animal products and preserved meats	All raw, smoked-dried, and pickled sausage, salami, bacon, ham, sausage, and pork
Preservatives and additives	Tartrazine, benzoates, sulfites, BHA, BHT, MSG, nitrates, and food colorings
Seafood	Tuna, mackerel, sardines, anchovies, crustaceans (e.g., lobster, crab, shrimp), herring; preserved, marinated, salted, or dried fish; rolled, pickled herring; fish sauces
Cheese and dairy products	Cheese of all kinds, milk, yogurt, kefir, cream, and buttermilk
Breads and cereals	Yeast, baking powder, bleached flours, and leavening agents
Vegetables and legumes	Tomatoes, soy and soy products, pickles, olives, avocados, eggplant, mushrooms, pumpkin, spinach, sauerkraut, and vegetables marinated in vinegar-based products
Juices, beer, and wine	Fruit juices, beer, wine, and champagne
Medications	Muscle relaxants, antibiotics, antidepressants, antihypertensive agents, diuretics, and more

The preceding page contains an expanded list of common foods, food additives, and medications known to increase histamine burden or inhibit the DAO enzyme. As you can see, many healthy foods, such as fruits and seafood, are on the list. If you experience symptoms of histamine intolerance or leaky gut, minimize your intake of the least healthy items (e.g., breads, preserved meats, alcohol, dairy, etc.) to see if your symptoms improve. If you feel that you may be sensitive to histamine, avoid the foods listed below and try supplemental DAO in capsule form with meals. I recommend a few capsules of DAO when consuming alcohol.

Boutique clinical testing laboratories can assess your body's DAO level to give you an idea whether histamine is the cause of your sensitive and intolerant immune system. Please see www.DunWoodyLabs. com for more details.

REVERSING INFLAMMATION

During the quest to achieve a state of immune balance, the surveying cells of the immune system that monitor the gut for danger and strange molecules trigger the breakdown of tryptophan, the amino acid that acts as a building block for the happy brain chemicals serotonin and melatonin.[96] During chronic inflammatory states, immune mediators trigger the enzyme IDO (indoleamine 2,3-dioxygenase), which has been linked to psychological disorders.[97] Although IDO is increased by inflammation, leading to neurotransmitter precursor breakdown, the enzyme may actually be attempting to increase activity of the immune centennial T regulatory cells that combat chronic inflammation.[98] A specialized urine test called Organic Acid screens for elevated levels of *kynurenate* and *quinolinate*, which suggest inflammation, namely from the intestine. Elevated levels are an indication of inflammation, possibly from an imbalance of gut microflora.[99,100]

The inflammation caused by IDO can be reduced naturally with the amino acid taurine (500–1,000 mg/day) and broad-spectrum polyphenolic support, including curcumin (95% curcuminoids) and quercetin.[101,102,103] Since curcumin is poorly absorbed, it's best taken alongside piperine.

RESTORING IMMUNE TOLERANCE

The main way to restore balance among the cells of the intestine is to eat ample amounts of prebiotics and probiotics, polyphenol-rich foods, and supplements of vitamins A and D.[104,105,106,107] Research suggests that vitamins A and D are deficient in most people, particularly those who are overweight and obese.[108,109,110,111] Additionally, these two fat-soluble vitamins have pronounced anti-inflammatory effects on the immune system and are known to increase T regulatory cells.

I suggest a minimum of 5,000 IU a day of vitamin D for maintenance, and after two months have a blood test for 25(OH) vitamin D3 to ensure that your levels are higher than 65 ng/mL. Even in sunny states, such as Colorado and Arizona, many people display suboptimal vitamin D levels.[112,113] Since the vitamin is involved in so many aspects of immune regulation, it's important to maintain serum levels above 65 ng/mL.

Vitamin A is an equally important immunomodulator. Foods rich in vitamin A include liver, carrots, and sweet potatoes. The vitamin is in nutritional supplements as retinyl palmitate or beta-carotene, and a blend of both is ideal.

Vitamin A deficiency promotes imbalances of T helper cells. More specifically, insufficient vitamin A skews the T lymphocyte population toward an inflammatory T helper type 1 and type 17.[114] In contrast, vitamin A supplementation has been shown to restore immune tolerance by pivoting T lymphocytes in favor of the balancing Treg cells.

Pregnant women should avoid high doses of vitamin A, but others can benefit from 10,000 to 20,0000 IU a day for three to four weeks, then decreasing to a maintenance dose of 5,000 IU per day.

OMEGA-3 FATTY ACIDS AND T REGULATORY CELLS

The omega-3 fatty acids *docosahexaenoic acid* (DHA) and *eicosapentaenoic acid* (EPA) and their derivatives offer many anti-inflammatory properties. The list of health benefits associated with taking DHA and EPA is extensive. Tissue culture and animal model studies suggest that DHA in particular favors the formation of the anti-inflammatory T lymphocytes—that is, increased T regulatory cell at the expense of reduced Th1 and Th17 cells.[115,116,117] Ideally, one would take 1,500-2,000 mg of a high-quality, pharmaceutical-grade DHA per day with meals. As discussed in Chapter 4, enteric-coated soft gels have been shown to offer greater anti-inflammatory action in the small intestine, so I often recommend choosing enteric-coated omega-3 fatty acids over non-enteric coated versions and liquids.

POWERFUL PROBIOTICS

A preponderance of scientific reports confirms that oral bacteria supplements, or probiotics, have broad-spectrum health effects.[118,119,120,121] A recent study showed that oral *Bifidobacterium*, *Streptococcus thermophiles*, and *Lactobacillus* affect neuronal connections in the brain involved in processing emotions and sensations.[122]

The effects of probiotics, however, appear to vary according to the specific strain and its associated DNA.[123,124] Take, for example, two different strains belonging to the identical genus and species of *Escherichia coli*. *E. coli* O157:H7 is a lethal pathogen-associated with blood disorders.[125] In contrast, *E. coli* Nissle 1917 is as much or more effective than mesalazine for treating ulcerative colitis (UC). It's sold as a probiotic called Mutaflor.[126]

With that in context, the available scientific research overwhelmingly suggests that species and strains belonging to the *Bifidobacterium* genera exhibit the greatest health benefits. Studies suggest that the presence of just the DNA from *Bifidobacterium* is enough to induce anti-inflammatory effects inside cells of the gut immune system.[127] Other major anti-inflammatory strains include *B. lactis*, *B. longum*, *B. bifidum*, *B. infantis*, *B. breve* and *LGG*, *Lactobacillus plantarum*, *L. reuteri*, *L. casei Shirota*, and *L. acidophilus*.[128,129,130,131]

Of all the *Bifidobacterium* strains available, *Bifidobacterium lactis* HN019 appears to have been the most studied with regard to safety, ability to colonize, and immune enhancement.[132,133,134,135,136] From preventing iron deficiency in children to increasing natural killer cells (NK cells) in the elderly to normalizing gut ecology, *Bifidobacterium lactis* HN019 is robust and effective.[137,138,139]

Be sure to check with the manufacturer of the probiotic you choose that it has been grown on media that is free of dairy and wheat. Most nutritional manufacturers should be able tell you the genera, species, and strain of your probiotic as well. If not, look for a manufacturer that does.

Additionally, new studies suggest that acid-resistant vegetable capsules are superior delivery systems for probiotics because they preserve the viability of the organisms as they pass through the intestinal tract. Researchers recently published a study using probiotics delivered in acid-resistant capsules to patients embarking on colon cancer surgery.[140] The probiotics were shown to reduce gut permeability and decrease zonulin signaling.

The minimum effective dose for probiotics, according to many recent published studies, is thirty billion CFU (colony forming units), although some studies use up to one trillion CFU per dose. Enhanced manufacturing stability and delivery systems may negate the need to dose at such extreme levels. Probiotics best colonize when taken with meals, such as prebiotic fiber.

INTESTINAL IMMUNOGLOBULINS AS INFLAMMATION FIGHTERS

Proteins released from the gut immune system called *immunoglobulins* help the body achieve the desirable quiescent immune tone.[141] By releasing these antimicrobial peptides, the immune system can better defend itself and control which microbes colonize the gut.[142,143] Intestinal immunoglobulins also minimize leakages of immune stimulatory proteins, such as bacterial endotoxin, through the gut wall, preventing the immune system from overreacting to both potentially pathogenic and otherwise healthy gut bacteria.[144]

People with low levels of gut immunoglobulins, particularly IgA, tend to have increased microbial translocation across the gut wall.[145] This increases inflammation and places a burden on the systemic immune system.

There are three ways to increase the production of anti-inflammatory immunoglobulins in the gut: practicing stress reduction techniques (see Chapter 6), taking the probiotic *Saccharomyces boulardii*, and supplementing with immunoglobulins..

Saccharomyces boulardii.

This probiotic yeast is quite impressive. In addition to boosting the secretion of secretory IgA and exerting anti-inflammatory and rebuilding effects on the gut wall, the beneficial yeast is very stable, is resistant to antibiotics, and prevents *Clostridium difficile* and travelers' diarrhea.[146,147] Also, research shows it protects against Crohn's disease.[148] New data also suggests that this probiotic yeast may block the inflammatory effects of bacterial endotoxin.[149] Additionally, *Saccharomyces boulardii* has been found to increase healthy levels of *short-chain fatty acids* (SCFA), decrease leaky gut, and increase activity of T regulatory cells.[150]

Unpublished studies presented at a poster session by scientists at an Italian biotechnology company, Gnosis, suggest that *Saccharomyces boulardii* may reduce leptin levels, prevent absorption of endotoxin, and increase levels of various anti-inflammatory mediators in the intestine. All of these effects are favorable in reducing body fat and improving blood-sugar handling. Research suggests taking ten billion CFU of *Saccharomyces boulardii* a day with a meal.

Oral immunoglobulins.

Bioactive proteins such as immunoglobulins successfully offset intestinal endotoxin absorption, reduce intestinal inflammation, and ameliorate the cachexia normally accompanying cancer chemotherapy.[151,152,153,154] Sources include bovine serum immunoglobulins and colostrum. They're great for people who experience low energy, fatigue, chronic infections, intestinal inflammation, and high leptin levels. People who take oral immunoglobulin generally note its benefits within one week of beginning therapy. Typical doses are 2.5-5 grams daily.

YOU ARE WHAT YOUR
GUT BUGS FERMENT

There are many variations on the adage, "You are what you eat." To some that means, "You are what you eat, digest, and absorb." I say, "You are what you eat and what your gut bugs ferment." If trillions of microbes didn't colonize your intestine, your ability to digest, absorb, and synthesize various nutrients and healthy metabolites would be compromised.

The innumerable bacteria harbor eight million protein-coding genes, compared to the 22,000 genes of the human genome.[155,156] This extra surrogate genetic material fosters more than six thousand functions that humans otherwise do not have genetic information for. Engendering extra digestive and metabolic functions, our old bacterial friends enhance our ability to survive in many ways, including extracting more energy from foods; synthesizing anti-inflammatory products, such as SCFA; increasing gut-derived metabolic hormones (GLP-1, for example); producing vitamins; and protecting against intestinal infection by disease-causing bacteria.[157,158]

The proper balance of gut bacteria is needed to optimize all of these functions and more. Poor food choices, improper chewing, digestive-altering medications, and an unhealthy lifestyle can inadvertently exploit this primitive symbiotic relationship.[159,160,161] Instead of protecting us, our gut microbes can make us fat.

Fermentation is one main way that bacteria have evolved to help us get more mileage from the food we eat. Otherwise, indigestible carbohydrate-type fibers are fermented in the gut into SCFA, which can then be used for energy.[162] For example, 10–30 percent of the calories consumed as protein and carbohydrates are acted on by gut microflora of the colon.[163] Although humans don't have all the proper enzymes for digesting complex plant-based carbohydrates, the trillions of our gut bacteria offer digestive assistance. By piggybacking on the extra genetic material in bacteria, we can extract energy out of otherwise indigestible food.

This fermentation process can work for you, and help to burn fat. Eating high-fiber, colorful fruits and vegetables creates healthy food for the trillions of microbes in your gut, forming fermentation products that do not have deleterious health problems.[164]

In contrast, consumption of excessive and processed fat, sugars, and alcohol, as found in the Western diet, not only perturbs the balance of gut microbes, affecting barrier status and immunity, but also leads to the formation of toxic gases and metabolites known to increase fat storage.[165] That's because gut bacteria imbalances and poor food choices can cause those microbial friends to extract even more energy from food, increasing fat storage and altering blood-sugar metabolism, which is undesirable.[166]

SHORT-CHAIN FATTY ACIDS

Short-chain fatty acids (SCFA) epitomize the notion that when we eat, our microbes are eating too. The bacteria in our gut ferment our food, synthesizing three main types of SCFA—acetate, propionate, and butyrate—in roughly a 70:20:10 ratio.[167] The ratio and amount of SCFA produced is contingent upon the type of microbes in the intestine as well as the type of foods eaten.[168] Both, of course, vary from one person to another. Butyrate is the primary fuel supply for the cells of the colon, while propionate and acetate readily cross pass through the wall of the large intestine to be converted into carbohydrates and fats, including cholesterol.

SCFA are indirect nutrients, and they have immune and metabolic roles.[169] Acetate, for example, is involved in stimulating the liver to make lipids, while propionate blocks lipid metabolism to favor carbohydrate (*gluconeogenesis*) synthesis.[170] While butyrate is involved in changing the pH of the colon to prevent bad bacteria from growing, it also suppresses inflammation of the colon. Butyrate keeps NF-κβ (*nuclear factor kappa Beta*) from driving inflammation.

Microbial synthesized SCFA also have fat-fighting properties. They can latch onto G protein-coupled receptors (GPR43 and GPR41), which are found on immune cells and fat cells. Acetate, for example, is known to suppress intestinal inflammation by docking onto GPR43 in the gut.[171] Omega-3s exert their anti-inflammatory effects, in part, by docking onto the G protein-coupled receptors.

The main way that high-fiber diets reduce appetite and lower body weight is by increasing SCFA binding to GPR41, which then bind to endocrine cells of the gut.[172,173] Simultaneously, this action reduces intestinal inflammation and fat storage, improves blood-sugar regulation, and improves appetite. Animal and human studies have shown how prebiotic dietary fiber, such as inulin, is able to increase levels of incretins PYY and GLP-1.

A recent study compared levels of SCFA and fecal microbiota between European children and children who live in a rural African village and eat a diet rich in plant fibers with no processed carbohydrates. Among the many differences between these groups, it was observed that children of rural Africa have increased levels of gut microbes, including *Bacteroides* and *Faecalibacterium*, which are known to produce healthy SCFA. These children had nearly double the amount of these anti-inflammatory SCFA in their intestines and in a more balanced ratio among the different fatty acids compared to European children. European children had increased acetate-to-propionate ratio; acetate being a main substrate to synthesize cholesterol and other lipids.

Studies in humans suggest that overweight and obese people have an imbalance of SCFA, possibly too much propionate, which is involved in forming fat cells.[174,175] This may be due to the high saturated-fat content of the diet, which skews the gut microflora balance. Research does suggest that such a diet reduces the number of bacteria in the gut, while decreasing production of healthy SCFA.[176]

In contrast, studies suggest that propionate and butyrate may offer protection against obesity by increasing gut satiety hormones and reducing inflammation.[177] Butyric acid and acetic acid, on the other hand, are anti-inflammatory, inhibiting the growth of pathogenic *E. coli* O157:H7 and decreasing cancer risk.[178]

Lastly, SCFA in the intestine may increase leptin.[179] Fat cells can sense increased SCFA from the diet, leading to increased leptin levels, which may drive inflammation and boost appetite.

Some of the best ways to simultaneously increase the release of fat-fighting intestinal metabolic hormones, such as GLP-1, and balance the gut microflora to prevent absorption of endotoxin and increase healthy levels of SCFA are to consume plant-based polyphenol compounds, prebiotic fiber, probiotics, and pea and whey protein.[180,181,182]

FERMENTATION GETS NASTY

Two recent studies have showed that changes in the composition of gut microbes in obese persons are linked with high levels of toxic metabolites known as *volatile organic compounds* (VOCs).[183] One study associated increased levels of *Proteobacteria, Firmicutes,* and *Clostridia* with increased levels of these secondary metabolites in obese people with liver disease. Similarly, obese children were found to exhale more than fifty significantly fermented compounds compared to non-obese children.[184] Among these compounds are ammonia, hydrogen sulfide, and various alcohol-like substances.

While it's not fully understood which secondary compounds cause obesity, ammonia is linked with colon cancer, and various amine-like metabolites are associated with other diseases, including heart disease.[185] So it's best to make lifestyle choices that promote healthy gut microflora, such as eating prebiotic fibers and colorful foods and to avoid those that alter gut microbes, including processed carbs and excessive fats.

Excessively high-protein diets, for example, increase microbial fermentation of proteins and lead to the formation of metabolites (ammonia, polyamines, and N nitroso compounds) known to be deleterious to intestinal health.[186] High-heat cooking and frying can lead to altered nitrogen (amine) type compounds, such as nitrosamines and heterocyclic amines, that may readily be modified to more toxic metabolites.

WESTERN DIETS ALTER GUT MICROBE BALANCE

With continual and intimate cross talk between gut microbes and the majority of the body's immune system, many of the metabolic and immune problems associated with meals can be traced back to various changes in the composition of the gastrointestinal microflora.[187,188] This occurs even in metabolically healthy people who eat high-carbohydrate, high-fat meals.[189]

Gut microbes are remarkably changeable: high-carb, high-fat foods rapidly shift the structure of the gut microflora, altering both the expression of bacterial genes and metabolic pathways, which influence metabolism.[190]

Bacteria tend to proliferate on foodstuffs best suited to their growth. For example, *Clostridia* and *Bacteroides* may have an easier time flourishing in environments devoid of carbohydrates.[191] As a result they are present in greater numbers in the intestines of meat eaters. European children, for example, have significantly more gut bacteria of the *Escherichia*, *Salmonella*, *Shigella*, and *Klebsiella* type compared to children raised in rural African villages.

Children of rural Africa have increased levels of microbes containing enzymes known to digest fibers, while European children have a more imbalanced intestinal bacterial profile, which likely arises from both diet and aspects of the urban lifestyle—including Cesarean-section birthing, reduced breast-feeding, increased hygiene, and greater antibiotic exposure. (Antibiotic exposure has been shown to reduce healthy levels of *Bifidobacterium* and *Faecalibacterium*.[192])

Lastly, African children had increased bacteria of the *Bacteroidetes* phyla group and fewer bacteria from the *Firmicutes* phyla, a microbial signature common to obesity, compared to their Italian counterparts.

GO GRAIN-FREE TO BALANCE YOUR GUT MICROBES

The key to reducing belly fat, lowering leptin, and balancing gut microbes is to avoid grains altogether. I recommend a grain-free diet, consisting of moderate levels of healthy fats and high quantities of plant fibers, rich in colorful polyphenol compounds from vegetables and fruit.[193,194,195]

Diets high in processed fats, sugars, and other easy-to-digest carbohydrates favor an unhealthy gut microflora profile as well as increased transfer of inflammatory endotoxin.[196,197]

Increased levels of anti-nutrients such as lectins, saponins, and gliadin present in grain-based foods and the synthetic chemicals in processed foods also perturb gut microflora.[198] These compounds reduce the function of the gut barrier, increase leakage of both food and bacterial particulate matter, such as endotoxin, and more. That's why it's best to avoid grains altogether, particularly if you're concerned about weight gain.

GO FOR COLOR

Eating the right foods is the best way to ensure that healthy gut bacteria flourish. Nature combines the healthiest fiber sources and plant polyphenol compounds for a reason—both increase the metabolic health of the intestine and balance gut microflora.[199] Some of the healthiest foods on the planet contain both fibers and lignans paired with colorful polyphenols, such as anthocyanidins and ellagic acid in blueberries and raspberries. Since the foods we eat have been shown to powerfully affect the type of bacteria in our gut, it's important that we remember to make food choices that favor healthy, butyrate-producing bacteria such as *Faecalibacterium praunsnitzii* and *Bifidobacteria*.

Polyphenols are also in herbs and spices that help protect you from the sun's damaging UV rays.[200] (These pigmented compounds also protect animals and insects in the wild from being eaten.[201]) Polyphenols act like mild, positive stressors that reduce inflammation. They mimic the beneficial effects of exercise and improve lipid and glucose metabolism for overall metabolic improvements and disease-fighting capabilities.[202,203]

Many of the secondary compounds created after polyphenols that are acted on by the gut microflora have anti-inflammatory and anti-cancer effects.[204] Now we know that the many health benefits ascribed to polyphenols may also be due to improvements in the microbial composition of the gut. In fact, polyphenols have been shown to interact with the intestinal microflora, suppressing the growth of endotoxin-containing bacteria in the gut.

It's important to have a high and varied polyphenol-rich diet, because the compounds have been shown to be selective with regard to the type of microbial compounds they encourage. One study found black tea polyphenols increased some protective gut microbes, while red wine polyphenols were found to change another type.[205] Indeed, each polyphenol may act like its own prebiotic, or bacterial-promoting compound, while also having its own specific antibiotic properties.[206] A recent study found that the polyphenols from green tea and grapes (*epigallocatechin gallate* and resveratrol) decreased the zonulin-signaling pathway that is involved in the development of leaky gut.[207]

Polyphenols from cruciferous vegetables also indirectly influence the microbes in the intestine by modulating the immune system.[208,209] These *Brassica*-containing vegetables stimulate an immune aryl hydrocarbon receptor (AhR) that may exclude pathogens such as *Citrobacter rodentium*.[210] Mice devoid of this organism exhibit extensive inflammation.[211] Curcumin (of turmeric) and the amino metabolites of the amino acid tryptophan bind to the AhR, inducing a more "tolerogenic" state inside the intestine, congruent with reducing inflammation by increasing Treg cell function.[212]

FAT-BURNING FOODS

The metabolically healthy, fat-fighting *Bacteroidetes* in the gut contain a significant amount of enzymes that are involved in the breakdown of polyphenol from colorful foods such as berries, green vegetables, and teas. In contrast, *Firmicutes* bacteria, which increase in obesity, contain a smaller proportion of enzymes known to degrade these polyphenols. Therefore, these bacteria don't flourish in the presence of polyphenol foods. Moreover, polyphenols may have suppressive effects on the growth of fat-promoting Firmicutes in the gut. So by eating a diet rich in colorful vegetables and fruits, one is going to favor the proper balance of gut microbes—that is, a high *Bacteroidetes/Firmicutes* ratio—optimal levels of healthy SCFA, a sufficient gut barrier function, and few endotoxin.[213]

There are no polyphenols in processed cereal grains. By eating processed grains, you enhance the growth of bacteria that thrive on carbohydrates and risk creating inflammation, gastrointestinal permeability, leptin resistance, and obesity.

PREBIOTIC FIBER

Prebiotics are the non-digestible fibers that fuel the growth of healthy intestinal bacteria, namely the *Bifidobacterium* species. Breast milk, for example, features more than two hundred different oligosaccharides that stimulate healthy bacterial growth in the infant intestine.[214] The main prebiotic compound present in foods and supplements is inulin, which is rich in onions, garlic, chicory, artichoke, and bananas.

Other available forms of prebiotics are fructo-oligosaccharides (FOS), galacto-oligosaccharides (GOS), and xylo-oligosaccharides (XOS). Inulin and GOS have the most positive research. Scientists have long known that inulin and oligofructose prevent obesity caused by a high-fat diet as well as many of the gastrointestinal complications that normally follow, such as intestinal bacteria imbalances and leaky gut.[215,216] Through reviving gastrointestinal barrier function, researchers have shown that prebiotic fiber reduces the absorption of endotoxin.

Many recent human studies have confirmed animal studies of this phenomenon.[217,218,219,220] Scientists in France used a low-dose combination of inulin (3 grams) and XOS (1 gram) per day; the results noted were in serum endotoxin levels and intestinal inflammation and increases in healthy *Bifidobacterium*. Other studies have used higher levels, showing that sixteen grams of inulin-rich prebiotic fiber each day increases levels of two protective bacterial strains (*Bifidobacterium* and *Faecalibacterium prausnitzii*) that are known to increase healthy SCFA.[221]

One study showed that prebiotic fiber reduced intestinal endotoxin and improved blood-sugar control. Researchers have also found that daily inulin (10 grams) improves blood-sugar control and antioxidant status in people with type 2 diabetes.[222]

Lastly, the prebiotic inulin may help offset the formation of leaky gut. Italian scientists showed that inulin-enriched pasta (14 grams/day) reduces zonulin signaling—the peptide involved in leaky gut development—and also increases the gut hormone GLP-2, which is involved in the maintenance of gut barrier function.[223] I suggest eating ample amounts of food rich in prebiotics, including leeks, tubers (yams, turnips, and sweet potatoes), onions, okra, and artichokes.

To minimize your burden of endotoxin, drink a high-quality protein shake that delivers 8–12 grams of inulin daily. Drinking extra inulin is especially protective before consuming high-fat foods when you dine out or when you drink alcohol.

EAT THIS (NOT THAT)

Carbohydrate choices: Yams and sweet potatoes; soaked black or red rice; any green or red, purple, yellow, white, or orange vegetables; berries; oranges; and grapefruits. Eat as many vegetables and fruits as you wish, and one or two servings of yams or soaked rice early in the day.

Protein choices: Always choose wild-caught fish, free-range game and poultry, and eggs from fowl that are allowed to roam freely. Avoid grain-fed animal products and farm-raised fish, since their fatty acid profiles are unfavorable and probably inflammatory. I suggest one 3–5 ounce serving of protein three times per day, particularly on days when you exercise.
Tip: Supplement with non-GMO pea protein and whey protein smoothies.

Fat choices: 1–2 tablespoons of organic, cold-pressed coconut oil daily, half an avocado, and a handful of soaked nuts and seeds as a snack.
Tip: It's best to soak nuts overnight in water prior to eating as this releases some of their anti-nutrient and preservative factors and increases absorption.

KEY TAKEAWAYS

The proper balance of your resident gut microflora is imperative for fat loss and blood-sugar regulation. Overwhelming scientific evidence suggests that poor food choices and eating too many processed carbohydrates and fats negatively influences the type of microbes in your intestinal tract.

Imbalanced gut microbes affect body composition, inflammation, and metabolism in many different ways. The dysbiosis that the imbalance creates weakens your intestinal barrier and increases the burden of inflammatory molecules. Imbalanced gut microbes also increase the levels of unfavorable secondary metabolites, such as short-chain fatty acids and volatile organic compounds.

Healthy digestion and diets of colorful, high-fiber vegetables, fruits, herbs and spices, such as curcumin, and resveratrol have been shown to favor the proliferation of healthy, fat-fighting gut microbes.

Prebiotic compounds from inulin in foods such as onions, leeks, and root vegetables are highly protective because they act like fertilizer for intestinal microflora.

Oral immunoglobulins and probiotics, particularly strains of the *Bifidobacterium*, reduce intestinal inflammation, improve gut integrity, and reduce endotoxin absorption.

ACKNOWLEDGMENTS

I'd like to thank my beautiful and supportive wife, Deanna, and daughter, Inez. The time spent away from them researching and synthesizing concepts was instrumental in writing this book.

I am thankful for the support of my parents and brothers, whom I frequently leaned on for guidance. I am grateful for their ongoing belief in my vision and goals.

We owe a great deal of gratitude to the scientists and researchers who conducted much of the work that has been explored in this book. I'd like to acknowledge Gökhan S. Hotamisligil, MD, PhD; José Manuel Fernández-Real, MD, PhD; John Pickup, MD; Carey N. Lumeng, MD, PhD; Henk S. Schipper, MD; Justin I. Odegaard, MD, PhD; Ajay Chawla, MD, PhD; Jerrold M. Olefsky, MD; Garry Egger, MPH, PhD; Alistair V. W. Nunn, BSc, PhD; Jesse Roth, MD; and Rainer H. Straub, MD, PhD, for the groundbreaking research that illuminates the links between metabolism and immunity. We are deeply indebted to the ongoing research and discoveries in the field of gut microflora endotoxin and intestinal health due to contributions from Patrice D. Cani, PhD; Nathalie M. Delzenne, PhD; Peter J. Turnbaugh, PhD; Jeffrey I. Gordon, MD; Fredrik Bäckhed, PhD; Jacques Amar, PhD; Rémy Burcelin, PhD; Liping Zhao, PhD; Matteo Serino, PhD; José María Moreno-Navarrete, PhD; Martin J. Blaser, MD; Lora V. Hooper, PhD; and Alessio Fasano, MD. Last but not least, the contributions and works from evolutionary biologists Loren Cordain, PhD; S. Boyd Eaton, MD; James H. O'Keefe, MD; Pedro Carrera-Bastos, MA, MS, PhD; and Ian Spreadbury, PhD have been instrumental in enhancing our knowledge of the ways we can modify our nutrition and lifestyle to emulate that of our ancestors for improved health.

I am indebted to the inspiration and teachings of my early mentors, who include Harry Eidenier, PhD; Daniel Boenning; Gerard Guillory, MD; Bettina Newman, RD; Deanna Minich, PhD; Kim Celmer, ND; Bob Rose, RN; Jeffery Moss, DDS; David Brady, ND, DC; Ryan Frace; Fred Grover, MD; Shawn Naylor, DO; Alex Vasquez, DO; David Haase, MD; Sheri Fox, PA; Denver Hager, Pac; Joseph L Evans, PhD; Robert Rountree, MD; Patrick Donovan, ND; David Musnick, MD; Cheryl Burdette, ND; Mike Antonelli; Ben Lynch, ND; Matt Angove, ND; John Catanzaro, ND; Kris Fobes; Kathyrn Retzler, ND; Daniel Soule; Athena Paradise, DC; Carrie Jones, ND; Maggy Yu, MD; Sarah Ashlager; Kasra Pournadeali, ND; Mark Clark, RPh; John Brimhall, DC; Richard Horowitz, MD; and David Perlmutter, MD.

I'd like to offer thanks to Brian and Stephanie Blackburn, Mike Mahoney, Daniel Gulick, Ryan Frace, Rachelle Tomey, Matt Grabau, Todd Hilvitz, Amy Salerno, Sela Aguglia, Clay Crossan, DD Ames, Denisha Sefcik, Nina Stout, Joell Daniel, Eula Seyda, Todd Handel, Seth Adams, and the entire XYMOGEN family. I wholeheartedly embrace their continued support. Last but not least, I'm grateful for the efforts of my graphic designer Sean Swope and editors Dianne Lange, Ely White, Rose Angove, Bettina Newman, and Elaine and Bud Fawcett.

The wonderful medical illustrations were works by Molly Borman-Pullen (www.mborman.com) and Laurie O'Keefe (www.laurieokeefe.com).

RESOURCES

SUGGESTED RESOURCES FOR CONTINUING EDUCATION

Belly Fat Effect
www.BellyFatEffect.com

Institute for Functional Medicine
www.functionalmedicine.org

International Conference on Human Nutrition
and Functional Medicine
www.ichnfm.org

Institute of HeartMath
www.heartmath.org

Seeking Health Educational Institute
www.seekinghealth.org

The Bulletproof Executive — The State of High Performance
www.bulletproofexec.com

LABORATORY TESTING

Genova Diagnostics
www.gdx.net

Dunwoody Labs
www.dunwoodylabs.com

OmegaQuant
www.omegaquant.com

SpectraCell Laboratories
www.spectracell.com

Doctor's Data
www.doctorsdata.com

Cyrex Laboratories
www.cyrexlabs.com

NATURAL PRODUCTS AND THERAPIES

Health Coach 7
www.healthcoach7.com

Hormone Synergy
www.hormonesynergy.com

MCT Foods
www.mctfoods.com

Seeking Health
www.seekinghealth.com

XYMOGEN Exclusive Professional Formulas
www.xymogen.com

REFERENCES

PREFACE

1. Turnbaugh, P. J., Ridaura, V. K., Faith, J. J., Rey, F. E., Knight, R., & Gordon, J. I. (2009). The effect of diet on the human gut microbiome: a metagenomic analysis in humanized gnotobiotic mice. *Science Translational Medicine*, *1*(6), 6ra14. doi:10.1126/scitranslmed.3000322

2. Ghanim, H., Sia, C. L., Korzeniewski, K., Lohano, T., Abuaysheh, S., Marumganti, A., et al. (2011). A resveratrol and polyphenol preparation suppresses oxidative and inflammatory stress response to a high-fat, high-carbohydrate meal. *The Journal of Clinical Endocrinology and Metabolism*, *96*(5), 1409–1414. doi:10.1210/jc.2010-1812

3. Kolehmainen, M., Mykkänen, O., Kirjavainen, P. V., Leppänen, T., Moilanen, E., Adriaens, M., et al. (2012). Bilberries reduce low-grade inflammation in individuals with features of metabolic syndrome. *Molecular Nutrition & Food Research*, n/a–n/a. doi:10.1002/mnfr.201200195

4. Harte, A. L., Varma, M. C., Tripathi, G., McGee, K. C., Al-Daghri, N. M., Al-Attas, O. S., et al. (2012). High Fat Intake Leads to Acute Postprandial Exposure to Circulating Endotoxin in Type 2 Diabetic Subjects. *Diabetes Care*, *35*(2), 375–382. doi:10.2337/dc11-1593

5. Erridge, C., Attina, T., Spickett, C. M., & Webb, D. J. (2007). A high-fat meal induces low-grade endotoxemia: evidence of a novel mechanism of postprandial inflammation. *Am J Clin Nutr*, *86*(5), 1286–1292.

6. Cani, P. D., Osto, M., Geurts, L., & Everard, A. (2012). Involvement of gut microbiota in the development of low-grade inflammation and type 2 diabetes associated with obesity. *Gut Microbes*, *3*(4), 1–10. doi:10.4161/gmic.19625

7. Bäckhed, F., & Crawford, P. A. (2010). Coordinated regulation of the metabolome and lipidome at the host-microbial interface. *Biochimica et Biophysica Acta*, *1801*(3), 240–245. doi:10.1016/j.bbalip.2009.09.009

8. Johnson, A. R., Milner, J. J., & Makowski, L. (2012). The inflammation highway: metabolism accelerates inflammatory traffic in obesity. *Immunological Reviews*, *249*(1), 218–238. doi:10.1111/j.1600-065X.2012.01151.x

9. Straub, R. H., Cutolo, M., Buttgereit, F., & Pongratz, G. (2010). Review: Energy regulation and neuroendocrine-immune control in chronic inflammatory diseases. *Journal of Internal Medicine*, *267*(6), 543–560. doi:10.1111/j.1365-2796.2010.02218.x

10. Shapiro, H., Lutaty, A., & Ariel, A. (2011). Macrophages, meta-inflammation, and immuno-metabolism. *The Scientific World Journal*, *11*, 2509–2529. doi:10.1100/2011/397971

11. Heikamp, E. B., & Powell, J. D. (2013). Sensing the immune microenvironment to coordinate T cell metabolism, differentiation & function. *Seminars in Immunology*, *24*(6), 414–420. doi:10.1016/j.smim.2012.12.003

12. Johnson, A. R., Milner, J. J., & Makowski, L. (2012). The inflammation highway: metabolism accelerates inflammatory traffic in obesity. *Immunological Reviews*, *249*(1), 218–238. doi:10.1111/j.1600-065X.2012.01151.x

13. Nakarai, H., Yamashita, A., Nagayasu, S., Iwashita, M., Kumamoto, S., Ohyama, H., et al. (2012). Adipocyte-macrophage interaction may mediate LPS-induced low-grade inflammation: Potential link with metabolic complications. *Innate Immunity*, *18*(1), 164–170. doi:10.1177/1753425910393370

14. Flegal, K. M., Carroll, M. D., Kit, B. K., & Ogden, C. L. (2012). Prevalence of Obesity and Trends in the Distribution of Body Mass Index Among US Adults, 1999-2010. *JAMA*, *307*(5), 491–497. doi:10.1001/jama.2012.39

15. Ogden, C. L., Carroll, M. D., Kit, B. K., & Flegal, K. M. (2012). Prevalence of obesity and trends in body mass index among US children and adolescents, 1999-2010. *JAMA*, *307*(5), 483–490. doi:10.1001/jama.2012.40

16. Shah, N. R., & Braverman, E. R. (2012). Measuring Adiposity in Patients: The Utility of Body Mass Index (BMI), Percent Body Fat, and Leptin. (Q. Nizami, Ed.)*PLoS ONE*, *7*(4), e33308. doi:10.1371/journal.pone.0033308.t004

17. Reaven, G. M. (1993). Role of Insulin Resistance in Human Disease (Syndrome X): An Expanded Definition. *Annual Review of Medicine*, *44*(1), 121–131. doi:10.1146/annurev.me.44.020193.001005

18. Thorpe, K. E., & Philyaw, M. (2012). The Medicalization of Chronic Disease and Costs. *Annual Review of Public Health*, *33*(1), 409–423. doi:10.1146/annurev-publhealth-031811-124652

19. Wang, Y., McPherson, K., Marsh, T., Gortmaker, S. L., & Brown, M. (2011). Health and economic burden of the projected obesity trends in the USA and the UK. *The Lancet, 378*(9793), 815–825. doi:10.1016/S0140-6736(11)60814-3

20. Marvasti, F., & Stafford, R. S. (2012). From Sick Care to health Care — reengineering Prevention into the U.S. System. *New England Journal of Medicine, 367*(10), 889–891. doi:10.1056/nEjMp1206230

21. Robles, S., Adrion, E., & Anderson, G. F. (2012). Premature adult mortality from non-communicable diseases (NCD) in three middle-income countries: do NCD programmes matter? *Health policy and planning, 27*(6), 487–498. doi:10.1093/heapol/czr073

22. Chronic Diseases The Power To Prevent, The Call To Control: At A Glance (2009).*Center for Disease Control and Prevention.*

23. Pearson, W. S., Bhat-Schelbert, K., & Probst, J. C. (2012). Multiple chronic conditions and the aging of america: challenge for primary care physicians. *Journal of primary care & community health, 3*(1), 51–56. doi:10.1177/2150131911414577

24. Bussche, H. V. D., Koller, D., Kolonko, T., Hansen, H., Wegscheider, K., Glaeske, G., et al. (2011). Which chronic diseases and disease combinations are specific to multimorbidity in the elderly? Results of a claims data based cross-sectional study in Germany. *BMC Public Health, 11*(1), 101. doi:10.1186/1471-2458-11-101

25. Preston, S. H., & Stokes, A. (2011). Contribution of obesity to international differences in life expectancy. *American Journal of Public Health, 101*(11), 2137–2143. doi:10.2105/AJPH.2011.300219

26. Jones, D.S. (2010). Textbook of functional medicine. *Institute for Functional Medicine.* ISBN-13: 978-0-9773713-7-2

27. Bodenheimer, T., Lorig, K., Holman, H., & Grumbach, K. (2002). Patient Self-management of Chronic Disease in Primary Care. *JAMA, 288*(19), 2469–2475. doi:10.1001/jama.288.19.2469

28. Egger, G., & Dixon, J. (2009). Should obesity be the main game? Or do we need an environmental makeover to combat the inflammatory and chronic disease epidemics? *Obesity reviews : an official journal of the International Association for the Study of Obesity, 10*(2), 237–249. doi:10.1111/j.1467-789X.2008.00542.x

29. Fani Marvasti, F., & Stafford, R. S. (2012). From Sick Care to Health Care — Reengineering Prevention into the U.S. System. *New England Journal of Medicine, 367*(10), 889–891. doi:10.1056/NEJMp1206230

30. Cani, P. D., & Delzenne, N. M. (2009). Interplay between obesity and associated metabolic disorders: new insights into the gut microbiota. *Current Opinion in Pharmacology, 9*(6), 737–743. doi:10.1016/j.coph.2009.06.016

31. Round, J. L., & Mazmanian, S. K. (2009). The gut microbiota shapes intestinal immune responses during health and disease. *Nature Reviews Immunology, 9*(5), 313–323.

32. Bäckhed, F., Ley, R. E., Sonnenburg, J. L., Peterson, D. A., & Gordon, J. I. (2005). Host-bacterial mutualism in the human intestine. *Science, 307*(5717), 1915–1920. doi:10.1126/science.1104816

33. Cani, P. D., & Delzenne, N. M. (2011). The gut microbiome as therapeutic target. *Pharmacology and Therapeutics, 130*(2), 202–212. doi:10.1016/j.pharmthera.2011.01.012

34. Krajmalnik-Brown, R., Ilhan, Z.-E., Kang, D.-W., & DiBaise, J. K. (2012). Effects of gut microbes on nutrient absorption and energy regulation. *Nutrition in Clinical Practice, 27*(2), 201–214. doi:10.1177/0884533611436116

35. Jumpertz, R., Le, D. S., Turnbaugh, P. J., Trinidad, C., Bogardus, C., Gordon, J. I., & Krakoff, J. (2011). Energy-balance studies reveal associations between gut microbes, caloric load, and nutrient absorption in humans. *American Journal of Clinical Nutrition, 94*(1), 58–65. doi:10.3945/ajcn.110.010132

36. Kussmann, M., & Van Bladeren, P. J. (2011). The extended nutrigenomics–understanding the interplay between the genomes of food, gut microbes, and human host. *Frontiers in genetics, 2.* doi:10.3389/fgene.2011.00021/abstract

37. Xiao, S., Fei, N., Pang, X., Shen, J., Wang, L., Zhang, B., et al. (2013). A gut microbiota-targeted dietary intervention for amelioration of chronic inflammation underlying metabolic syndrome. *FEMS Microbiology Ecology.* doi:10.1111/1574-6941.12228

38. Walker, A. W., & Lawley, T. D. (2013). Therapeutic modulation of intestinal dysbiosis. *Pharmacological Research: the Official Journal of the Italian Pharmacological Society, 69*(1), 75–86. doi:10.1016/j.phrs.2012.09.008

39. Hawkesworth, S., Moore, S. E., Fulford, A. J. C., Barclay, G. R., Darboe, A. A., Mark, H., et al. (2013). Evidence for metabolic endotoxemia in obese and diabetic Gambian women. *Nutrition and Diabetes, 3*(8), e83–6. doi:10.1038/nutd.2013.24

40. Vrieze, A., Van Nood, E., Holleman, F., Salojärvi, J., Kootte, R. S., Bartelsman, J. F. W. M., et al. (2012). Transfer of Intestinal Microbiota From Lean Donors Increases Insulin Sensitivity in Individuals With Metabolic Syndrome. *Gastroenterology, 143*(4), 913–916.e7. doi:10.1053/j.gastro.2012.06.031

41. Yoshikawa, I., Nagato, M., Yamasaki, M., Kume, K., & Otsuki, M. (2009). Long-term treatment with proton pump inhibitor is associated with undesired weight gain. *World Journal of Gastroenterology, 15*(38), 4794–4798. doi:10.3748/wjg.15.4794

42. Vael, C., Verhulst, S. L., Nelen, V., Goossens, H., & Desager, K. N. (2011). Intestinal microflora and body mass index during the first three years of life: an observational study. *Gut Pathogens*, 3(1), 8. doi:10.1186/1757-4749-3-8

43. Thuny, F., Richet, H., Casalta, J.P., Angelakis, E., Habib, G., & Raoult, D. (2010). Vancomycin Treatment of Infective Endocarditis Is Linked with Recently Acquired Obesity. (S. Bereswill, Ed.)*PLoS ONE*, 5(2), e9074. doi:10.1371/journal.pone.0009074.t003

44. Mesquita, D. N., Barbieri, M. A., Goldani, H., & Cardoso, V. C. (2013). Cesarean Section Is Associated with Increased Peripheral and Central Adiposity in Young Adulthood: Cohort Study. *PLoS ONE*, 8(6), e66827.

45. Huh, S. Y., Rifas-Shiman, S. L., Zera, C. A., Edwards, J. W. R., Oken, E., Weiss, S. T., & Gillman, M. W. (2012). Delivery by caesarean section and risk of obesity in preschool age children: a prospective cohort study. *Archives of Disease in Childhood*, 97(7), 610–616. doi:10.1136/archdischild-2011-301141

46. Ajslev, T. A., Andersen, C. S., Gamborg, M., Sørensen, T. I. A., & Jess, T. (2011). Childhood overweight after establishment of the gut microbiota: the role of delivery mode, pre-pregnancy weight and early administration of antibiotics. *International Journal of Obesity*, 35(4), 522–529. doi:10.1038/ijo.2011.27

47. Pflughoeft, K. J., & Versalovic, J. (2012). Human Microbiome in Health and Disease. *Annual Review of Pathology: Mechanisms of Disease*, 7(1), 99–122. doi:10.1146/annurev-pathol-011811-132421

48. Cummings, J. H., Antoine, J.-M., Azpiroz, F., Bourdet-Sicard, R., Brandtzaeg, P., Calder, P. C., et al. (2004). PASSCLAIM--gut health and immunity. *European Journal of Nutrition*, 43 Suppl 2,II8–II173. doi:10.1007/s00394-004-1205-4

49. Greiner, T., & Bäckhed, F. (2011). Effects of the gut microbiota on obesity and glucose homeostasis. *Trends in Endocrinology & Metabolism*, 22(4), 117–123. doi:10.1016/j.tem.2011.01.002

50. Hvistendahl, M. (2012). *My microbiome and me. Science.*Vol. 336, pp. 1248–1250. doi:10.1126/science.336.6086.1248

51. Diamant, M., Blaak, E. E., & de Vos, W. M. (2011). Do nutrient-gut-microbiota interactions play a role in human obesity, insulin resistance and type 2 diabetes? *Obesity reviews : an official journal of the International Association for the Study of Obesity*, 12(4), 272–281. doi:10.1111/j.1467-789X.2010.00797.x

52. Calay, E. S., & Hotamisligil, G. S. (2013). Turning off the inflammatory, but not the metabolic, flames. *Nature Medicine*, 19(3), 265–267. doi:10.1038/nm.3114

53. Cox, L. M., & Blaser, M. J. (2013). Pathways in microbe-induced obesity. *Cell Metabolism*, 17(6), 883–894. doi:10.1016/j.cmet.2013.05.004

54. Zhang, H., DiBaise, J. K., Zuccolo, A., Kudrna, D., Braidotti, M., Yu, Y., et al. (2009). Human gut microbiota in obesity and after gastric bypass. *Proceedings of the National Academy of Sciences*, *106*(7), 2365–2370. doi:10.1073/pnas.0812600106

55. Rubino, F., Shukla, A., Pomp, A., Moreira, M., Ahn, S. M., & Dakin, G. (2013). Bariatric, Metabolic, and Diabetes Surgery. *Annals of Surgery*, 1. doi:10.1097/SLA.0b013e3182759656

56. Falken, Y., Hellstrom, P. M., Holst, J. J., & Naslund, E. (2011). Changes in Glucose Homeostasis after Roux-en-Y Gastric Bypass Surgery for Obesity at Day Three, Two Months, and One Year after Surgery: Role of Gut Peptides. *Journal of Clinical Endocrinology & Metabolism*, *96*(7), 2227–2235. doi:10.1210/jc.2010-2876

57. Wickremesekera, K., Miller, G., Naotunne, T. D., Knowles, G., & Stubbs, R. S. (2005). Loss of Insulin Resistance after Roux-en-Y Gastric Bypass Surgery: a Time Course Study. *Obesity Surgery*, *15*(4), 474–481. doi:10.1381/0960892053723402

58. Larsen, N., Vogensen, F. K., van den Berg, F. W. J., Nielsen, D. S., Andreasen, A. S., Pedersen, B. K., et al. (2010). Gut Microbiota in Human Adults with Type 2 Diabetes Differs from Non-Diabetic Adults. (S. Bereswill, Ed.) *PLoS ONE*, *5*(2), e9085. doi:10.1371/journal.pone.0009085.t003

59. Furet, J.-P., Kong, L.-C., Tap, J., Poitou, C., Basdevant, A., Bouillot, J.-L., et al. (2010). Differential adaptation of human gut microbiota to bariatric surgery-induced weight loss: links with metabolic and low-grade inflammation markers. *Diabetes*, *59*(12), 3049–3057. doi:10.2337/db10-0253

60. Li, J. V., Ashrafian, H., Bueter, M., Kinross, J., Sands, C., le Roux, C. W., et al. (2011). Metabolic surgery profoundly influences gut microbial-host metabolic cross-talk. *Gut*, *60*(9), 1214–1223. doi:10.1136/gut.2010.234708

61. Shillitoe, E., weinstock, r., kim, T., Simon, h., Planer, j., noonan, S., & Cooney, r. (2012). The oral microflora in obesity and type-2 diabetes. *Journal of Oral Microbiology*, *4*(0), 956. doi:10.1016/j.

62. Koromantzos, P. A., Makrilakis, K., Dereka, X., Offenbacher, S., Katsilambros, N., Vrotsos, I. A., & Madianos, P. N. (2012). Effect of Non-Surgical Periodontal Therapy on C-Reactive Protein, Oxidative Stress, and Matrix Metalloproteinase (MMP)-9 and MMP-2 Levels in Patients With Type 2 Diabetes: A Randomized Controlled Study. *Journal of Periodontology*, *83*(1), 3–10. doi:10.1902/jop.2011.110148

63. Koren, O., Spor, A., Felin, J., Fåk, F., Stombaugh, J., Tremaroli, V., et al. (2011). Colloquium Paper: Human oral, gut, and plaque microbiota in patients with atherosclerosis. *Proceedings of the National Academy of Sciences*, *108*(Supplement_1), 4592–4598. doi:10.1073/pnas.1011383107

64. Gunstad, J., Strain, G., Devlin, M. J., Wing, R., Cohen, R. A., Paul, R. H., et al. (2011). Improved memory function 12 weeks after bariatric surgery. *Surgery for Obesity and Related Diseases*, 7(4), 465–472. doi:10.1016/j. soard.2010.09.015

65. Ghanim, H., Monte, S. V., Sia, C. L., Abuaysheh, S., Green, K., Caruana, J. A., & Dandona, P. (2012). Reduction in Inflammation and the Expression of Amyloid Precursor Protein and Other Proteins Related to Alzheimer's Disease following Gastric Bypass Surgery. *Journal of Clinical Endocrinology & Metabolism*, 97(7), E1197–E1201. doi:10.1210/jc.2011-3284

66. Tadross, J. A., & le Roux, C. W. (2009). The mechanisms of weight loss after bariatric surgery. *International Journal of Obesity*, 33(S1), S28–S32. doi:10.1038/ijo.2009.14

67. Huerta, S., Kohan, D., Siddiqui, A., Anthony, T., & Livingston, E. H. (2007). Assessment of comorbid conditions in veteran patients after Roux-en-Y gastric bypass. *The American Journal of Surgery*, 194(1), 48–52. doi:10.1016/j.amjsurg.2006.11.017

68. Kelly, C. J., Colgan, S. P., & Frank, D. N. (2012). Of microbes and meals: the health consequences of dietary endotoxemia. *Nutrition in Clinical Practice*, 27(2), 215–225. doi:10.1177/0884533611434934 Hellström, P. M. (2013). Satiety signals and obesity. *Current Opinion in Gastroenterology*, 29(2), 222–227. doi:10.1097/MOG.0b013e32835d9ff8

69. Erridge, C., Attina, T., Spickett, C. M., & Webb, D. J. (2007). A high-fat meal induces low-grade endotoxemia: evidence of a novel mechanism of postprandial inflammation. *Am J Clin Nutr*, 86(5), 1286–1292.

70. Harte, A. L., Varma, M. C., Tripathi, G., McGee, K. C., Al-Daghri, N. M., Al-Attas, O. S., et al. (2012). High Fat Intake Leads to Acute Postprandial Exposure to Circulating Endotoxin in Type 2 Diabetic Subjects. *Diabetes Care*, 35(2), 375–382. doi:10.2337/dc11-1593

71. Deopurkar, R., Ghanim, H., Friedman, J., Abuaysheh, S., Sia, C. L., Mohanty, P., et al. (2010). Differential Effects of Cream, Glucose, and Orange Juice on Inflammation, Endotoxin, and the Expression of Toll-Like Receptor-4 and Suppressor of Cytokine Signaling-3. *Diabetes Care*, 33(5), 991–997. doi:10.2337/dc09-1630

72. Ghanim, H., Sia, C. L., Upadhyay, M., Korzeniewski, K., Viswanathan, P., Abuaysheh, S., et al. (2010). Orange juice neutralizes the proinflammatory effect of a high-fat, high-carbohydrate meal and prevents endotoxin increase and Toll-like receptor expression. *American Journal of Clinical Nutrition*, 91(4), 940–949. doi:10.3945/ajcn.2009.28584

73. Fei, N., & Zhao, L. (2012). An opportunistic pathogen isolated from the gut of an obese human causes obesity in germfree mice. *The ISME Journal*, 7(4), 880–884. doi:10.1038/ismej.2012.153

74. Mohammed, N., Tang, L., Jahangiri, A., de Villiers, W., & Eckhardt, E. (2012). Elevated IgG levels against specific bacterial antigens in obese patients with diabetes and in mice with diet-induced obesity and glucose intolerance. *Metabolism: clinical and experimental, 61*(9), 1211–1214. doi:10.1016/j.metabol.2012.02.007

75. Lassenius, M. I., Pietilainen, K. H., Kaartinen, K., Pussinen, P. J., Syrjanen, J., Forsblom, C., et al. (2011). Bacterial Endotoxin Activity in Human Serum Is Associated With Dyslipidemia, Insulin Resistance, Obesity, and Chronic Inflammation. *Diabetes Care, 34*(8), 1809–1815. doi:10.2337/dc10-2197

76. Pussinen, P. J., Havulinna, A. S., Lehto, M., Sundvall, J., & Salomaa, V. (2011). Endotoxemia is associated with an increased risk of incident diabetes. *Diabetes Care, 34*(2), 392–397. doi:10.2337/dc10-1676

77. Chang, S., & Li, L. (2011). Metabolic endotoxemia: a novel concept in chronic disease pathology. *J Med Sci, 3*, 191–209.

78. Carrera-Bastos, P., Fontes-Villalba, M., O'Keefe, J. H., Lindeberg, S., & Cordain, L. (2011). The western diet and lifestyle and diseases of civilization. *Res Rep Clin Cardiol, 2*, 15–35.

79. Erridge, C. (2011). Diet, commensals and the intestine as sources of pathogen-associated molecular patterns in atherosclerosis, type 2 diabetes and non-alcoholic fatty liver disease. *Atherosclerosis, 216*(1), 1–6. doi:10.1016/j.atherosclerosis.2011.02.043

80. Burcelin, R., Serino, M., Chabo, C., Blasco-Baque, V., & Amar, J. (2011). Gut microbiota and diabetes: from pathogenesis to therapeutic perspective. *Acta Diabetologica, 48*(4), 257–273. doi:10.1007/s00592-011-0333-6

81. Spreadbury, I. (2012). Comparison with ancestral diets suggests dense acellular carbohydrates promote an inflammatory microbiota, and may be the primary dietary cause of leptin resistance and obesity. *Diabetes, Metabolic Syndrome and Obesity: Targets and Therapy, 5*, 175–189. doi:10.2147/DMSO.S33473

82. Wolowczuk, I., Verwaerde, C., Viltart, O., Delanoye, A., Delacre, M., Pot, B., & Grangette, C. (2008). Feeding our immune system: impact on metabolism. *Clinical and Developmental Immunology, 2008*, 639803. doi:10.1155/2008/639803

83. Könner, A. C., & Brüning, J. C. (2011). Toll-like receptors: linking inflammation to metabolism. *Trends in endocrinology and metabolism: TEM, 22*(1), 16–23. doi:10.1016/j.tem.2010.08.007

84. Medzhitov, R. (2010). Inflammation 2010: New Adventures of an Old Flame. *Cell, 140*(6), 771–776. doi:10.1016/j.cell.2010.03.006

85. Chawla, A., Nguyen, K. D., & Goh, Y. P. S. (2011). Macrophage-mediated inflammation in metabolic disease. *Nature Reviews Immunology, 11*(11), 738–749. doi:10.1038/nri3071

86. Tanti, J.-F., Ceppo, F., Jager, J., & Berthou, F. (2012). Implication of inflammatory signaling pathways in obesity-induced insulin resistance. *Frontiers in endocrinology, 3*, 181. doi:10.3389/fendo.2012.00181

87. Schipper, H. S., Prakken, B., Kalkhoven, E., & Boes, M. (2012). Adipose tissue-resident immune cells: key players in immunometabolism. *Trends in Endocrinology & Metabolism, 23*(8), 407–415. doi:10.1016/j.tem.2012.05.011

00. Johnson, A. M. F., & Olefsky, J. M. (2013). The Origins and Drivers of Insulin Resistance. *Cell, 152*(4), 673–684. doi:10.1016/j.cell.2013.01.041

89. Shu, C. J., Benoist, C., & Mathis, D. (2012). The immune system's involvement in obesity-driven type 2 diabetes. *Seminars in Immunology, 24*(6), 436–442. doi:10.1016/j.smim.2012.12.001

90. Hotamisligil, G. S., & Erbay, E. (2008). Nutrient sensing and inflammation in metabolic diseases. *Nature Reviews Immunology, 8*(12), 923–934. doi:10.1038/nri2449

91. Batra, A., & Siegmund, B. (2012). The Role of Visceral Fat. *Digestive Diseases, 30*(1), 70–74. doi:10.1159/000335722

92. Caricilli, A. M., & Saad, M. J. A. (2013). The role of gut microbiota on insulin resistance. *Nutrients, 5*(3), 829–851. doi:10.3390/nu5030829

93. Mehta, N. N., McGillicuddy, F. C., Anderson, P. D., Hinkle, C. C., Shah, R., Pruscino, L., et al. (2010). Experimental endotoxemia induces adipose inflammation and insulin resistance in humans. *Diabetes, 59*(1), 172–181. doi:10.2337/db09-0367

94. Kemp, D. M. (2013). Does chronic low-grade endotoxemia define susceptibility of obese humans to insulin resistance via dietary effects on gut microbiota? *Adipocyte, 2*(3), 188–190. doi:10.4161/adip.24776

95. Spreadbury, I. (2012). Comparison with ancestral diets suggests dense acellular carbohydrates promote an inflammatory microbiota, and may be the primary dietary cause of leptin resistance and obesity. *Diabetes, Metabolic Syndrome and Obesity: Targets and Therapy, 5*, 175–189. doi:10.2147/DMSO.S33473

96. Meier, J. J. (2009). The contribution of incretin hormones to the pathogenesis of type 2 diabetes. *Best Practice & Research Clinical Endocrinology & Metabolism, 23*(4), 433–441. doi:10.1016/j.beem.2009.03.007

97. Hellström, P. M. (2013). Satiety signals and obesity. *Current Opinion in Gastroenterology, 29*(2), 222–227 doi:10.1097/MOG.0b013e32835d9ff8

98. Beckman, L. M., Beckman, T. R., Sibley, S. D., Thomas, W., Ikramuddin, S., Kellogg, T. A., et al. (2011). Changes in Gastrointestinal Hormones and Leptin After Roux-en-Y Gastric Bypass Surgery. *Journal of Parenteral and Enteral Nutrition, 35*(2), 169–180. doi:10.1177/0148607110381403

99. Salehi, M., Prigeon, R. L., & D'Alessio, D. A. (2011). Gastric Bypass Surgery Enhances Glucagon-Like Peptide 1-Stimulated Postprandial Insulin Secretion in Humans. *Diabetes, 60*(9), 2308–2314. doi:10.2337/db11-0203

100. Dao, T.-M. A., Waget, A., Klopp, P., Serino, M., Vachoux, C., Pechere, L., et al. (2011). Resveratrol Increases Glucose Induced GLP-1 Secretion in Mice: A Mechanism which Contributes to the Glycemic Control. *PLoS ONE*, *6*(6), e20700. doi:10.1371/journal.pone.0020700

101. Panickar, K. S. (2013). Effects of dietary polyphenols on neuroregulatory factors and pathways that mediate food intake and energy regulation in obesity. *Molecular Nutrition & Food Research*, *57*(1), 34–47. doi:10.1002/mnfr.201200431

102. Geraedts, M. C. P., Troost, F. J., Munsters, M. J. M., Stegen, J. H. C. H., de Ridder, R. J., Conchillo, J. M., et al. (2011). Intraduodenal Administration of Intact Pea Protein Effectively Reduces Food Intake in Both Lean and Obese Male Subjects. (J.-M. A. Lobaccaro, Ed.)*PLoS ONE*, *6*(9), e24878. doi:10.1371/journal.pone.0024878.t001

CHAPTER 1: BEYOND CALORIES

1. Odegaard, J. I., & Chawla, A. (2013). Pleiotropic actions of insulin resistance and inflammation in metabolic homeostasis. *Science*, *339*(6116), 172–177. doi:10.1126/science.1230721

2. Lazar, M. A. (2005). How obesity causes diabetes: not a tall tale. *Science*, *307*(5708), 373–375. doi:10.1126/science.1104342

3. Liou, A. P., & Turnbaugh, P. J. (2012). Antibiotic Exposure Promotes Fat Gain. *Cell Metab.*, *16*(4), 408–410. doi:10.1016/j.cmet.2012.09.009

4. Trasande, L., Blustein, J., Liu, M., Corwin, E., Cox, L. M., & Blaser, M. J. (2013). Infant antibiotic exposures and early-life body mass. *International Journal of Obesity*, *37*(1), 16–23. doi:10.1038/ijo.2012.132

5. Thuny, F., Richet, H., Casalta, J.-P., Angelakis, E., Habib, G., & Raoult, D. (2010). Vancomycin Treatment of Infective Endocarditis Is Linked with Recently Acquired Obesity. (S. Bereswill, Ed.)*PLoS ONE*, *5*(2), e9074. doi:10.1371/journal.pone.0009074.t003

6. Barros, F. C., Matijasevich, A., Hallal, P. C., Horta, B. L., Barros, A. J., Menezes, A. B., et al. (2012). Cesarean section and risk of obesity in childhood, adolescence, and early adulthood: evidence from 3 Brazilian birth cohorts. *American Journal of Clinical Nutrition*, *95*(2), 465–470. doi:10.3945/ajcn.111.026401

7. Mesquita, D. N., Barbieri, M. A., Goldani, H., & Cardoso, V. C. (2013). Cesarean Section Is Associated with Increased Peripheral and Central Adiposity in Young Adulthood: Cohort Study. *PLoS ONE*, *8*(6), e66827.

8. Liu, X., Lagoy, A., Discenza, I., Papineau, G., Lewis, E., Braden, G., et al. (2012). Metabolic and Neuroendocrine Responses to Roux-en-Y Gastric Bypass. I: Energy Balance, Metabolic Changes, and Fat Loss. *Journal of Clinical Endocrinology & Metabolism*. doi:10.1210/jc.2012-1016

9.   Monte, S. V., Caruana, J. A., Ghanim, H., Sia, C. L., Korzeniewski, K., Schentag, J. J., & Dandona, P. (2012). Reduction in endotoxemia, oxidative and inflammatory stress, and insulin resistance after Roux-en-Y gastric bypass surgery in patients with morbid obesity and type 2 diabetes mellitus. *Surgery, 151*(4), 587–593. doi:10.1016/j.surg.2011.09.038

10. Bose, M., Teixeira, J., Oliván, B., Bawa, B., Arias, S., Machineni, S., et al. (2010). Weight loss and incretin responsiveness improve glucose control independently after gastric bypass surgery. *Journal of diabetes, 2*(1), 47–55. doi:10.1111/j.1753-0407.2009.00064.x

11. Hansen, E. N., Tamboli, R. A., Isbell, J. M., Saliba, J., Dunn, J. P., Marks-Shulman, P. A., & Abumrad, N. N. (2011). Role of the foregut in the early improvement in glucose tolerance and insulin sensitivity following Roux-en-Y gastric bypass surgery. *AJP: Gastrointestinal and Liver Physiology, 300*(5), G795–G802. doi:10.1152/ajpgi.00019.2011

12. Laferrère, B. (2011). Do we really know why diabetes remits after gastric bypass surgery? *Endocrine, 40*(2), 162–167. doi:10.1007/s12020-011-9514-x

13. Bradley, D., Magkos, F., & Klein, S. (2012). Effects of Bariatric Surgery on Glucose Homeostasis and Type 2 Diabetes. *Gastroenterology, 143*(4), 897–912.

14. Goktas, Z., Moustaid-Moussa, N., Shen, C.-L., Boylan, M., Mo, H., & Wang, S. (2013). Effects of bariatric surgery on adipokine-induced inflammation and insulin resistance. *Frontiers in endocrinology, 4*, 69. doi:10.3389/fendo.2013.00069

15. Egger, G. (2011). Obesity, Chronic Disease, and Economic Growth: A Case for "Big Picture" Prevention. *Advances in Preventive Medicine, 2011*, 1–6. doi:10.4061/2011/149158

16. Egger, G., & Dixon, J. (2011). Non-nutrient causes of low-grade, systemic inflammation: support for a "canary in the mineshaft" view of obesity in chronic disease. *Obesity reviews : an official journal of the International Association for the Study of Obesity, 12*(5), 339–345. doi:10.1111/j.1467-789X.2010.00795.x

17. Bäckhed, F., Ding, H., Wang, T., Hooper, L. V., Koh, G. Y., Nagy, A., et al. (2004). The gut microbiota as an environmental factor that regulates fat storage. *Proceedings of the National Academy of Sciences of the United States of America, 101*(44), 15718–15715723. doi:10.1073/pnas.0407076101

18. Lake, A., & Townshend, T. (2006). Obesogenic environments: exploring the built and food environments. *The Journal of the Royal Society for the Promotion of Health, 126*(6), 262–267. doi:10.1177/1466424006070487

19. Ajslev, T. A., Andersen, C. S., Gamborg, M., Sørensen, T. I. A., & Jess, T. (2011). Childhood overweight after establishment of the gut microbiota: the role of delivery mode, pre-pregnancy weight and early administration of antibiotics. *International Journal of Obesity, 35*(4), 522–529. doi:10.1038/ijo.2011.27

20. Snedeker, S. M., & Hay, A. G. (2011). Do Interactions Between Gut Ecology and Environmental Chemicals Contribute to Obesity and Diabetes? *Environmental Health Perspectives, 120*(3), 332–339. doi:10.1289/ehp.1104204

21. Snedeker, S. M., & Hay, A. G. (2011). Do Interactions Between Gut Ecology and Environmental Chemicals Contribute to Obesity and Diabetes? *Environmental Health Perspectives, 120*(3), 332–339. doi:10.1289/ehp.1104204

22. Thompson, A. L. (2012). Developmental origins of obesity: Early feeding environments, infant growth, and the intestinal microbiome. *American Journal of Human Biology, 24*(3), 350–360. doi:10.1002/ajhb.22254

23. Janesick, A., & Blumberg, B. (n.d.). *The Role of Environmental Obesogens in the Obesity Epidemic. link.springer.com* (pp. 383–399). Springer US. doi:10.1007/978-1-4419-7034-3_19

24. Johnson, A. R., Milner, J. J., & Makowski, L. (2012). The inflammation highway: metabolism accelerates inflammatory traffic in obesity. *Immunological Reviews, 249*(1), 218–238. doi:10.1111/j.1600-065X.2012.01151.x

25. Larder, R., & O'Rahilly, S. (2012). Guts over glory—why diets fail. *Nature Medicine, 18*(5), 666–667. doi:10.1038/nm.2747

26. Seidell, J. (2000). Obesity, insulin resistance and diabetes – a worldwide epidemic. *British Journal of Nutrition, 83*, S5–S8.

27. Eaton, S. B. (2007). The ancestral human diet: what was it and should it be a paradigm for contemporary nutrition? *Proceedings of the Nutrition Society, 65*(01), 1–6. doi:10.1079/PNS2005471

28. Carrera-Bastos, P., Fontes-Villalba, M., O'Keefe, J. H., Lindeberg, S., & Cordain, L. (2011). The western diet and lifestyle and diseases of civilization. *Research Reports in Clinical Cardiology, 2*, 15–35. doi:10.2147/RRCC.S16919

29. Spreadbury, I., & Samis, A. J. W. (2013). Evolutionary Aspects of Obesity, Insulin Resistance, and Cardiovascular Risk. *Current Cardiovascular Risk Reports, 7*(2), 136–146. doi:10.1007/s12170-013-0293-1

30. Cordain, L., Eaton, S. B., Brand Miller, J., Mann, N., & Hill, K. (2002). Original Communications-The paradoxical nature of hunter-gatherer diets: Meat-based, yet non-atherogenic. *European Journal of Clinical Nutrition, 56*(1), S42.

31. Nunn, A. V., Bell, J. D., & Guy, G. W. (2009). Lifestyle-induced metabolic inflexibility and accelerated ageing syndrome: insulin resistance, friend or foe? *Nutrition & Metabolism, 6*(1), 16. doi:10.1186/1743-7075-6-16

32. Zafon, C., & Simó, R. (2011). The Current Obesity Epidemic: Unravelling the Evolutionary Legacy of Adipose Tissue. *The Open Obesity Journal, 3*, 98–106.

33. Wells, J. C. K. (2013). Obesity as malnutrition: the dimensions beyond energy balance. *European Journal of Clinical Nutrition, 67*(5), 507–512. doi:10.1038/ejcn.2013.31

34. Wells, J., & Siervo, M. (2011). Obesity and energy balance: is the tail wagging the dog? *European Journal of Clinical Nutrition, 65*(11), 1173–1189. doi:10.1038/ejcn.2011.132

35. Thomas, D. M., Bouchard, C., Church, T., Slentz, C., Kraus, W. E., Redman, L. M., et al. (2012). Why do individuals not lose more weight from an exercise intervention at a defined dose? An energy balance analysis. *Obesity reviews : an official journal of the International Association for the Study of Obesity, 13*(10), 835–847. doi:10.1111/j.1467-789X.2012.01012.x

36. Bo, S., Ciccone, G., Durazzo, M., Ghinamo, L., Villois, P., Canil, S., et al. (2011). Contributors to the obesity and hyperglycemia epidemics. A prospective study in a population-based cohort. *International Journal of Obesity, 35*(11), 1442–1449. doi:10.1038/ijo.2011.5

37. Ford, E. S., & Dietz, W. H. (2013). Trends in energy intake among adults in the United States: findings from NHANES. *American Journal of Clinical Nutrition, 97*(4), 848–853. doi:10.3945/ajcn.112.052662

38. Hill, J. O. (2012). Energy Balance and Obesity. *Circulation, 126*(126), 126–132. doi:10.1161/Circulationaha.111.087213

39. Rosenkilde, M., Auerbach, P., Reichkendler, M. H., Ploug, T., Stallknecht, B. M., & Sjodin, A. (2012). Body fat loss and compensatory mechanisms in response to different doses of aerobic exercise--a randomized controlled trial in overweight sedentary males. *AJP: Regulatory, Integrative and Comparative Physiology, 303*(6), R571–R579. doi:10.1152/ajpregu.00141.2012

40. Ross, R., & Bradshaw, A. J. (2009). The future of obesity reduction: beyond weight loss. *Nature Reviews | Endocrinology, 5*(6), 319–326. doi:10.1038/nrendo.2009.78

41. Little, J. P., Safdar, A., Bishop, D., Tarnopolsky, M. A., & Gibala, M. J. (2011). An acute bout of high-intensity interval training increases the nuclear abundance of PGC-1α and activates mitochondrial biogenesis in human skeletal muscle. *AJP: Regulatory, Integrative and Comparative Physiology, 300*(6), R1303–10. doi:10.1152/ajpregu.00538.2010

42. Gibala, M. J., & McGee, S. L. (2008). Metabolic adaptations to short-term high-intensity interval training: a little pain for a lot of gain? *Exercise and sport sciences reviews, 36*(2), 58–63. doi:10.1097/JES.0b013e318168ec1f

43. Hamilton, M. T., Hamilton, D. G., & Zderic, T. W. (2007). Role of Low Energy Expenditure and Sitting in Obesity, Metabolic Syndrome, Type 2 Diabetes, and Cardiovascular Disease. *Diabetes, 56*(11), 2655–2667. doi:10.2337/db07-0882

44. Yates, T., Khunti, K., Wilmot, E. G., Brady, E., Webb, D., Srinivasan, B., et al. (2012). Self-Reported Sitting Time and Markers of Inflammation, Insulin Resistance, and Adiposity. *American Journal of Preventive Medicine, 42*(1), 1–7. doi:10.1016/j.amepre.2011.09.022

45. Pietiläinen, K. H., Naukkarinen, J., Rissanen, A., Saharinen, J., Ellonen, P., Keränen, H., et al. (2008). Global transcript profiles of fat in monozygotic twins discordant for BMI: pathways behind acquired obesity. *PLOS Medicine*, *5*(3), e51.

46. Sommer, F., & Bäckhed, F. (2013). The gut microbiota--masters of host development and physiology. *Nature Reviews Microbiology*, *11*(4), 227–238. doi:10.1038/nrmicro2974

47. Roos, V., Rönn, M., Salihovic, S., Lind, L., van Bavel, B., Kullberg, J., et al. (2013). Circulating levels of persistent organic pollutants in relation to visceral and subcutaneous adipose tissue by abdominal MRI. *Obesity*, *21*(2), 413–418. doi:10.1002/oby.20267

48. Lee, D.-H. (2012). Persistent Organic Pollutants and Obesity-Related Metabolic Dysfunction: Focusing on Type 2 Diabetes. *Epidemiology and Health*, *34*. doi:10.4178/epih/e2012002

49. Holtcamp, W. (2012, February). Obesogens: an environmental link to obesity. *Environmental Health Perspectives*, pp. a62–8. doi:10.1289/ehp.120-a62

50. Morino, K., Petersen, K. F., & Shulman, G. I. (2006). Molecular mechanisms of insulin resistance in humans and their potential links with mitochondrial dysfunction. *Diabetes*, *55*(Supplement 2), S9–S15. doi:10.2337/db06-S002

51. Ye, J. (2008). Emerging role of adipose tissue hypoxia in obesity and insulin resistance. *International Journal of Obesity*, *33*(1), 54–66. doi:10.1038/ijo.2008.229

52. Schwartz, R. S., Eltzschig, H. K., & Carmeliet, P. (2011). Hypoxia and inflammation. *N Engl J Med*, *364*(7), 656–665.

53. Ebbeling, C. B., Swain, J. F., Feldman, H. A., Wong, W. W., Hachey, D. L., Garcia-Lago, E., & Ludwig, D. S. (2012). Effects of dietary composition on energy expenditure during weight-loss maintenance. *JAMA*, *307*(24), 2627–2634.

54. Manuel-y-Keenoy, B., & Perez-Gallardo, L. (2012). Metabolic Impact of the Amount and Type of Dietary Carbohydrates on the Risk of Obesity and Diabetes. *Open Nutrition Journal*, 6, 21–34.

55. Bäckhed, F. (2011). Programming of host metabolism by the gut microbiota. *Annals of nutrition & metabolism*, 58 (Suppl 2), 44–52. doi:10.1159/000328042

56. Bray, G. A. (2007). How bad is fructose? *Am J Clin Nutr*, *86*(4), 895–896.

57. Shimer, S. (2012). Effects of Differentially Sweetened Beverages on Hepatic and Adipose De Novo Lipogenesis in Healthy Young Adults. n.p.: *ProQuest*, UMI Dissertations Publishing.

58. Stanhope, K. L., Griffen, S. C., Bremer, A. A., Vink, R. G., Schaefer, E. J., Nakajima, K., et al. (2011). Metabolic responses to prolonged consumption of glucose-and fructose-sweetened beverages are not associated with postprandial or 24-h glucose and insulin excursions. *Am J Clin Nutr*, *94*(1), 112–119. doi:10.3945/ajcn.110.002246

59. Stanhope, K. L., Schwarz, J.-M., Keim, N. L., Griffen, S. C., Bremer, A. A., Graham, J. L., et al. (2009). Consuming fructose-sweetened, not glucose-sweetened, beverages increases visceral adiposity and lipids and decreases insulin sensitivity in overweight/obese humans. *The Journal of Clinical Investigation,119*(5), 1322.

60. Lustig, R. H. (2010). Fructose: Metabolic, Hedonic, and Societal Parallels with Ethanol. *YJADA, 110*(9), 1307–1321. doi:10.1016/j.jada.2010.06.008

61. Purnell, J. Q., & Fair, D. A. (2013). Fructose Ingestion and Cerebral, Metabolic, and Satiety Responses of Fructose Ingestion and Satiety Responses. *JAMA, 309*(1), 85–86. doi:10.1001/jama.2012.190505

62. Vos, M. B., & McClain, C. J. (2009). Fructose takes a toll. *Hepatology, 50*(4), 1004–1006. doi:10.1002/hep.23212

63. Spruss, A., & Bergheim, I. (2009). Dietary fructose and intestinal barrier: potential risk factor in the pathogenesis of nonalcoholic fatty liver disease. *The Journal of Nutritional Biochemistry, 20*(9), 657–662. doi:10.1016/j.jnutbio.2009.05.006

64. Spreadbury, I. (2012). Comparison with ancestral diets suggests dense acellular carbohydrates promote an inflammatory microbiota, and may be the primary dietary cause of leptin resistance and obesity. *Diabetes, Metabolic Syndrome and Obesity: Targets and Therapy, 5*, 175–189. doi:10.2147/DMSO.S33473

65. Eaton, S. B. (2007). The ancestral human diet: what was it and should it be a paradigm for contemporary nutrition? *Proceedings of the Nutrition Society, 65*(01), 1–6. doi:10.1079/PNS2005471

66. Price, W. A. (1998). *Nutrition and physical degeneration.* Keats. ISBN: 9780879838164

67. Low, F. M., Gluckman, P. D., & Hanson, M. A. (2012). Developmental plasticity, epigenetics and human health. *Evolutionary Biology, 39*(4), 650–665. doi:10.1007/s11692-011-9157-0

68. Vandegehuchte, M. B., & Janssen, C. R. (2011). Epigenetics and its implications for ecotoxicology. *Ecotoxicology (London, England), 20*(3), 607–624. doi:10.1007/s10646-011-0634-0

69. Rodenhiser, D., & Mann, M. (2006). Epigenetics and human disease: translating basic biology into clinical applications. *Canadian Medical Association Journal, 174*(3), 341–348. doi:10.1503/cmaj.050774

70. Jirtle, R. L. (2008, March 19). Randy L. Jirtle, PhD: epigenetics a window on gene dysregulation, disease. Interview by Bridget M. Kuehn. *JAMA*, pp. 1249–1250. doi:10.1001/jama.299.11.1249

71. Zhang, X., & Ho, S. M. (2010). Epigenetics meets endocrinology. *Journal of Molecular Endocrinology, 46*(1), R11–R32. doi:10.1677/JME-10-0053

72. Slomko, H., Heo, H. J., & Einstein, F. H. (2012). Minireview: Epigenetics of Obesity and Diabetes in Humans. *Endocrinology, 153*(3), 1025–1030. doi:10.1210/en.2011-1759

73. Adamo, K. B., Ferraro, Z. M., & Brett, K. E. (2012). Can We Modify the Intrauterine Environment to Halt the Intergenerational Cycle of Obesity? *International Journal of Environmental Research and Public Health, 9*(4), 1263–1307. doi:10.3390/ijerph9041263

74. Rao, K. R., Padmavathi, I. J. N., & Raghunath, M. (2012). Maternal micronutrient restriction programs the body adiposity, adipocyte function and lipid metabolism in offspring: A review. *Reviews in Endocrine and Metabolic Disorders, 13*(2), 103–108. doi:10.1007/s11154-012-9211-y

75. Portha, B., Chavey, A., & Movassat, J. (2011). Early-life origins of type 2 diabetes: fetal programming of the beta-cell mass. *Experimental Diabetes Research, 2011*, 105076. doi:10.1155/2011/105076

76. Shillitoe, E., Weinstock, R., Kim, T., Simon, H., Planer, J., Noonan, S., & Cooney, R. (2012). The oral microflora in obesity and type-2 diabetes. *Journal of Oral Microbiology, 4*(0), 956. doi:10.1016/j.femsre.2004.01.003

77. Koren, O., Spor, A., Felin, J., Fåk, F., Stombaugh, J., Tremaroli, V., et al. (2011). Colloquium Paper: Human oral, gut, and plaque microbiota in patients with atherosclerosis. *Proceedings of the National Academy of Sciences, 108*(Supplement_1), 4592–4598. doi:10.1073/pnas.1011383107

78. Gürgan, C. A., Altay, U., & Ağbaht, K. (2012). Changes in Inflammatory and Metabolic Parameters After Periodontal Treatment in Obese and Non-Obese Patients. *Journal of Periodontology*. doi:10.1902/jop.2012.110646

79. Correa, F. O. B., Gonçalves, D., Figueredo, C. M. S., Bastos, A. S., Gustafsson, A., & Orrico, S. R. P. (2010). Effect of periodontal treatment on metabolic control, systemic inflammation and cytokines in patients with type 2 diabetes. *Journal of Clinical Periodontology, 37*(1), 53–58. doi:10.1111/j.1600-051X.2009.01498.x

80. Vidal, F., Figueredo, C. M. S., Cordovil, I., & Fischer, R. G. (2009). Periodontal therapy reduces plasma levels of interleukin-6, C-reactive protein, and fibrinogen in patients with severe periodontitis and refractory arterial hypertension. *Journal of Periodontology, 80*(5), 786–791. doi:10.1902/jop.2009.080471

81. Pottenger, F. M. (1995). *Pottenger's cats: a study in nutrition. 2nd Edition.* Price-Pottenger Nutrition Foundation. ISBN-13: 978-0916764067

82. Cordain, L., Toohey, L., Smith, M. J., & Hickey, M. S. (2000). Modulation of immune function by dietary lectins in rheumatoid arthritis. *The British journal of nutrition, 83*(3), 207–217.

83. Cordain, L., Eaton, S. B., Sebastian, A., Mann, N., Lindeberg, S., Watkins, B. A., et al. (2005). Origins and evolution of the Western diet: health implications for the 21st century. *Am J Clin Nutr, 81*(2), 341–354.

84. Nunn, A. V. W., Bell, J., & Barter, P. (2007). The integration of lipid-sensing and anti-inflammatory effects: how the PPARs play a role in metabolic balance. *Nuclear receptor, 5*(1), 1. doi:10.1186/1478-1336-5-1

CHAPTER 2: WHAT IS SICK FAT?

1. Tilg, H., & Moschen, A. R. (2006). Adipocytokines: mediators linking adipose tissue, inflammation and immunity. *Nature Reviews Immunology*, 6(10), 772–783. doi:10.1038/nri1937

2. FIX: Adipose Tissue as an Endocrine Organ. (2000). Adipose Tissue as an Endocrine Organ. *Trends in Endocrinology & Metabolism*, 6.

3. Zhang, H., & Zhang, C. (2009). Adipose "Talks" to Distant Organs to Regulate Insulin Sensitivity and Vascular Function. *Obesity*, 18(11), 2071–2076. doi:10.1038/oby.2010.91

4. Lee, J. (2013). Adipose tissue macrophages in the development of obesity-induced inflammation, insulin resistance and type 2 Diabetes. *Archives of Pharmacal Research*, 36(2), 208–222. doi:10.1007/s12272-013-0023-8

5. Caspar-Bauguil, S., Cousin, B., Galinier, A., Segafredo, C., Nibbelink, M., André, M., et al. (2005). Adipose tissues as an ancestral immune organ: Site-specific change in obesity. *FEBS Letters*, 579(17), 3487–3492. doi:10.1016/j.febslet.2005.05.031

6. Vissers, D., Hens, W., Taeymans, J., Baeyens, J.-P., Poortmans, J., & Van Gaal, L. (2013). The Effect of Exercise on Visceral Adipose Tissue in Overweight Adults: A Systematic Review and Meta-Analysis. (S. B. Votruba,Ed.)*PLoS ONE*, 8(2), e56415. doi:10.1371/journal.pone.0056415.s002

7. Bays, H., Blonde, L., & Rosenson, R. (2006). Adiposopathy: how do diet, exercise and weight loss drug therapies improve metabolic disease in overweight patients? *Expert Rev Cardiovasc Ther*, 4(6), 871–895. doi:10.1586/14779072.4.6.871

8. Ye, J. (2008). Emerging role of adipose tissue hypoxia in obesity and insulin resistance. *International Journal of Obesity*, 33(1), 54–66. doi:10.1038/ijo.2008.229

9   Ouchi, N., Parker, J. L., Lugus, J. J., & Walsh, K. (2011). Adipokines in inflammation and metabolic disease. *Nature Reviews Immunology*, 11(2), 85–97. doi:10.1038/nri2921

10. Gokalp, D., Bahceci, M., Ozmen, S., Arikan, S., Tuzcu, A., & Danıs, R. (2008). Adipocyte volumes and levels of adipokines in diabetes and obesity. *Diabetes and Metabolic Syndrome: Clinical Research and Reviews*, 2(4), 253–258. doi:10.1016/j.dsx.2008.07.001

11. Després, J.-P., & Lemieux, I. (2006). Abdominal obesity and metabolic syndrome. *Nature*, 444(7121), 881–887. doi:10.1038/nature05488

12. Chaldakov, G. N., Tonchev, A. B., Georgieva, Z., Ghenev, P. I., & Stankulov, I. S. (2005). Adipobiology of inflammation. *Biomedical Reviews*, 16, 83–88.

13. Drouet, M., Dubuquoy, L., Desreumaux, P., & Bertin, B. (2012). Visceral fat and gut inflammation. *Nutrition*, 28(2), 113–117. doi:10.1016/j.nut.2011.09.009

14. Unger, R. H. (2003). Minireview: weapons of lean body mass destruction: the role of ectopic lipids in the metabolic syndrome. *Endocrinology, 144*(12), 5159–5165. doi:10.1210/en.2003-0870

15. Bennett, B., Larson-Meyer, D. E., Ravussin, E., Volaufova, J., Soros, A., Cefalu, W. T., et al. (2009). Impaired Insulin Sensitivity and Elevated Ectopic Fat in Healthy Obese vs. Nonobese Prepubertal Children. *Obesity, 20*(2), 371–375. doi:10.1038/oby.2011.264

16. Juge-Aubry, C. E., Henrichot, E., & Meier, C. A. (2005). Adipose tissue: a regulator of inflammation. *Best Practice & Research Clinical Endocrinology & Metabolism, 19*(4), 547–566. doi:10.1016/j.beem.2005.07.009

17. Schipper, H. S., Prakken, B., Kalkhoven, E., & Boes, M. (2012). Adipose tissue-resident immune cells: key players in immunometabolism. *Trends in Endocrinology & Metabolism, 23*(8), 407–415. doi:10.1016/j. tem.2012.05.011

18. Odegaard, J. I., & Chawla, A. (2011). Alternative macrophage activation and metabolism. *Annual review of pathology, 6*, 275. doi:10.1146/annurev-pathol-011110-130138

19. Kominsky, D. J., Campbell, E. L., & Colgan, S. P. (2010). Metabolic Shifts in Immunity and Inflammation. *The Journal of Immunology, 184*(8), 4062–4068. doi:10.4049/jimmunol.0903002

20. Singla, P., Bardoloi, A., & Parkash, A. A. (2010). Metabolic effects of obesity: A review. *World Journal of Diabetes, 1*(3), 76. doi:10.4239/wjd.v1.i3.76

21. Laugerette, F., Vors, C., Peretti, N., & Michalski, M.-C. (2011). Complex links between dietary lipids, endogenous endotoxins and metabolic inflammation. *Biochimie, 93*(1), 39–45. doi:10.1016/j.biochi.2010.04.016

22. Vague J. La différenciation sexuelle: facteur déterminant des formes de l'obesité. Presse Med 1947; 339-40.

23. Haslam, D. (2007). Obesity: a medical history. *Obesity reviews : an official journal of the International Association for the Study of Obesity, 8 Suppl 1*, 31–36. doi:10.1111/j.1467-789X.2007.00314.x

24. Wajchenberg, B. L. (2000). Subcutaneous and visceral adipose tissue: their relation to the metabolic syndrome. *Endocrine Reviews, 21*(6), 697–738.

25. Harwood, H. J., Jr. (2012). The adipocyte as an endocrine organ in the regulation of metabolic homeostasis. *Neuropharmacology, 63*(1), 57–75. doi:10.1016/j.neuropharm.2011.12.010

26. Egger, G., & Dixon, J. (2008). Should obesity be the main game? Or do we need an environmental makeover to combat the inflammatory and chronic disease epidemics? *Obesity reviews : an official journal of the International Association for the Study of Obesity, 10*(2), 237–249. doi:10.1111/j.1467-789X.2008.00542.x

27. Weisberg, S. P., McCann, D., Desai, M., Rosenbaum, M., Leibel, R. L., & Ferrante, A. W. (2003). Obesity is associated with macrophage accumulation in adipose tissue. *Journal of Clinical Investigation, 112*(12), 1796–1808. doi:10.1172/JCI200319246

28. Lumeng, C. N., Deyoung, S. M., Bodzin, J. L., & Saltiel, A. R. (2007). Increased inflammatory properties of adipose tissue macrophages recruited during diet-induced obesity. *Diabetes*, *56*(1), 16–23. doi:10.2337/db06-1076

29. Wellen, K. E., & Hotamisligil, G. S. (2003). Obesity-induced inflammatory changes in adipose tissue. *Journal of Clinical Investigation*, *112*(12), 1785–1788. doi:10.1172/JCI20514

30. Curat, C. A., Wegner, V., Sengenes, C., Miranville, A., Tonus, C., Busse, R., & Bouloumié, A. (2006). Macrophages in human visceral adipose tissue: increased accumulation in obesity and a source of resistin and visfatin. *Diabetologia*, *49*(4), 744–747. doi:10.1007/s00125-006-0173-z

31. Lafontan, M. (2013). Adipose tissue and adipocyte dysregulation. *Diabetes & Metabolism*. doi:10.1016/j.diabet.2013.08.002 [Epub ahead of print]

32. Mitrou, P., Raptis, S. A., & Dimitriadis, G. (2013). Insulin action in morbid obesity: a focus on muscle and adipose tissue. *Hormones (Athens, Greece)*, *12*(2), 201–213.

33. Cancello, R., Tordjman, J., Poitou, C., Guilhem, G., Bouillot, J.-L., Hugol, D., et al. (2006). Increased infiltration of macrophages in omental adipose tissue is associated with marked hepatic lesions in morbid human obesity. *Diabetes*, *55*(6), 1554–1561. doi:10.2337/db06-0133

34. Ahlin, S., Sjöholm, K., Jacobson, P., Andersson-Assarsson, J. C., Walley, A., Tordjman, J., et al. (2013). Macrophage Gene Expression in Adipose Tissue is Associated with Insulin Sensitivity and Serum Lipid Levels Independent of Obesity. *Obesity*, n/a–n/a. doi:10.1002/oby.20443

35. Beutler, B., & Cerami, A. (1988). Tumor Necrosis, Cachexia, Shock, and Inflammation: A Common Mediator. *Annual Review of Biochemistry*, *57*, 505–518.

36. Shah, N. R., & Braverman, E. R. (2012). Measuring Adiposity in Patients: The Utility of Body Mass Index (BMI), Percent Body Fat, and Leptin. (Q. Nizami, Ed.)*PLoS ONE*, *7*(4), e33308. doi:10.1371/journal.pone.0033308.t004

37. Carpenter, C. L., Yan, E., Chen, S., Hong, K., Arechiga, A., Kim, W. S., et al. (2013). Body Fat and Body-Mass Index among a Multiethnic Sample of College-Age Men and Women. *Journal of Obesity*, *2013*(5), 1–7. doi:10.1152/japplphysiol.00086.2009

38. Kruschitz, R., Wallner-Liebmann, S. J., Hamlin, M. J., Moser, M., Ludvik, B., Schnedl, W. J., & Tafeit, E. (2013). Detecting Body Fat–A Weighty Problem BMI versus Subcutaneous Fat Patterns in Athletes and Non-Athletes. (A. A. Romanovsky, Ed.)*PLoS ONE*, *8*(8), e72002. doi:10.1371/journal.pone.0072002.s001

39. Kennedy, A. P., Shea, J. L., & Sun, G. (2009). Comparison of the Classification of Obesity by BMI vs. Dual-energy X-ray Absorptiometry in the Newfoundland Population. *Obesity*, *17*(11), 2094–2099. doi:10.1038/oby.2009.101

40. Yajnik, C. S. (2004). A critical evaluation of the fetal origins hypothesis and its implications for developing countries. *J. Nutr.*, *134*(205), 10.

41. Donini, L. M., Poggiogalle, E., Migliaccio, S., Aversa, A., & Pinto, A. (2013). Body composition in sarcopenic obesity: systematic review of the literature. *Mediterranean Journal of Nutrition and Metabolism*. doi:10.1007/s12349-013-0135-1

42. Sbarbati, A., Osculati, F., Silvagni, D., Benati, D., Galiè, M., Camoglio, F. S., et al. (2006). Obesity and inflammation: evidence for an elementary lesion. *PEDIATRICS*, *117*(1), 220–223. doi:10.1542/peds.2004-2854

43. Chatzigeorgiou, A., karalis, k. P., bornstein, S. r., & Chavakis, T. (2012). lymphocytes in obesity-related adipose tissue inflammation. *Diabetologia*, *55*(10), 2583–2592. doi:10.1007/s00125-012-2607-0

44. Maffeis, C., Silvagni, D., Bonadonna, R., Grezzani, A., Banzato, C., & Tatò, L. (2007). Fat Cell Size, Insulin Sensitivity, and Inflammation in Obese Children. *The Journal of Pediatrics*, *151*(6), 647–652. doi:10.1016/j.jpeds.2007.04.053

45. Nikolajczyk, B. S., Jagannathan-Bogdan, M., & Denis, G. V. (2012). The outliers become a stampede as immunometabolism reaches a tipping point. *Immunological Reviews*, *249*(1), 253–275. doi:10.1111/j.1600-065X.2012.01142.x

46. Michaud, A., Drolet, R., Noël, S., Paris, G., & Tchernof, A. (2012). Visceral fat accumulation is an indicator of adipose tissue macrophage infiltration in women. *Metabolism*, *61*(5), 689–698. doi:10.1016/j.metabol.2011.10.004

47. Batsis, J. A., Sahakyan, K. R., Rodriguez-Escudero, J. P., Bartels, S. J., Somers, V. K., & Lopez-Jimenez, F. (2013). Normal Weight Obesity and Mortality in United States Subjects ≥60 Years of Age (from the Third National Health and Nutrition Examination Survey). *The American Journal of Cardiology*, *112*(10), 1592–1598. doi:10.1016/j.amjcard.2013.07.014

48 Janssen, I., Katzmarzyk, P. T., & Ross, R. (2004). Waist circumference and not body mass index explains obesity-related health risk. *Am J Clin Nutr*, *79*(3), 379–384.

49. Brambilla, P., Bedogni, G., Heo, M., & Pietrobelli, A. (2013). Waist circumference-to-height ratio predicts adiposity better than body mass index in children and adolescents. *International Journal of Obesity*, *37*(7), 943–946. doi:10.1038/ijo.2013.32

50. Janssen, I., Katzmarzyk, P. T., & Ross, R. (2004). Waist circumference and not body mass index explains obesity-related health risk. *Am J Clin Nutr*, *79*(3), 379–384.

51. Carmienke, S., Freitag, M. H., Pischon, T., Schlattmann, P., Fankhaenel, T., Goebel, H., & Gensichen, J. (2013). General and abdominal obesity parameters and their combination in relation to mortality: a systematic review and meta-regression analysis. *European Journal of Clinical Nutrition*, *67*(6), 573–585. doi:10.1038/ejcn.2013.61

52. De Schutter, A., Lavie, C. J., Arce, K., Menéndez, J. A., & Milani, R. V. (2013). Correlation and discrepancies between obesity by body mass index and body fat in patients with coronary heart disease. *Journal of Cardiopulmonary Rehabilitation and Prevention*, *33*(2), 77–83. doi:10.1097/HCR.0b013e31828254fc

53. Donini, L. M., Poggiogalle, E., del Balzo, V., Lubrano, C., Faliva, M., Opizzi, A., et al. (2013). How to estimate fat mass in overweight and obese subjects. *International Journal of Endocrinology*, 2013, 285680. doi:10.1155/2013/285680

54. Wildman, R. P., Gu, D., Reynolds, K., Duan, X., & He, J. (2004). Appropriate body mass index and waist circumference cutoffs for categorization of overweight and central adiposity among Chinese adults. *Am J Clin Nutr*, *80*(5), 1129–1136.

55. Lopez-Miranda, J., & Perez-Martinez, P. (2013). It is time to define metabolically obese but normal-weight (MONW) individuals. *Clinical Endocrinology*, *79*(3), 314–315. doi:10.1111/cen.12181

56. Ruderman, N., Chisholm, D., Pi-Sunyer, X., & Schneider, S. (1998). The metabolically obese, normal-weight individual revisited. *Diabetes*, *47*(5), 699–713.

57. Gesta, S., Tseng, Y.-H., & Kahn, C. R. (2007). Developmental Origin of Fat: Tracking Obesity to Its Source. *Cell*, *131*(2), 242–256. doi:10.1016/j.cell.2007.10.004

58. Bordicchia, M., Liu, D., Amri, E.-Z., Ailhaud, G., Dessì-Fulgheri, P., Zhang, C., et al. (2012). Cardiac natriuretic peptides act via p38 MAPK to induce the brown fat thermogenic program in mouse and human adipocytes. *Journal of Clinical Investigation*, *122*(3), 1022–1036. doi:10.1172/JCI59701DS1

59. Bartelt, A., Merkel, M., & Heeren, J. (2012). A new, powerful player in lipoprotein metabolism: brown adipose tissue. *Journal of Molecular Medicine*, *90*(8), 887–893. doi:10.1007/s00109-012-0858-3

60. Wang, Q., Zhang, M., Ning, G., Gu, W., Su, T., Xu, M., et al. (2011). Brown Adipose Tissue in Humans Is Activated by Elevated Plasma Catecholamines Levels and Is Inversely Related to Central Obesity. (M. Ludgate, Ed.)*PLoS ONE*, *6*(6), e21006. doi:10.1371/journal.pone.0021006.t002

61. van Marken Lichtenbelt, W. D., Vanhommerig, J. W., Smulders, N. M., Drossaerts, J. M. A. F. L., Kemerink, G. J., Bouvy, N. D., et al. (2009). Cold-activated brown adipose tissue in healthy men. *New England Journal of Medicine*, *360*(15), 1500–1508. doi:10.1056/NEJMoa0808718

62. Bo, S., Ciccone, G., Durazzo, M., Ghinamo, L., Villois, P., Canil, S., et al. (2011). Contributors to the obesity and hyperglycemia epidemics. A prospective study in a population-based cohort. *International Journal of Obesity*, *35*(11), 1442–1449. doi:10.1038/ijo.2011.5

63. Tremblay, A., Royer, M.-M., Chaput, J. P., & Doucet, É. (2012). Adaptive thermogenesis can make a difference in the ability of obese individuals to lose body weight. *International Journal of Obesity, 37*(6), 759–764. doi:10.1038/ijo.2012.124

64. Schipper, H. S., Nuboer, R., Prop, S., van den Ham, H. J., de Boer, F. K., Kesmir, Ç., et al. (2012). Systemic inflammation in childhood obesity: circulating inflammatory mediators and activated CD14++ monocytes. *Diabetologia, 55*(10), 2800–2810. doi:10.1007/s00125-012-2641-y

65. Lumeng, C. N. (2013). Innate immune activation in obesity. *Molecular Aspects of Medicine, 34*(1), 12–29. doi:10.1016/j.mam.2012.10.002

66. Lumeng, C. N., & Saltiel, A. R. (2011). Inflammatory links between obesity and metabolic disease. *The Journal of Clinical Investigation, 121*(6), 2111–2117. doi:10.1172/JCI57132

67. Hotamisligil, G., Shargill, N., & Spiegelman, B. (1993). Adipose expression of tumor necrosis factor-alpha: direct role in obesity-linked insulin resistance. *Science, 259*(5091), 87–91. doi:10.1126/science.7678183

68. Hotamisligil, G. S., Arner, P., Caro, J. F., Atkinson, R. L., & Spiegelman, B. M. (1995). Increased adipose tissue expression of tumor necrosis factor-alpha in human obesity and insulin resistance. *Journal of Clinical Investigation, 95*(5), 2409–2415. doi:10.1172/JCI117936

69. Hotamisligil, G. S. (2006). Inflammation and metabolic disorders. *Nature, 444*(7121), 860–867. doi:10.1038/nature05485

70. Wellen, K. E., & Hotamisligil, G. S. (2005). Inflammation, stress, and diabetes. *Journal of Clinical Investigation, 115*(5), 1111–1119. doi:10.1172/JCI200525102DS1

71. Lord, G. M., Matarese, G., Howard, J. K., Baker, R. J., Bloom, S. R., & Lechler, R. I. (1998). Leptin modulates the T-cell immune response and reverses starvation-induced immunosuppression. *Nature, 394*(6696), 897–901.

72. Matarese, G., Procaccini, C., De Rosa, V., Horvath, T. L., & La Cava, A. (2010). Regulatory T cells in obesity: the leptin connection. *Trends in Molecular Medicine, 16*(6), 247–256. doi:10.1016/j.molmed.2010.04.002

73. Viikari, L. A., Huupponen, R. K., Viikari, J. S. A., Marniemi, J., Eklund, C., Hurme, M., et al. (2007). Relationship between Leptin and C-Reactive Protein in Young Finnish Adults. *Journal of Clinical Endocrinology & Metabolism, 92*(12), 4753–4758. doi:10.1210/jc.2007-0103

74. Park, J. S., Cho, M. H., Nam, J. S., Ahn, C. W., Cha, B. S., Lee, E. J., et al. (2009). Visceral adiposity and leptin are independently associated with C-reactive protein in Korean type 2 diabetic patients. *Acta Diabetologica, 47*(2), 113–118. doi:10.1007/s00592-009-0125-4

75. Matarese, G., & La Cava, A. (2004). The intricate interface between immune system and metabolism. *Trends in Immunology, 25*(4), 193–200. doi:10.1016/j.it.2004.02.009

76. Lago, R., Gómez, R., Lago, F., Gómez-Reino, J., & Gualillo, O. (2008). Leptin beyond body weight regulation—Current concepts concerning its role in immune function and inflammation. *Cellular Immunology, 252*(1-2), 139–145. doi:10.1016/j.cellimm.2007.09.004

77. Maachi, M., Pieroni, L., Bruckert, E., Jardel, C., Fellahi, S., Hainque, B., et al. (2004). Systemic low-grade inflammation is related to both circulating and adipose tissue TNF-α, leptin and IL-6 levels in obese women. *International Journal of Obesity, 28*(8), 993–997.

78. Bulló, M., García-Lorda, P., Megias, I., & Salas-Salvadó, J. (2003). Systemic inflammation, adipose tissue tumor necrosis factor, and leptin expression. *Obesity research, 11*(4), 525–531. doi:10.1038/oby.2003.74

79. Haiyan Xu, G. T. B. Q. Y. G. T. D. Y. C. J. C. J. S. A. N. J. S. R. L. A. T. H. C. (2003). Chronic inflammation in fat plays a crucial role in the development of obesity-related insulin resistance. *Journal of Clinical Investigation, 112*(12), 1821–1830. doi:10.1172/JCI19451

80. Cowie, C. C., Rust, K. F., Ford, E. S., Eberhardt, M. S., Byrd-Holt, D. D., Li, C., et al. (2009). Full accounting of diabetes and prediabetes in the US population in 1988–1994 and 2005–2006. *Diabetes Care, 32*(2), 287–294.

81. Hosler, A. S. (2009). Prevalence of self-reported prediabetes among adults participating in a community-based health awareness program, New York State. *Preventing Chronic Disease, 6*(2), A48.

82. Tabák, A. G., Herder, C., Rathmann, W., Brunner, E. J., & Kivimäki, M. (2012). Prediabetes: a high-risk state for diabetes development. *Lancet, 379*(9833), 2279–2290. doi:10.1016/S0140-6736(12)60283-9

83. Sliem, H., & Nasr, G. (2010). Aortic stiffness in prediabetic adults: relationship to insulin resistance. *Journal of clinical medicine research, 2*(2), 62–67. doi:10.4021/jocmr2010.03.269w

84. Nolan, C. J., Damm, P., & Prentki, M. (2011). Type 2 diabetes across generations: from pathophysiology to prevention and management. *Lancet, 378*(9786), 169–181. doi:10.1016/S0140-6736(11)60614-4

85. Boyle, J. P., Thompson, T. J., Gregg, E. W., Barker, L. E., & Williamson, D. F. (2010). Projection of the year 2050 burden of diabetes in the US adult population: dynamic modeling of incidence, mortality, and prediabetes prevalence. *Population Health Metrics, 8*(1), 29. doi:10.1186/1478-7954-8-29

86. Grundy, S. M. (2012). Prediabetes, metabolic syndrome, and cardiovascular risk. *JAC, 59*(7), 635–643.

87. Diabetes Overview. National Diabetes Information Clearinghouse. *National Diabetes Education Program*. Retrieved August 23, 2013, from http://diabetes.niddk.nih.gov/dm/pubs/overview/

88. Levi, J., Vinter, S., St Laurent, R., Segal, L., Lang, A., & Rayburn, J. (2013). F as in Fat. *Trust for America's Health* (The Robert Wood Johnson Foundation). Issue Report, August 2013.

89. Glickman, D., & Shalala, D. *Lots to Lose: How America's Health and Obesity crisis Threatens our Economic Future* (pp. 1–110). Bipartisan Policy Center. http://bipartisanpolicy.org/projects/lots-lose

90. Zimmet, P., Alberti, K., & Shaw, J. (2001). Global and societal implications of the diabetes epidemic. *Nature, 414*(6865), 782–787.

91. Lancet, T. (2012). Prediabetes and the potential to prevent diabetes. *The Lancet, 379*(9833), 2213. doi:10.1016/S0140-6736(12)60960-X

92. Scully, T. (2012). Diabetes in numbers. *Nature, 485*(7398), S2–3.

93. Ludwig, D. S. (2007). Childhood obesity—the shape of things to come. *N Engl J Med, 357*(23), 2325–2327.

94. Marvasti, F., & Stafford, R. S. (2012). From Sick Care to health Care — reengineering Prevention into the U.S. System. *New England Journal of Medicine, 367*(10), 889–891. doi:10.1056/nEjMp1206230

95. McCage, S., Albanese-O'Neill, A., & Everette, T. D. (2013). The Special Diabetes Program: Past Success, Future Promise. *Clinical Diabetes.*

96. Centers for Disease Control and Prevention. National Diabetes Fact Sheet: national estimates and general information on diabetes and prediabetes in the United States, 2011. Atlanta, GA: U.S. Department of Health and Human Services, Centers for Disease Control and Prevention, 2011.

97. Chen, L., Magliano, D. J., & Zimmet, P. Z. (2011). The worldwide epidemiology of type 2 diabetes mellitus—present and future perspectives. *Nature Reviews | Endocrinology, 8*(4), 228–236. doi:10.1038/nrendo.2011.183

98. Stringhini, S., Tabak, A. G., Akbaraly, T. N., Sabia, S., Shipley, M. J., Marmot, M. G., et al. (2012). Contribution of modifiable risk factors to social inequalities in type 2 diabetes: prospective Whitehall II cohort study. *BMJ, 345*(aug21 1), e5452–e5452. doi:10.1136/bmj.e5452

99. Freedman, D. H. (2012, February 1). How to Fix the Obesity Crisis: Scientific American. *Scientific American*, 40–47.

100. Sambataro, M., Perseghin, G., Lattuada, G., Beltramello, G., Luzi, L., & Pacini, G. (2012). Lipid accumulation in overweight type 2 diabetic subjects: relationships with insulin sensitivity and adipokines. *Acta Diabetologica*. doi:10.1007/s00592-011-0366-x

101. Wlodek, M. G. (2011). Development of a Standardized Clinical Protocol for Ranking Foods and Meals Based on Postprandial Triglyceride Responses: The Lipemic Index. *ISRN Vascular Medicine, 2011*. doi:10.5402/2011/936974

102. Kolovou, G. D., Mikhailidis, D. P., Kovar, J., Lairon, D., Nordestgaard, B. G., Ooi, T. C., et al. (2011). Assessment and clinical relevance of non-fasting and postprandial triglycerides: an expert panel statement. *Current vascular pharmacology, 9*(3), 258–270.

103. Brownlee, M. M. (1995). Advanced protein glycosylation in diabetes and aging. *Annual Review of Medicine, 46*(1), 223–234.

104. Nathan, D. M. (2009). International Expert Committee Report on the Role of the A1C Assay in the Diagnosis of Diabetes Response to Kilpatrick, Bloomgarden, and Zimmet. *Diabetes Care, 32*(12), e160–e160.

105. Cerami, A. (2012). The unexpected pathway to the creation of the HbA1c test and the discovery of AGE's. *Journal of Internal Medicine, 271*(3), 219–226.

106. Irshad, S., Riaz, R., & Ghafoor, F. (2012). Value of Serum Glycated Albumin in Prediction of Coronary Artery Disease in Type 2 Diabetes Mellitus. *Public Health Research, 2*(3), 37–42. doi:10.5923/j.phr.20120203.01

107. Cave, M. C., Hurt, R. T., Frazier, T. H., Matheson, P. J., Garrison, R. N., McClain, C. J., & McClave, S. A. (2008). Obesity, inflammation, and the potential application of pharmaconutrition. *Nutrition in Clinical Practice, 23*(1), 16–34.

108. Tahara, N., Yamagishi, S.-I., Matsui, T., Takeuchi, M., Nitta, Y., Kodama, N., et al. (2012). Serum levels of advanced glycation end products (AGEs) are independent correlates of insulin resistance in nondiabetic subjects. *Cardiovascular therapeutics, 30*(1), 42–48. doi:10.1111/j.1755-5922.2010.00177.x

109. Win, M. T. T., Yamamoto, Y., Munesue, S., Saito, H., Han, D., Motoyoshi, S., et al. (2011). Regulation of RAGE for attenuating progression of diabetic vascular complications. *Experimental Diabetes Research, 2012.* doi:10.1155/2012/894605

110. Rojas, A., González, I., Morales, E., Pérez-Castro, R., Romero, J., & Figueroa, H. (2011). Diabetes and cancer: Looking at the multiligand/RAGE axis. *World Journal of Diabetes, 2*(7), 108–113. doi:10.4239/wjd.v2.i7.108

111. Goldberg, T., Cai, W., Peppa, M., Dardaine, V., Baliga, B. S., Uribarri, J., & Vlassara, H. (2004). Advanced glycoxidation end products in commonly consumed foods. *YJADA, 104*(8), 1287–1291. doi:10.1016/j.jada.2004.05.214

112. URIBARRI, J. (2005). Diet-Derived Advanced Glycation End Products Are Major Contributors to the Body's AGE Pool and Induce Inflammation in Healthy Subjects. *Annals of the New York Academy of Sciences, 1043*(1), 461–466. doi:10.1196/annals.1333.052

113. Forbes, J. M., Cowan, S. P., Andrikopoulos, S., Morley, A. L., Ward, L. C., Walker, K. Z., et al. (2013). Glucose homeostasis can be differentially modulated by varying individual components of a western diet. *The Journal of Nutritional Biochemistry, 24*(7), 1251–1257. doi:10.1016/j.jnutbio.2012.09.009

114. Šebeková, K., & Somoza, V. (2007). Dietary advanced glycation endproducts (AGEs) and their health effects – PRO. *Molecular Nutrition & Food Research, 51*(9), 1079–1084. doi:10.1002/mnfr.200700035

115. Unoki, H., & Yamagishi, S.-I. (2008). Advanced Glycation End Products and Insulin Resistance. *Current Pharmaceutical Design, 14*(10), 987–989. doi:10.2174/138161208784139747

116. Willemsen, S., Hartog, J. W. L., Heiner-Fokkema, M. R., van Veldhuisen, D. J., & Voors, A. A. (2012). Advanced glycation end-products, a pathophysiological pathway in the cardiorenal syndrome. *Heart failure reviews*, *17*(2), 221–228. doi:10.1007/s10741-010-9225-z

117. Piarulli, F., Sartore, G., & Lapolla, A. (2013). Glyco-oxidation and cardiovascular complications in type 2 diabetes: a clinical update. *Acta Diabetologica*, *50*(2), 101–110. doi:10.1007/s00592-012-0412-3

118. Pincock, S. (2006). Paul Zimmet: fighting the "diabesity" pandemic. *The Lancet*, *368*(9548), 1643. doi:10.1016/S0140-6736(06)69682-7

119. Astrup, A., & Finer, N. (2000). Redefining type 2 diabetes:'diabesity' or 'obesity dependent diabetes mellitus'? *Obesity Reviews*, *1*(2), 57–59.

120. Bozorgmanesh, M., Hadaegh, F., & Azizi, F. (2011). Predictive performance of the visceral adiposity index for a visceral adiposity-related risk: Type 2 Diabetes. *Lipids in Health and Disease*, *10*(1), 88. doi:10.1186/1476-511X-10-88

121. Shafrir, E. (1997). Development and consequences of insulin resistance : Lessons from animals with hyperinsulinaemia. *Diabète et métabolisme*, *22*(2), 122–131.

122. Wang, G., Liu, X., Christoffel, K. K., Zhang, S., Wang, B., Liu, R., et al. (2010). Prediabetes is not all about obesity: association between plasma leptin and prediabetes in lean rural Chinese adults. *European Journal of Endocrinology*, *163*(2), 243–249. doi:10.1530/EJE-10-0145

123. McGill, H. C., McMahan, C. A., Herderick, E. E., Zieske, A. W., Malcom, G. T., Tracy, R. E., & Strong, J. P. (2002). Obesity accelerates the progression of coronary atherosclerosis in young men. *Circulation*, *105*(23), 2712–2718. doi:10.1161/01.CIR.0000018121.67607.CE

124. Bajraktari, G. (2012). Abnormal myocardial systolic and diastolic myocardial function in obese asymptomatic adolescents. *European Journal of Heart Failure Supplements*, *11*(S1), S142.

125. Olshansky, S. J., Passaro, D. J., Hershow, R. C., Layden, J., Carnes, B. A., Brody, J., et al. (2005). A potential decline in life expectancy in the United States in the 21st century. *N Engl J Med*, *352*(11), 1138–1145.

126. Rountree, R. (2010). Roundoc Rx: A Functional Medicine Approach to Metabolic Syndrome: Part 1—*Metabolic Syndrome Explained. Alternative and Complementary Therapies*, *16*(6), 319–323. doi:10.1089/act.2010.16605

127. Reaven, G. M. (1988). Banting lecture 1988. Role of insulin resistance in human disease. *Diabetes*, *37*(12), 1595–1607.

128. Reaven, G. M. (1993). Role of Insulin Resistance in Human Disease (Syndrome X): An Expanded Definition. *Annual Review of Medicine*, *44*(1), 121–131. doi:10.1146/annurev.me.44.020193.001005

129. Povel, C. M., Beulens, J. W., van der Schouw, Y. T., Dolle, M. E. T., Spijkerman, A. M. W., Verschuren, W. M. M., et al. (2013). Metabolic Syndrome Model Definitions Predicting Type 2 Diabetes and Cardiovascular Disease. *Diabetes Care, 36*(2), 362–368. doi:10.2337/dc11-2546

130. Kayaniyil, S., Harris, S. B., Retnakaran, R., Vieth, R., Knight, J. A., Gerstein, H. C., et al. (2013). Prospective association of 25(OH)D with metabolic syndrome. *Clinical Endocrinology*, n/a–n/a. doi:10.1111/cen.12190

131. Invitti, C., Maffeis, C., Gilardini, L., Pontiggia, B., Mazzilli, G., Girola, A., et al. (2006). Metabolic syndrome in obese Caucasian children: prevalence using WHO-derived criteria and association with nontraditional cardiovascular risk factors. *International Journal of Obesity, 30*(4), 627–633. doi:10.1038/sj.ijo.0803151

132. Ervin, R. B. (2009). Prevalence of metabolic syndrome among adults 20 years of age and over, by sex, age, race and ethnicity, and body mass index: United States. *National health statistics reports, 13*, 1–8.

133. Viggiano, D., De Filippo, G., Rendina, D., Fasolino, A., D'Alessio, N., Avellino, N., et al. (2009). Screening of Metabolic Syndrome in Obese Children: A Primary Care Concern. *Journal of Pediatric Gastroenterology and Nutrition, 49*(3), 329–334. doi:10.1097/MPG.0b013e31819b54b7

134. Saffari, F., Jalilolghadr, S., Esmailzadehha, N., & Azinfar, P. (2012). Metabolic syndrome in a sample of the 6-to 16-year-old overweight or obese pediatric population: a comparison of two definitions. *Therapeutics and Clinical Risk Management, 8*, 55. doi:10.2147/TCRM.S26673

135. Croymans, D. M., Sanchez, A., Barth, J. D., & Roberts, C. K. (2010). Carotid intima-media thickness, dietary intake, and cardiovascular phenotypes in adolescents: relation to metabolic syndrome. *Cell Metabolism, 59*(4), 533–539. doi:10.1016/j.metabol.2009.08.016

136. Stern, M. P. (1995). Diabetes and Cardiovascular Disease: The "Common Soil" Hypothesis. *Diabetes, 44*(4), 369–374.

137. Roth, J., Qiang, X., Marbán, S. L., Redelt, H., & Lowell, B. C. (2004). The Obesity Pandemic: Where Have We Been and Where Are We Going? *Obesity, 12*, 88S–101S. doi:10.1038/oby.2004.273

138. Collaboration, P. S. (2009). Body-mass index and cause-specific mortality in 900 000 adults: collaborative analyses of 57 prospective studies. *The Lancet, 373*(9669), 1083–1096. doi:10.1016/S0140-6736(09)60318-4

139. Wai, W. S., Dhami, R. S., Gelaye, B., Girma, B., Lemma, S., Berhane, Y., et al. (2012). Comparison of Measures of Adiposity in Identifying Cardiovascular Disease Risk Among Ethiopian Adults. *Obesity, 20*(9), 1887–1895. doi:10.1038/oby.2011.103

140. Peyrin-Biroulet, L., Gonzalez, F., Dubuquoy, L., Rousseaux, C., Dubuquoy, C., Decourcelle, C., et al. (2011). Mesenteric fat as a source of C reactive protein and as a target for bacterial translocation in Crohn's disease. *Gut, 61*(1), 78–85. doi:10.1136/gutjnl-2011-300370

141. Calabrò, P., Golia, E., Maddaloni, V., Malvezzi, M., Casillo, B., Marotta, C., et al. (2008). Adipose tissue-mediated inflammation: the missing link between obesity and cardiovascular disease? *Internal and Emergency Medicine, 4*(1), 25–34. doi:10.1007/s11739-008-0207-2

142. Bibbins-Domingo, K., Coxson, P., Pletcher, M. J., Lightwood, J., & Goldman, L. (2007). Adolescent overweight and future adult coronary heart disease. *N Engl J Med, 357*(23), 2371–2379.

143. Bombelli, M., Facchetti, R., Fodri, D., Brambilla, G., Sega, R., Grassi, G., & Mancia, G. (2013). Impact of body mass index and waist circumference on the cardiovascular risk and all-cause death in a general population: Data from the PAMELA study. *Nutrition, Metabolism and Cardiovascular Diseases, 23*(7), 650–656. doi:10.1016/j.numecd.2012.01.004

144. Ritchie, S. A., & Connell, J. M. C. (2007). The link between abdominal obesity, metabolic syndrome and cardiovascular disease. *Nutrition, Metabolism and Cardiovascular Diseases, 17*(4), 319–326. doi:10.1016/j.numecd.2006.07.005

145. Skinner, A. C., Steiner, M. J., Henderson, F. W., & Perrin, E. M. (2010, April 1). Multiple Markers of Inflammation and Weight Status: Cross-sectional Analyses Throughout Childhood. *Pediatrics.* doi:10.1542/peds.2009-2182

147. Di Bonito, P., Moio, N., Scilla, C., Cavuto, L., Sibilio, G., Forziato, C., et al. (2010). Preclinical manifestations of organ damage-associated with the metabolic syndrome and its factors in outpatient children. *Atherosclerosis, 213*(2), 611–615. doi:10.1016/j.atherosclerosis.2010.09.017

CHAPTER 3: METABOLISM MEETS IMMUNITY

1. Haslam, D. (2011). The history of obesity. *Clinical Obesity, 1*(4-6), 189–197.

2. Kershaw, E. E., & Flier, J. S. (2004). Adipose tissue as an endocrine organ. *Journal of Clinical Endocrinology & Metabolism, 89*(6), 2548–2556. doi:10.1210/jc.2004-0395

3. Samaras, K., Botelho, N. K., Chisholm, D. J., & Lord, R. V. (2009). Subcutaneous and Visceral Adipose Tissue Gene Expression of Serum Adipokines That Predict Type 2 Diabetes. *Obesity, 18*(5), 884–889. doi:10.1038/oby.2009.443

4. Harford, K. A., Reynolds, C. M., McGillicuddy, F. C., & Roche, H. M. (2011). Fats, inflammation and insulin resistance: insights to the role of macrophage and T-cell accumulation in adipose tissue. *Proceedings of the Nutrition Society,* 1–10. doi:10.1017/S0029665111000565

5. Kaminski, D. A., & Randall, T. D. (2010). Adaptive immunity and adipose tissue biology. *TRENDS in Immunology, 31*(10), 384–390. doi:10.1016/j.it.2010.08.001

6. Schäffler, A., & Schölmerich, J. (2010). Innate immunity and adipose tissue biology. *Trends in Immunology, 31*(6), 228–235. doi:10.1016/j.it.2010.03.001

7. Weisberg, S. P., McCann, D., Desai, M., Rosenbaum, M., Leibel, R. L., & Ferrante, A. W. (2003). Obesity is associated with macrophage accumulation in adipose tissue. *Journal of Clinical Investigation, 112*(12), 1796–1808. doi:10.1172/JCI200319246

8. Ghanim, H., Abuaysheh, S., Sia, C. L., Korzeniewski, K., Chaudhuri, A., Fernandez-Real, J. M., & Dandona, P. (2009). Increase in Plasma Endotoxin Concentrations and the Expression of Toll-Like Receptors and Suppressor of Cytokine Signaling-3 in Mononuclear Cells After a High-Fat, High-Carbohydrate Meal: Implications for insulin resistance. *Diabetes Care, 32*(12), 2281–2287. doi:10.2337/dc09-0979

9. Lionetti, L., Mollica, M. P., Lombardi, A., Cavaliere, G., Gifuni, G., & Barletta, A. (2009). From chronic overnutrition to insulin resistance: The role of fat-storing capacity and inflammation. *Nutrition, Metabolism and Cardiovascular Diseases, 19*(2), 146–152. doi:10.1016/j.numecd.2008.10.010

10. Lee, J. (2013). Adipose tissue macrophages in the development of obesity-induced inflammation, insulin resistance and type 2 Diabetes. *Archives of Pharmacal Research, 36*(2), 208–222. doi:10.1007/s12272-013-0023-8

11. Oh, D. Y., Morinaga, H., Talukdar, S., Bae, E. J., & Olefsky, J. M. (2012). Increased Macrophage Migration Into Adipose Tissue in Obese Mice. *Diabetes, 61*(2), 346–354. doi:10.2337/db11-0860

12. Nishimura, S., Manabe, I., Nagasaki, M., Eto, K., Yamashita, H., Ohsugi, M., et al. (2009). CD8+ effector T cells contribute to macrophage recruitment and adipose tissue inflammation in obesity. *Nature Medicine, 15*(8), 914–920. doi:10.1038/nm.1964

13. Wu, H., Ghosh, S., Perrard, X. D., Feng, L., Garcia, G. E., Perrard, J. L., et al. (2007). T-Cell Accumulation and Regulated on Activation, Normal T Cell Expressed and Secreted Upregulation in Adipose Tissue in Obesity. *Circulation, 115*(8), 1029–1038. doi:10.1161/Circulationaha.106.638379

14. Bruun, J. M., Lihn, A. S., Pedersen, S. B., & Richelsen, B. (2005). Monocyte chemoattractant protein-1 release is higher in visceral than subcutaneous human adipose tissue (AT): implication of macrophages resident in the AT. *Journal of Clinical Endocrinology & Metabolism, 90*(4), 2282–2289. doi:10.1210/jc.2004-1696

15. Schipper, H. S., Nuboer, R., Prop, S., van den Ham, H. J., de Boer, F. K., Kesmir, Ç., et al. (2012). Systemic inflammation in childhood obesity: circulating inflammatory mediators and activated CD14++ monocytes. *Diabetologia, 55*(10), 2800–2810. doi:10.1007/s00125-012-2641-y

16. Gui, T., Shimokado, A., Sun, Y., Akasaka, T., & Muragaki, Y. (2012). Diverse roles of macrophages in atherosclerosis: from inflammatory biology to biomarker discovery. *Mediators of Inflammation, 2012*, 693083. doi:10.1155/2012/693083

17. Creely, S. J., McTernan, P. G., Kusminski, C. M., Fisher, F. M., Da Silva, N. F., Khanolkar, M., et al. (2006). Lipopolysaccharide activates an innate immune system response in human adipose tissue in obesity and type 2 diabetes. *AJP: Endocrinology and Metabolism, 292*(3), E740–E747. doi:10.1152/ajpendo.00302.2006

18. Theoharides, T. C., Sismanopoulos, N., Delivanis, D.-A., Zhang, B., Hatziagelaki, E. E., & Kalogeromitros, D. (2011). Mast cells squeeze the heart and stretch the gird: their role in atherosclerosis and obesity. *Trends in Pharmacological Sciences, 32*(9), 534–542. doi:10.1016/j.tips.2011.05.005

19. Lloyd, C. M., & Saglani, S. (2013). Eosinophils in the Spotlight: Finding the link between obesity and asthma. *Nature Medicine, 19*(8), 976–977. doi:doi:10.1038/nm.3296

20. Aroor, A. R., McKarns, S., DeMarco, V. G., Jia, G., & Sowers, J. R. (2013). Maladaptive immune and inflammatory pathways lead to cardiovascular insulin resistance. *Metabolism*, 1–10. doi:10.1016/j.metabol.2013.07.001

21. Nishimura, S., Manabe, I., Nagasaki, M., Eto, K., Yamashita, H., Ohsugi, M., et al. (2009). CD8+ effector T cells contribute to macrophage recruitment and adipose tissue inflammation in obesity. *Nature Medicine, 15*(8), 914–920. doi:10.1038/nm.1964

22. Thewissen, M. M., Damoiseaux, J. G., Duijvestijn, A. M., van Greevenbroek, M. M., van der Kallen, C. J., Feskens, E. J., et al. (2009). Abdominal Fat Mass Is Associated With Adaptive Immune Activation: The CODAM Study. *Obesity, 19*(8), 1690–1698. doi:10.1038/oby.2010.337

23. Oh, D. Y., Morinaga, H., Talukdar, S., Bae, E. J., & Olefsky, J. M. (2012). Increased Macrophage Migration Into Adipose Tissue in Obese Mice. *Diabetes, 61*(2), 346–354. doi:10.2337/db11-0860

24. Winer, S., & Winer, D. A. (2012). The adaptive immune system as a fundamental regulator of adipose tissue inflammation and insulin resistance. *Immunology and Cell Biology, 90*(8), 755–762. doi:10.1038/icb.2011.110

25. Schulzke, J.-D., Günzel, D., John, L. J., & Fromm, M. (2012). Perspectives on tight junction research. *Annals of the New York Academy of Sciences, 1257*(1), 1–19. doi:10.1111/j.1749-6632.2012.06485.x

26. Yu, L. C.-H. (2012). Intestinal Epithelial Barrier Dysfunction in Food Hypersensitivity. *Journal of Allergy, 2012*, 1–11. doi:10.1155/2012/596081

27. Barrett, K. E. (2012). Epithelial biology in the gastrointestinal system: insights into normal physiology and disease pathogenesis. *The Journal of Physiology, 590*(Pt 3), 419–420. doi:10.1113/jphysiol.2011.227058

28. Teixeira, T. F. S., Souza, N. C. S., Chiarello, P. G., Franceschini, S. C. C., Bressan, J., Ferreira, C. L. L. F., & do Carmo G Peluzio, M. (2012). Intestinal permeability parameters in obese patients are correlated with metabolic syndrome risk factors. *Clinical Nutrition, 31*(5), 735–740. doi:10.1016/j.clnu.2012.02.009

29. Yu, L. C.-H., Wang, J.-T., Wei, S.-C., & Ni, Y.-H. (2012). Host-microbial interactions and regulation of intestinal epithelial barrier function: From physiology to pathology. *World Journal of Gastrointestinal Pathophysiology*, *3*(1), 27–43. doi:10.4291/wjgp.v3.i1.27

30. Hooper, L. V., Littman, D. R., & Macpherson, A. J. (2012). Interactions Between the Microbiota and the Immune System. *Science*, *336*(6086), 1268–1273. doi:10.1126/science.1223490

31. Jin, B., Sun, T., Yu, X.-H., Yang, Y.-X., & Yeo, A. E. T. (2012). The Effects of TLR Activation on T-Cell Development and Differentiation. *Clinical and Developmental Immunology*, *2012*, 1–32. doi:10.1155/2012/836485

32. Gewirtz, A. (2011). Physiological Interactions Between Toll-Like Receptors and the Microbiome. *Annual Review of Physiology*, *74*(1), 110301101907077. doi:10.1146/annurev-physiol-020911-153330

33. Wolowczuk, I., Verwaerde, C., Viltart, O., Delanoye, A., Delacre, M., Pot, B., & Grangette, C. (2008). Feeding our immune system: impact on metabolism. *Clinical and Developmental Immunology*, *2008*, 639803. doi:10.1155/2008/639803

34. Fu, C.-P., Sheu, W. H. H., Lee, I.-T., Tsai, I.-C., Lee, W.-J., Liang, K.-W., et al. (2013). Effects of weight loss on epicardial adipose tissue thickness and its relationship between serum soluble CD40 ligand levels in obese men. *Clinica Chimica Acta*, *421*, 98–103. doi:10.1016/j.cca.2013.03.005

35. Fournier, B. M., & Parkos, C. A. (2012). The role of neutrophils during intestinal inflammation. *Mucosal Immunology*, *5*(4), 354–366. doi:10.1038/mi.2012.24

36. Könner, A. C., & Brüning, J. C. (2011). Toll-like receptors: linking inflammation to metabolism. *Trends in endocrinology and metabolism: TEM*, *22*(1), 16–23. doi:10.1016/j.tem.2010.08.007

37. Shi, H., Kokoeva, M. V., Inouye, K., Tzameli, I., Yin, H., & Flier, J. S. (2006). TLR4 links innate immunity and fatty acid-induced insulin resistance. *Journal of Clinical Investigation*, *116*(11), 3015–3025. doi:10.1172/JCI28898

38. Abreu, M. T., Fukata, M., & Arditi, M. (2005). TLR signaling in the gut in health and disease. *J Immunol*, *174*(8), 4453–4460.

39. Curat, C. A., Miranville, A., Sengenes, C., Diehl, M., Tonus, C., Busse, R., & Bouloumié, A. (2004). From Blood Monocytes to Adipose Tissue-Resident Macrophages: Induction of Diapedesis by Human Mature Adipocytes. *Diabetes*, *53*(5), 1285–1292. doi:10.2337/diabetes.53.5.1285

40. Cox, C. L., Stanhope, K. L., Schwarz, J. M., Graham, J. L., Hatcher, B., Griffen, S. C., et al. (2011). Circulating Concentrations of Monocyte Chemoattractant Protein-1, Plasminogen Activator Inhibitor-1, and Soluble Leukocyte Adhesion Molecule-1 in Overweight/Obese Men and Women Consuming Fructose- or Glucose-Sweetened Beverages for 10 Weeks. *Journal of Clinical Endocrinology & Metabolism*, *96*(12), E2034–E2038. doi:10.1210/jc.2011-1050

41. Jin, C., & Flavell, R. A. (2013). Innate sensors of pathogen and stress: linking inflammation to obesity. *J Allergy Clin Immunol*, *132*(2), 287–294. doi:10.1016/j.jaci.2013.06.022

42. Vaishnava, S., & Hooper, L. V. (2011). Eat your carrots! T cells are RARing to go. *Immunity*, *34*(3), 290–292. doi:10.1016/j.immuni.2011.03.007

43. Sell, H., Habich, C., & Eckel, J. (2012). Adaptive immunity in obesity and insulin resistance. *Nature Reviews | Endocrinology*, *8*(12), 709–716. doi:10.1038/nrendo.2012.114

44. Pacifico, L., Di Renzo, L., Anania, C., Osborn, J. F., Ippoliti, F., Schiavo, E., & Chiesa, C. (2006). Increased T-helper interferon-γ-secreting cells in obese children. *European Journal of Endocrinology*, *154*(5), 691–697. doi:10.1530/eje.1.02138

45. Sumarac-Dumanovic, M., Stevanovic, D., Ljubic, A., Jorga, J., Simic, M., Stamenkovic-Pejkovic, D., et al. (2008). Increased activity of interleukin-23/interleukin-17 proinflammatory axis in obese women. International Journal of Obesity, 33(1), 151–156. doi:10.1038/ijo.2008.216

46. Winer, S., Paltser, G., Chan, Y., Tsui, H., Engleman, E., Winer, D., & Dosch, H.-M. (2009). Obesity predisposes to Th17 bias. *European Journal of Immunology*, *39*(9), 2629–2635. doi:10.1002/eji.200838893

47. O'rourke, R. W., & Lumeng, C. N. (2013). Editorials. *YGAST*, *145*(2), 282–285. doi:10.1053/j.gastro.2013.06.026

48. Heikamp, E. B., & Powell, J. D. (2013). Sensing the immune microenvironment to coordinate T cell metabolism, differentiation & function. *Seminars in Immunology*, *24*(6), 414–420. doi:10.1016/j.smim.2012.12.003

49. Liu, T. F., Brown, C. M., Gazzar, El, M., McPhail, L., Millet, P., Rao, A., et al. (2012). Fueling the flame: bioenergy couples metabolism and inflammation. *Journal of Leukocyte Biology*, *92*(3), 499–507. doi:10.1189/jlb.0212078

50. Wang, R., & Green, D. R. (2012). The immune diet: meeting the metabolic demands of lymphocyte activation. *F1000 biology reports*, *4*, 9. doi:10.3410/B4-9

51. Bertola, A., Ciucci, T., Rousseau, D., Bourlier, V., Duffaut, C., Bonnafous, S., et al. (2012). Identification of Adipose Tissue Dendritic Cells Correlated With Obesity-Associated Insulin-Resistance and Inducing Th17 Responses in Mice and Patients. *Diabetes*, *61*(9), 2238–2247. doi:10.2337/db11-1274

52. DeFuria, J., Belkina, A. C., Jagannathan-Bogdan, M., Snyder-Cappione, J., Carr, J. D., Nersesova, Y. R., et al. (2013). B cells promote inflammation in obesity and type 2 diabetes through regulation of T-cell function and an inflammatory cytokine profile. *Proceedings of the National Academy of Sciences of the United States of America*, *110*(13), 5133–5138. doi:10.1073/pnas.1215840110/-/DCSupplemental/pnas.201215840SI.pdf

53. Cildir, G., Akıncılar, S. C., & Tergaonkar, V. (2013). Chronic adipose tissue inflammation: all immune cells on the stage. *Trends in Molecular Medicine, 19*(8), 487–500. doi:10.1016/j.molmed.2013.05.001

54. Richardson, V. R., Smith, K. A., & Carter, A. M. (2013). Immunobiology. *Immunobiology, 218*(12), 1497–1504. doi:10.1016/j.imbio.2013.05.002

55. Xu, H. (2013). Obesity and metabolic inflammation. *Drug Discovery Today: Disease Mechanisms, 10*(1-2), e21–e25. doi:10.1016/j.ddmec.2013.03.006

56. Brooks-Worrell, B., & Palmer, J. P. (2011). Immunology in the Clinic Review Series; focus on metabolic diseases: development of islet autoimmune disease in type 2 diabetes patients: potential sequelae of chronic inflammation. *Clinical and Experimental Immunology, 167*(1), 40–46. doi:10.1111/j.1365-2249.2011.04501.x

57. McArdle, M. A., Finucane, O. M., Connaughton, R. M., McMorrow, A. M., & Roche, H. M. (2013). Mechanisms of obesity-induced inflammation and insulin resistance: insights into the emerging role of nutritional strategies. *Frontiers in endocrinology, 4*, 52. doi:10.3389/fendo.2013.00052

58. Ferrante, A. W., Jr. (2013). The immune cells in adipose tissue. *Diabetes, Obesity and Metabolism, 15*(s3), 34–38. doi:10.1111/dom.12154

59. Fan, H., Liu, Z., & Jiang, S. (2011). Th17 and regulatory T cell subsets in diseases and clinical application. *International Immunopharmacology, 11*(5), 533–535. doi:10.1016/j.intimp.2011.02.020

60. Bollrath, J., & Powrie, F. (2013). Feed Your Tregs More Fiber. *Science, 341*(6145), 463–464. doi:10.1126/science.1242674

61. Lee, B.-C., & Lee, J. (2013). Biochimica et Biophysica Acta. *BBA - Molecular Basis of Disease*, 1–17. doi:10.1016/j.bbadis.2013.05.017

62. Karelis, A. D. (2011, December). To be obese--does it matter if you are metabolically healthy? *Nature Reviews | Endocrinology,*, pp. 699–700. doi:10.1038/nrendo.2011.181

63. Lionetti, L., Mollica, M. P., Lombardi, A., Cavaliere, G., Gifuni, G., & Barletta, A. (2009). From chronic overnutrition to insulin resistance: the role of fat-storing capacity and inflammation. *Nutrition, metabolism, and cardiovascular diseases : NMCD, 19*(2), 146–152. doi:10.1016/j.numecd.2008.10.010

64. Fernández-Real, J.-M., & Pickup, J. C. (2008). Innate immunity, insulin resistance and type 2 diabetes. *Trends in Endocrinology and Metabolism: TEM, 19*(1), 10–16. doi:10.1016/j.tem.2007.10.004

65. Roth, J. (2009). Evolutionary speculation about tuberculosis and the metabolic and inflammatory processes of obesity. *JAMA: The Journal of the American Medical Association, 301*(24), 2586–2588.

66. Roth, J., Szulc, A. L., & Danoff, A. (2011). Energy, evolution, and human diseases: an overview. *American Journal of Clinical Nutrition, 93*(4), 875S–83. doi:10.3945/ajcn.110.001909

67. Hotamisligil, G. S. (2006). Inflammation and metabolic disorders. *Nature*, *444*(7121), 860–867. doi:10.1038/nature05485

68. Hotamisligil, G. S., & Erbay, E. (2008). Nutrient sensing and inflammation in metabolic diseases. *Nature Reviews Immunology*, *8*(12), 923–934. doi:10.1038/nri2449

69. Straub, R. H., Cutolo, M., Buttgereit, F., & Pongratz, G. (2010). Review: Energy regulation and neuroendocrine-immune control in chronic inflammatory diseases. *Journal of Internal Medicine*, *267*(6), 543–560. doi:10.1111/j.1365-2796.2010.02218.x

70. Spies, C. M., Straub, R. H., & Buttgereit, F. (2012). Energy metabolism and rheumatic diseases: from cell to organism. *Arthritis Research & Therapy*, *14*(3), 216. doi:10.1186/ar3885

71. Wellen, K. E., & Hotamisligil, G. S. (2005). Inflammation, stress, and diabetes. *Journal of Clinical Investigation*, *115*(5), 1111–1119. doi:10.1172/JCI200525102DS1

72. Conde, J., Scotece, M., Gómez, R., López, V., Gómez-Reino, J. J., Lago, F., & Gualillo, O. (2011). Adipokines: Biofactors from white adipose tissue. A complex hub among inflammation, metabolism, and immunity. *BioFactors*, *37*(6), 413–420. doi:10.1002/biof.185

73. Carbone, F., La Rocca, C., & Matarese, G. (2012). Immunological functions of leptin and adiponectin. *Biochimie*, *94*(10), 2082–2088. doi:10.1016/j.biochi.2012.05.018

74. Cava, A. L., & Matarese, G. (2004). The weight of leptin in immunity. *Nature Reviews Immunology*, *4*(5), 371–379. doi:10.1038/nri1350

75. Matarese, G., & La Cava, A. (2004). The intricate interface between immune system and metabolism. *TRENDS in Immunology*, *25*(4), 193–200. doi:10.1016/j.it.2004.02.009

76. Thomas, D. M., Bouchard, C., Church, T., Slentz, C., Kraus, W. E., Redman, L. M., et al. (2012). Why do individuals not lose more weight from an exercise intervention at a defined dose? An energy balance analysis. *Obesity reviews : an official journal of the International Association for the Study of Obesity*, *13*(10), 835–847. doi:10.1111/j.1467-789X.2012.01012.x

77. Volz, T., Kaesler, S., & Biedermann, T. (2012). Innate immune sensing 2.0 - from linear activation pathways to fine tuned and regulated innate immune networks. *Experimental Dermatology*, *21*(1), 61–69. doi:10.1111/j.1600-0625.2011.01393.x

78. Park, H., Bourla, A. B., Kastner, D. L., Colbert, R. A., & Siegel, R. M. (2012). Lighting the fires within: the cell biology of autoinflammatory diseases. *Nature Reviews Immunology*, *12*(8), 570–580. doi:10.1038/nri3261

79. Laugerette, F., Furet, J.-P., Debard, C., Daira, P., Loizon, E., Géloën, A., et al. (2012). Oil composition of high-fat diet affects metabolic inflammation differently in connection with endotoxin receptors in mice. *AJP: Endocrinology and Metabolism, 302*(3), E374–E386. doi:10.1152/ ajpendo.00314.2011

80. Lu, Y.-C., Yeh, W.-C., & Ohashi, P. S. (2008). LPS/TLR4 signal transduction pathway. *Cytokine, 42*(2), 145–151. doi:10.1016/j.cyto.2008.01.006

81. Manco, M., Putignani, L., & Bottazzo, G. F. (2010). Gut Microbiota, Lipopolysaccharides, and Innate Immunity in the Pathogenesis of Obesity and Cardiovascular Risk. *Endocrine Reviews, 31*(6), 817–844. doi:10.1210/ er.2009-0030

82. Miller, S. I., Ernst, R. K., & Bader, M. W. (2005). LPS, TLR4 and infectious disease diversity. *Nature Reviews Microbiology, 3*(1), 36–46. doi:10.1038/ nrmicro1068

83. Holland, W. L., Bikman, B. T., Wang, L.-P., Yuguang, G., Sargent, K. M., Bulchand, S., et al. (2011). Lipid-induced insulin resistance mediated by the proinflammatory receptor TLR4 requires saturated fatty acid–induced ceramide biosynthesis in mice. *The Journal of Clinical Investigation, 121*(5), 1858.

84. Piya, M. K., McTernan, P. G., & Kumar, S. (2013). Adipokine inflammation and insulin resistance: the role of glucose, lipids and endotoxin. *Journal of Endocrinology, 216*(1), T1–T15. doi:10.1530/JOE-12-0498

85. Tornatore, L., Thotakura, A. K., Bennett, J., Moretti, M., & Franzoso, G. (2012). The nuclear factor kappa B signaling pathway: integrating metabolism with inflammation. *Trends in Cell Biology*, 1–10. doi:10.1016/j. tcb.2012.08.001

86. Altman, B. J., & Dang, C. V. (2012). Normal and cancer cell metabolism: lymphocytes and lymphoma. *FEBS Journal, 279*(15), 2598–2609. doi:10.1111/j.1742-4658.2012.08651.x

87. Pearce, E. L., Poffenberger, M. C., Chang, C. H., & Jones, R. G. (2013). Fueling Immunity: Insights into Metabolism and Lymphocyte Function. *Science, 342*(6155), 1242454–1242454. doi:10.1126/science.1242454

88. Zeng H, Chi H. The interplay between regulatory T cells and metabolism in immune regulation. (2013) OncoImmunology; 2:e26586;

89. MacIver, N. J., Michalek, R. D., & Rathmell, J. C. (2013). Metabolic Regulation of T Lymphocytes. *Annual Review of Immunology, 31*(1), 259– 283. doi:10.1146/annurev-immunol-032712-095956

90. Schenk, S., Saberi, M., & Olefsky, J. M. (2008). Insulin sensitivity: modulation by nutrients and inflammation. *Journal of Clinical Investigation, 118*(9), 2992–3002. doi:10.1172/JCI34260

91. Saltiel, A. R. (2012). Insulin Resistance in the Defense against Obesity. *Cell Metab., 15*(6), 798–804. doi:10.1016/j.cmet.2012.03.001

92. Johnson, A. M. F., & Olefsky, J. M. (2013). The Origins and Drivers of Insulin Resistance. *Cell, 152*(4), 673–684. doi:10.1016/j.cell.2013.01.041

93. Dimitriadis, G., Mitron, P., Lambadiari, V., Maratou, E., & Raptis, S. A. (2011). Insulin effects in muscle and adipose tissue. *Diabetes Research and Clinical Practice*, *93*, S52–S59. doi:10.1016/S0168-8227(11)70014-6

94. Dhindsa, S., Tripathy, D., Mohanty, P., Ghanim, H., Syed, T., Aljada, A., & Dandona, P. (2004). Differential effects of glucose and alcohol on reactive oxygen species generation and intranuclear nuclear factor-κB in mononuclear cells. Metabolism, 53(3), 330–334. doi:10.1016/j.metabol.2003.10.013

95. Dickinson, S., Hancock, D. P., Petocz, P., Ceriello, A., & Brand-Miller, J. (2008). High-glycemic index carbohydrate increases nuclear factor-kappaB activation in mononuclear cells of young, lean healthy subjects. American Journal of Clinical Nutrition, 87(5), 1188–1193.

96. Ghanim, H., Mohanty, P., Pathak, R., Chaudhuri, A., Sia, C. L., & Dandona, P. (2007). Orange Juice or Fructose Intake Does Not Induce Oxidative and Inflammatory Response. Diabetes Care, 30(6), 1406–1411. doi:10.2337/dc06-1458

97. Aljada, A. A., Mohanty, P. P., Ghanim, H. H., Abdo, T. T., Tripathy, D. D., Chaudhuri, A. A., & Dandona, P. P. (2004). Increase in intranuclear nuclear factor kappaB and decrease in inhibitor kappaB in mononuclear cells after a mixed meal: evidence for a proinflammatory effect. American Journal of Clinical Nutrition, 79(4), 682–690.

98. Derosa, G., Ferrari, I., D'Angelo, A., Salvadeo, S. A. T., Fogari, E., Gravina, A., et al. (2009). Oral fat load effects on inflammation and endothelial stress markers in healthy subjects. *Heart and Vessels*, *24*(3), 204–210. doi:10.1007/s00380-008-1109-y

99. Peluso, I., Raguzzini, A., V Villano, D., Cesqui, E., Toti, E., Catasta, G., & Serafini, M. (2012). High Fat Meal Increase of IL-17 is Prevented by Ingestion of Fruit Juice Drink in Healthy Overweight Subjects. Current Pharmaceutical Design, 18(1), 85–90. doi:10.2174/138161212798919020

100. Skulas-Ray, A. C., Kris-Etherton, P. M., Teeter, D. L., Chen, C.-Y. O., Heuvel, J. P. V., & West, S. G. (2011). A High Antioxidant Spice Blend Attenuates Postprandial Insulin and Triglyceride Responses and Increases Some Plasma Measures of Antioxidant Activity in Healthy, Overweight Men. *Journal of Nutrition*, *141*(8), 1451–1457.

101. Ghanim, H., Sia, C. L., Korzeniewski, K., Lohano, T., Abuaysheh, S., Marumganti, A., et al. (2011). A Resveratrol and Polyphenol Preparation Suppresses Oxidative and Inflammatory Stress Response to a High-Fat, High-Carbohydrate Meal. *Journal of Clinical Endocrinology and Metabolism*, *96*(5), 1409–1414. doi:10.1210/jc.2010-1812

102. Kobayashi, M., Li, L., Iwamoto, N., Nakajima-Takagi, Y., Kaneko, H., Nakayama, Y., et al. (2009). The antioxidant defense system Keap1-Nrf2 comprises a multiple sensing mechanism for responding to a wide range of chemical compounds. *Molecular and Cellular Biology*, *29*(2), 493–502. doi:10.1128/MCB.01080-08

103. Singh, S., Vrishni, S., Singh, B. K., Rahman, I., & Kakkar, P. (2010). Nrf2-ARE stress response mechanism: A control point in oxidative stress-mediated dysfunctions and chronic inflammatory diseases. *Free Radical Research*, *44*(11), 1267–1288. doi:10.3109/10715762.2010.507670

104. Wang, R., & Green, D. R. (2012). Metabolic checkpoints in activated T cells. *Nature Publishing Group*, *13*(10), 907–915. doi:10.1038/ni.2386

105. Mohammed, N., Tang, L., Jahangiri, A., de Villiers, W., & Eckhardt, E. (2012). Elevated IgG levels against specific bacterial antigens in obese patients with diabetes and in mice with diet-induced obesity and glucose intolerance. *Metabolism: clinical and experimental*, *61*(9), 1211–1214. doi:10.1016/j.metabol.2012.02.007

106. Ailhaud, G. (2012). Is obesity an adaptative response to inflammation? *Obesity Reviews*, *13*(5), 480–481. doi:10.1111/j.1467-789X.2012.00995.x

107. Cani, P. D., Amar, J., Iglesias, M. A., Poggi, M., Knauf, C., Bastelica, D., et al. (2007). Metabolic Endotoxemia Initiates Obesity and Insulin Resistance. *Diabetes*, *56*(7), 1761–1772. doi:10.2337/db06-1491

108. Amar, J., Burcelin, R., Ruidavets, J. B., Cani, P. D., Fauvel, J., Alessi, M. C., et al. (2008). Energy intake is associated with endotoxemia in apparently healthy men. *American Journal of Clinical Nutrition*, *87*(5), 1219–1223.

109. Xiao, S., Fei, N., Pang, X., Shen, J., & Wang, L. (2013). A gut microbiota-targeted dietary intervention for amelioration of chronic inflammation underlying metabolic syndrome. *FEMS microbiology* doi:10.1111/1574-6941.12228

110. Fei, N., & Zhao, L. (2012). An opportunistic pathogen isolated from the gut of an obese human causes obesity in germfree mice. *The ISME Journal*, *7*(4), 880–884. doi:10.1038/ismej.2012.153

111. Hotamisligil, G. S. (2006). Inflammation and metabolic disorders. *Nature*, *444*(7121), 860–867. doi:10.1038/nature05485

112. Calay, E. S., & Hotamisligil, G. S. (2013). Turning off the inflammatory, but not the metabolic, flames. *Nature Medicine*, *19*(3), 265–267. doi:10.1038/nm.3114

113. Deng, T., Lyon, C. J., Minze, L. J., Lin, J., Zou, J., Liu, J. Z., et al. (2013). Class II Major Histocompatibility Complex Plays an Essential Role in Obesity-Induced Adipose Inflammation. *Cell Metabolism*, *17*(3), 411–422. doi:10.1016/j.cmet.2013.02.009

114. Pickup, J. C., Mattock, M. B., Chusney, G. D., & Burt, D. (1997). NIDDM as a disease of the innate immune system: association of acute-phase reactants and interleukin-6 with metabolic syndrome X. *Diabetologia*, *40*(11), 1286–1292. doi:10.1007/s001250050822

115. Pickup, J. C., & Crook, M. A. (1998). Is Type II diabetes mellitus a disease of the innate immune system? *Diabetologia*, *41*(10), 1241–1248. doi:10.1007/s001250051058

116. Tanti, J.-F., Ceppo, F., Jager, J., & Berthou, F. (2012). Implication of inflammatory signaling pathways in obesity-induced insulin resistance. *Frontiers in endocrinology*, *3*, 181. doi:10.3389/fendo.2012.00181

117. Straub, R. H. (2011). Concepts of evolutionary medicine and energy regulation contribute to the etiology of systemic chronic inflammatory diseases. *Brain, Behavior, and Immunity*, *25*(1), 1–5. doi:10.1016/j.bbi.2010.08.002

118. Straub, R. H. (2012). Evolutionary medicine and chronic inflammatory state—known and new concepts in pathophysiology. *Journal of Molecular Medicine*, *90*(5), 523–534. doi:10.1007/s00109-012-0861-8

119. Caro-Maldonado, A., Gerriets, V. A., & Rathmell, J. C. (2012). Matched and mismatched metabolic fuels in lymphocyte function. *Seminars in Immunology*, *24*(6), 405–413. doi:10.1016/j.smim.2012.12.002

120. A. Cynober et al. Nutrition and Critical Care: 8th Nestle Nutrition Series. Karger (2003) FIND MIKE

121. Kiecolt-Glaser, J. K., McGuire, L., Robles, T. F., & Glaser, R. (2002). Emotions, Morbidity, and Mortality: New Perspectives from Psychoneuroimmunology. *Annual Review of Psychology*, *53*, 83–107. doi:10.1146/annurev.psych.53.100901.135217

122. Chrousos, G. P. (2009). Stress and disorders of the stress system. *Nature Reviews | Endocrinology*, *5*(7), 374–381. doi:10.1038/nrendo.2009.106

123. Garg, A., Chren, M.-M., Sands, L. P., Matsui, M. S., Marenus, K. D., Feingold, K. R., & Elias, P. M. (2001). Psychological stress perturbs epidermal permeability barrier homeostasis: implications for the pathogenesis of stress-associated skin disorders. *Archives of Dermatology*, *137*(1), 53.

124. Brydon, L., Wright, C. E., O'Donnell, K., Zachary, I., Wardle, J., & Steptoe, A. (2007). Stress-induced cytokine responses and central adiposity in young women. *International Journal of Obesity*, *32*(3), 443–450.

125. Fleshner, M. (2012). Stress-evoked sterile inflammation, danger associated molecular patterns (DAMPs), microbial associated molecular patterns (MAMPs) and the inflammasome. *Brain, Behavior, and Immunity*, *27*(1), 1–7. doi:10.1016/j.bbi.2012.08.012

126. Bose, M., Oliván, B., & Laferrère, B. (2009). Stress and obesity: the role of the hypothalamic–pituitary–adrenal axis in metabolic disease. *Current Opinion in Endocrinology, Diabetes and Obesity*, *16*(5), 340. doi:10.1097/MED

127. Lupien, S. J., Mcewen, B. S., Gunnar, M. R., & Heim, C. (2009). Effects of stress throughout the lifespan on the brain, behaviour and cognition. *Nature Reviews Neuroscience*, *10*(6), 434–445. doi:10.1038/nrn2639

128. Heraclides, A. M., Chandola, T., Witte, D. R., & Brunner, E. J. (2012). Work stress, obesity and the risk of type 2 diabetes: gender-specific bidirectional effect in the Whitehall II study. *Obesity (Silver Spring)*, *20*(2), 428–433. doi:10.1038/oby.2011.95

129. Hajat, A., Diez-Roux, A. V., Sánchez, B. N., Holvoet, P., Lima, J. A., Merkin, S. S., et al. (2013). Examining the association between salivary cortisol levels and subclinical measures of atherosclerosis: The Multi-Ethnic Study of Atherosclerosis. *Psychoneuroendocrinology*, *38*(7), 1036–1046. doi:10.1016/j.psyneuen.2012.10.007

130. Flier, J. S., Underhill, L. H., & Chrousos, G. P. (1995). The hypothalamic–pituitary–adrenal axis and immune-mediated inflammation. *N Engl J Med*, *332*(20), 1351–1363.

131. Elenkov, I. J., & Chrousos, G. P. (2002). Stress hormones, proinflammatory and antiinflammatory cytokines, and autoimmunity. *Annals of the New York Academy of Sciences*, *966*(1), 290–303.

132. Black, P. H. (2003). The inflammatory response is an integral part of the stress response: Implications for atherosclerosis, insulin resistance, type II diabetes and metabolic syndrome X. *Brain, Behavior, and Immunity*, *17*(5), 350–364.

133. Otsuka, R., Yatsuya, H., Tamakoshi, K., Matsushita, K., Wada, K., & Toyoshima, H. (2006). Perceived psychological stress and serum leptin concentrations in Japanese men. *Obesity*, *14*(10), 1832–1838.

134. Martens, M. J., Rutters, F., Lemmens, S. G., Born, J. M., & Westerterp-Plantenga, M. S. (2010). Effects of single macronutrients on serum cortisol concentrations in normal weight men. *Physiology and Behavior*, *101*(5), 563–567. doi:10.1016/j.physbeh.2010.09.007

135. Gonzalez-Bono, E., Rohleder, N., Hellhammer, D. H., Salvador, A., & Kirschbaum, C. (2002). Glucose but Not Protein or Fat Load Amplifies the Cortisol Response to Psychosocial Stress. *Hormones and Behavior*, *41*(3), 328–333. doi:10.1006/hbeh.2002.1766

136. Macfarlane, D. P., Forbes, S., & Walker, B. R. (2008). Glucocorticoids and fatty acid metabolism in humans: fuelling fat redistribution in the metabolic syndrome. *Journal of Endocrinology*, *197*(2), 189–204. doi:10.1677/JOE-08-0054

137. Sanghez, V., Razzoli, M., Carobbio, S., Campbell, M., McCallum, J., Cero, C., et al. (2013). Psychosocial stress induces hyperphagia and exacerbates diet-induced insulin resistance and the manifestations of the Metabolic Syndrome. *Psychoneuroendocrinology*, *38*(12), 2933–2942. doi:10.1016/j.psyneuen.2013.07.022

138. Stimson, R. H., Andrew, R., McAvoy, N. C., Tripathi, D., Hayes, P. C., & Walker, B. R. (2011). Increased Whole-Body and Sustained Liver Cortisol Regeneration by 11 -Hydroxysteroid Dehydrogenase Type 1 in Obese Men With Type 2 Diabetes Provides a Target for Enzyme Inhibition. *Diabetes*, *60*(3), 720–725. doi:10.2337/db10-0726

139. Tomlinson, J. W., Finney, J., Hughes, B. A., Hughes, S. V., & Stewart, P. M. (2008). Reduced Glucocorticoid Production Rate, Decreased 5 -Reductase Activity, and Adipose Tissue Insulin Sensitization After Weight Loss. *Diabetes*, *57*(6), 1536–1543. doi:10.2337/db08-0094

140. Stimson, R. H., Johnstone, A. M., Homer, N. Z. M., Wake, D. J., Morton, N. M., Andrew, R., et al. (2007). Dietary Macronutrient Content Alters Cortisol Metabolism Independently of Body Weight Changes in Obese Men. *Journal of Clinical Endocrinology & Metabolism, 92*(11), 4480–4484. doi:10.1210/jc.2007-0692

141. Rutters, F., Fleur, S., Lemmens, S., Born, J., Martens, M., & Adam, T. (2012). The Hypothalamic-Pituitary-Adrenal Axis, Obesity, and Chronic Stress Exposure: Foods and HPA Axis. *Current Obesity Reports, 1*(4), 199–207. doi:10.1007/s13679-012-0024-9

142. Kyrou, I., Chrousos, G. P., & Tsigos, C. (2006). Stress, Visceral Obesity, and Metabolic Complications. *Annals of the New York Academy of Sciences, 1083*(1), 77–110. doi:10.1196/annals.1367.008

143. Novak, M., Björck, L., Giang, K. W., Heden-Ståhl, C., Wilhelmsen, L., & Rosengren, A. (2012). Perceived stress and incidence of Type 2 diabetes: a 35-year follow-up study of middle-aged Swedish men. *Diabetic Medicine, 30*(1), e8–e16. doi:10.1111/dme.12037

144. Scott, K. A., Melhorn, S. J., & Sakai, R. R. (2012). Effects of Chronic Social Stress on Obesity. *Current Obesity Reports, 1*(1), 16–25. doi:10.1007/s13679-011-0006-3

145. Amar, J., Serino, M., Lange, C., Chabo, C., Iacovoni, J., Mondot, S., et al. (2011). Involvement of tissue bacteria in the onset of diabetes in humans: evidence for a concept. *Diabetologia, 54*(12), 3055–3061. doi:10.1007/s00125-011-2329-8

146. Amar, J., Chabo, C., Waget, A., Klopp, P., Vachoux, C., Bermúdez-Humarán, L. G., et al. (2012). Intestinal mucosal adherence and translocation of commensal bacteria at the early onset of type 2 diabetes: molecular mechanisms and probiotic treatment. *EMBO Molecular Medicine, 3*(9), 559–572. doi:10.1002/emmm.201100159

147. Amar, J., Lange, C., Payros, G., Garret, C., Chabo, C., Lantieri, O., et al. (2013). Blood Microbiota Dysbiosis Is Associated with the Onset of Cardiovascular Events in a Large General Population: The D.E.S.I.R. Study. *PLoS ONE, 8*(1), e54461. doi:10.1371/journal.pone.0054461.t004

148. Erridge, C. (2011). Diet, commensals and the intestine as sources of pathogen-associated molecular patterns in atherosclerosis, type 2 diabetes and non-alcoholic fatty liver disease. *Atherosclerosis, 216*(1), 1–6. doi:10.1016/j.atherosclerosis.2011.02.043

149. Lumeng, C. N., & Saltiel, A. R. (2011). Inflammatory links between obesity and metabolic disease. *The Journal of Clinical Investigation, 121*(6), 2111–2117. doi:10.1172/JCI57132

150. Yin, J., Gao, Z., He, Q., Zhou, D., Guo, Z., & Ye, J. (2008). Role of hypoxia in obesity-induced disorders of glucose and lipid metabolism in adipose tissue. *AJP: Endocrinology and Metabolism, 296*(2), E333–E342. doi:10.1152/ajpendo.90760.2008

151. Blüher, M. (2013). Adipose tissue dysfunction contributes to obesity related metabolic diseases. *Best Practice & Research Clinical Endocrinology & Metabolism, 27*(2), 163–177. doi:10.1016/j.beem.2013.02.005

152. Kayser, B., & Verges, S. (2013). Hypoxia, energy balance and obesity: from pathophysiological mechanisms to new treatment strategies. *Obesity Reviews, 14*(7), 579–592. doi:10.1111/obr.12034

153. Zaldivar, F., McMurray, R. G., Nemet, D., Galassetti, P., Mills, P. J., & Cooper, D. M. (2006). Body fat and circulating leukocytes in children. *International Journal of Obesity, 30*(6), 906–911. doi:10.1038/sj.ijo.0803227

154. Mauras, N., DelGiorno, C., Kollman, C., Bird, K., Morgan, M., Sweeten, S., et al. (2010). Obesity without Established Comorbidities of the Metabolic Syndrome Is Associated with a Proinflammatory and Prothrombotic State, Even before the Onset of Puberty in Children. *Journal of Clinical Endocrinology & Metabolism, 95*(3), 1060–1068. doi:10.1210/jc.2009-1887

155. Giordano, P., Del Vecchio, G. C., Cecinati, V., Delvecchio, M., Altomare, M., De Palma, F., et al. (n.d.). Metabolic, inflammatory, endothelial and haemostatic markers in a group of Italian obese children and adolescents. *European Journal of Pediatrics, 170*(7), 845–850. doi:10.1007/s00431-010-1356-7

156. Galcheva, S. V., Iotova, V. M., Yotov, Y. T., Bernasconi, S., & Street, M. E. (2011). Circulating proinflammatory peptides related to abdominal adiposity and cardiometabolic risk factors in healthy prepubertal children. *European Journal of Endocrinology, 164*(4), 553–558. doi:10.1530/EJE-10-1124

157. Fadini, G. P., Marcuzzo, G., Marescotti, M. C., Kreutzenberg, S. V., & Avogaro, A. (2012). Elevated white blood cell count is associated with prevalence and development of the metabolic syndrome and its components in the general population. *Acta Diabetologica, 49*(6), 445–451. doi:10.1007/s00592-012-0402-5

158. Wu, C.-Z., Lin, J. D., Li, J.-C., Kuo, S.-W., Hsieh, C.-H., Lian, W.-C., et al. (2009). Association between white blood cell count and components of metabolic syndrome. *Pediatrics International, 51*(1), 14–18. doi:10.1111/j.1442-200X.2008.02658.x

159. Wu, C.-Z., Hsiao, F.-C., Lin, J.-D., Su, C.-C., Wang, K.-S., Chu, Y.-M., et al. (2009). Relationship between white blood cell count and components of metabolic syndrome among young adolescents. *Acta Diabetologica, 47*(1), 65–71. doi:10.1007/s00592-009-0101-z

160. McMurray, R. G., Zaldivar, F., Galassetti, P., Larson, J., Eliakim, A., Nemet, D., & Cooper, D. M. (2007). Cellular Immunity and Inflammatory Mediator Responses to Intense Exercise in Overweight Children and Adolescents. *Journal of Investigative Medicine, 55*(03), 120. doi:10.2310/6650.2007.06031

161. Meng, W., Zhang, C., Zhang, Q., Song, X., Lin, H., Zhang, D., et al. (2012). Association between Leukocyte and Metabolic Syndrome in Urban Han Chinese: A Longitudinal Cohort Study. *PLoS ONE*, *7*(11), e49875. doi:10.1371/journal.pone.0049875.s013

162. Schipper, H. S., Prakken, B., Kalkhoven, E., & Boes, M. (2012). Adipose tissue-resident immune cells: key players in immunometabolism. *Trends in Endocrinology & Metabolism*, *23*(8), 407–415. doi:10.1016/j.tem.2012.05.011

163. Kolb, H., & Mandrup-Poulsen, T. (2005). An immune origin of type 2 diabetes? *Diabetologia*, *48*(6), 1038–1050. doi:10.1007/s00125-005-1764-9

164. Nikolajczyk, B. S., Jagannathan-Bogdan, M., Shin, H., & Gyurko, R. (2011). State of the union between metabolism and the immune system in type 2 diabetes. *Genes and Immunity*, *12*(4), 239–250. doi:10.1038/gene.2011.14

165. Monteiro, R., & Azevedo, I. (2010). Chronic Inflammation in Obesity and the Metabolic Syndrome. *Mediators of Inflammation*, *2010*, 1–10. doi:10.1155/2010/289645

166. Dhurandhar, N. V. (2001). Infectobesity: obesity of infectious origin. *The Journal of Nutrition*, *131*(10), 2794S–2797S.

167. Na, H.-N., & Nam, J.-H. (2011). Infectobesity: a New Area for Microbiological and Virological Research. *Journal of Bacteriology and Virology*, *41*(2), 65. doi:10.4167/jbv.2011.41.2.65

168. Genoni, G., Prodam, F., Marolda, A., Giglione, E., Demarchi, I., Bellone, S., & Bona, G. (2013). Obesity and infection: two sides of one coin. *European Journal of Pediatrics*. doi:10.1007/s00431-013-2178-1

169. Gürgan, C. A., Altay, U., & Ağbaht, K. (2012). Changes in Inflammatory and Metabolic Parameters After Periodontal Treatment in Obese and Non-Obese Patients. *Journal of Periodontology*. doi:10.1902/jop.2012.110646

170. Correa, F. O. B., Gonçalves, D., Figueredo, C. M. S., Bastos, A. S., Gustafsson, A., & Orrico, S. R. P. (2010). Effect of periodontal treatment on metabolic control, systemic inflammation and cytokines in patients with type 2 diabetes. *Journal of Clinical Periodontology*, *37*(1), 53–58. doi:10.1111/j.1600-051X.2009.01498.x

171. Qin, J., Li, Y., Cai, Z., Li, S., Zhu, J., Zhang, F., et al. (2012). A metagenome-wide association study of gut microbiota in type 2 diabetes. *Nature*, *490*(7418), 55–60. doi:10.1038/nature11450

172. Burcelin, R., Garidou, L., & Pomié, C. (2012). Immuno-microbiota cross and talk: The new paradigm of metabolic diseases. *Seminars in Immunology*, 1–8. doi:10.1016/j.smim.2011.11.011

173. De Bandt, J.-P., Waligora-Dupriet, A.-J., & Butel, M.-J. (2011). Intestinal microbiota in inflammation and insulin resistance: relevance to humans. *Current Opinion in Clinical Nutrition and Metabolic Care*, *14*(4), 334–340. doi:10.1097/MCO.0b013e328347924a

174. Gabbert, C., Donohue, M., Arnold, J., & Schwimmer, J. B. (2010). Adenovirus 36 and Obesity in Children and Adolescents. *PEDIATRICS*, *126*(4), 721–726. doi:10.1542/peds.2009-3362

175. Atkinson, R. L., Dhurandhar, N. V., Allison, D. B., Bowen, R. L., Israel, B. A., Albu, J. B., & Augustus, A. S. (2004). Human adenovirus-36 is associated with increased body weight and paradoxical reduction of serum lipids. *International Journal of Obesity*, *29*(3), 281–286. doi:10.1038/sj.ijo.0802830

176. Desruisseaux, M. S., Trujillo, M. E., Tanowitz, H. B., & Scherer, P. E. (2007). Adipocyte, adipose tissue, and infectious disease. *Infection and Immunity*, *75*(3), 1066–1078.

177. Snyder-Cappione, J. E., & Nikolajczyk, B. S. (2013). When diet and exercise are not enough, think immunomodulation. *Molecular Aspects of Medicine*, *34*(1), 30–38. doi:10.1016/j.mam.2012.10.003

178. Lamas, O., Marti, A., & Martínez, J. A. (2002). Obesity and immunocompetence. *European Journal of Clinical Nutrition*, *56 Suppl 3*, S42–5. doi:10.1038/sj.ejcn.1601484

179. Nieman, D. C., Henson, D. A., Nehlsen-Cannarella,S. L., EKKENS, M., Utter, A. C., Butterworth, D. E., & Fagoaga, O. R. (1999). Influence of Obesity on Immune Function. *Journal of the American Dietetic Association*, *99*(3), 294–299. doi:10.1016/S0002-8223(99)00077-2

180. Falagas, M. E., & Kompoti, M. (2006). Obesity and infection. *The Lancet Infectious Diseases*, *6*(7), 438–446. doi:10.1016/S1473-3099(06)70523-0

181. Dhurandhar, N. V., Kulkarni, P. R., Ajinkya, S. M., Sherikar, A. A., & Atkinson, R. L. (1997). Association of adenovirus infection with human obesity. *Obesity research*, *5*(5), 464–469.

182. Trovato, G. M., Martines, G. F., Garozzo, A., Tonzuso, A., Timpanaro, R., Pirri, C., et al. (2010). Ad36 adipogenic adenovirus in human non-alcoholic fatty liver disease. *Liver International*, *30*(2), 184–190. doi:10.1111/j.1478-3231.2009.02127.x

183. Trovato, G. M., Castro, A., Tonzuso, A., Garozzo, A., Martines, G. F., Pirri, C., et al. (2009). Human obesity relationship with Ad36 adenovirus and insulin resistance. *International Journal of Obesity*, 1–8. doi:10.1038/ijo.2009.196

184. Fernández-Real, J.-M., Ferri, M.-J., Vendrell, J., & Ricart, W. (2007). Burden of infection and fat mass in healthy middle-aged men. *Obesity (Silver Spring)*, *15*(1), 245–252. doi:10.1038/oby.2007.541

185. Atkinson, R. L., Lee, I., Shin, H.-J., & He, J. (2010). Human adenovirus-36 antibody status is associated with obesity in children. *International Journal of Pediatric Obesity*, *5*(2), 157–160.

186. Morgan, O. W., Bramley, A., Fowlkes, A., Freedman, D. S., Taylor, T. H., Gargiullo, P., et al. (2010). Morbid Obesity as a Risk Factor for Hospitalization and Death Due to 2009 Pandemic Influenza A(H1N1) Disease. *PLoS ONE*, *5*(3), e9694. doi:10.1371/journal.pone.0009694.s001

187. Louie, J. K., Acosta, M., Samuel, M. C., Schechter, R., Vugia, D. J., Harriman, K., et al. (2011). A Novel Risk Factor for a Novel Virus: Obesity and 2009 Pandemic Influenza A (H1N1). *Clinical Infectious Diseases, 52*(3), 301–312. doi:10.1093/cid/ciq152

188. O'Shea, D., Cawood, T. J., O'Farrelly, C., & Lynch, L. (2010). Natural Killer Cells in Obesity: Impaired Function and Increased Susceptibility to the Effects of Cigarette Smoke. *PLoS ONE, 5*(1), e8660. doi:10.1371/journal.pone.0008660.g005

189. O'Shea, D., Corrigan, M., Dunne, M. R., Jackson, R., Woods, C., Gaoatswe, G., et al. (2013). Changes in human dendritic cell number and function in severe obesity may contribute to increased susceptibility to viral infection. *International Journal of Obesity, 37*(11), 1510–1513. doi:10.1038/ijo.2013.16

190. Nieman, D. C., Nehlsen-Cannalrella, S. L., Henson, D. A., Koch, A. J., Butterworth, D. E., Fagoaga, O. R., & Utter, A. (1998). Immune response to exercise training and/or energy restriction in obese women. *Medicine & Science in Sports & Exercise, 30*(5), 679–686.

191. Boroni Moreira, A. P., Fiche Salles Teixeira, T., do C Gouveia Peluzio, M., & de Cássia Gonçalves Alfenas, R. (2012). Gut microbiota and the development of obesity. *Nutrición hospitalaria, 27*(5), 1408–1414. doi:10.3305/nh.2012.27.5.5887

192. Lumeng, C. N. (2013). Innate immune activation in obesity. *Molecular Aspects of Medicine, 34*(1), 12–29.

CHAPTER 4: TURN ON FAT BURNING

1. Guilherme, A., Virbasius, J. V., Puri, V., & Czech, M. P. (2008). Adipocyte dysfunctions linking obesity to insulin resistance and type 2 diabetes. *Nature Reviews Molecular Cell Biology, 9*(5), 367–377. doi:10.1038/nrm2391

2. Corkey, B. E., & Shirihai, O. (2012). Metabolic master regulators: sharinginformation among multiple systems. *Trends in Endocrinology & Metabolism, 23*(12), 548–555. doi:10.1016/j.tem.2012.07.006

3. Biochem

4. Guttridge, K. H. F. D. G. D., Glass, D. J., & Guttridge, D. C. (2012). Cancer Cachexia:Mediators, Signaling, and Metabolic Pathways. *Cell Metab., 16*(2), 153–166. doi:10.1016/j.cmet.2012.06.011

5. Dominy, J. E., Jr, Lee, Y., Gerhart-Hines, Z., & Puigserver, P. (2010). Biochimica et Biophysica Acta. *BBA - Proteins and Proteomics, 1804*(8), 1676–1683. doi:10.1016/j.bbapap.2009.11.023

6. Schoultz, I., Söderholm, J. D., & McKay, D. M. (2011). Is metabolic stress a common denominator in inflammatory bowel disease? *Inflamm Bowel Dis, 17*(9), 2008–2018. doi:10.1002/ibd.21556

7. Lane, L. Power, Sex, Suicide *Mitochondria and the meaning of life*. 2005. Oxford University Press.: New York, New York, USA. 368p. ISBN: 0-192-80481-2 (hardcover).

8. Bjørndal, B., Burri, L., Staalesen, V., Skorve, J., & Berge, R. K. (2011). Different Adipose Depots: Their Role in the Development of Metabolic Syndrome and Mitochondrial Response to Hypolipidemic Agents. *Journal of Obesity*, *2011*(1), 1–15. doi:10.1016/j.bbalip.2005.02.011

9. Stephens, F. B., Constantin-Teodosiu, D., & Greenhaff, P. L. (2007). New insights concerning the role of carnitine in the regulation of fuel metabolism in skeletal muscle. *The Journal of Physiology*, *581*(2), 431–444. doi:10.1113/jphysiol.2006.125799

10. Wall, B. T., Stephens, F. B., Constantin-Teodosiu, D., Marimuthu, K., Macdonald, I. A., & Greenhaff, P. L. (2011). Chronic oral ingestion of L-carnitine and carbohydrate increases muscle carnitine content and alters muscle fuel metabolism during exercise in humans. *The Journal of Physiology*, *589*(4), 963–973. doi:10.1113/jphysiol.2010.201343

11. Nunn, A. V., Bell, J. D., & Guy, G. W. (2009). Lifestyle-induced metabolic inflexibility and accelerated ageing syndrome: insulin resistance, friend or foe? *Nutrition & Metabolism*, *6*, 16. doi:10.1186/1743-7075-6-16

12. Astrup, A. (2011). The relevance of increased fat oxidation for body-weight management: metabolic inflexibility in the predisposition to weight gain. *Obesity Reviews*, *12*(10), 859–865. doi:10.1111/j.1467-789X.2011.00894.x

13. Kelley, D. E., & Mandarino, L. J. (2000). Fuel selection in human skeletal muscle in insulin resistance: a reexamination. *Diabetes*, *49*(5), 677–683.

14. Aucouturier, J., Duche, P., & Timmons, B. W. (2011). Metabolic flexibility and obesity in children and youth. *Obesity Reviews*, *12*(5), e44–53. doi:10.1111/j.1467-789X.2010.00812.x

15. Kolehmainen, M., Vidal, H., Ohisalo, J. J., Pirinen, E., Alhava, E., & Uusitupa, M. I. J. (2002). Hormone sensitive lipase expression and adipose tissue metabolism show gender difference in obese subjects after weight loss. *International Journal of Obesity*, *26*(1), 6–16. doi:10.1038/sj.ijo.0801858

16. Guilherme, A., Virbasius, J. V., Puri, V., & Czech, M. P. (2008). Adipocyte dysfunctions linking obesity to insulin resistance and type 2 diabetes. *Nature Reviews Molecular Cell Biology*, *9*(5), 367–377. doi:10.1038/nrm2391

17. Dumas, J. F., Simard, G., Flamment, M., Ducluzeau, P. H., & Ritz, P. (2009). Is skeletal muscle mitochondrial dysfunction a cause or an indirect consequence of insulin resistance in humans? *Diabetes & Metabolism*, *35*(3), 159–167. doi:10.1016/j.diabet.2009.02.002

18. Lowell, B. B. (2005). Mitochondrial Dysfunction and Type 2 Diabetes. *Science*, *307*(5708), 384–387. doi:10.1126/science.1104343

19. Summers, S. A. (2006). Ceramides in insulin resistance and lipotoxicity. *Progress in Lipid Research*, *45*(1), 42–72. doi:10.1016/j.plipres.2005.11.002

20. Barazzoni, R., Zanetti, M., Cappellari, G. G., Semolic, A., Boschelle, M., Codarin, E., et al. (2011). Fatty acids acutely enhance insulin-induced oxidative stress and cause insulin resistance by increasing mitochondrial reactive oxygen species (ROS) generation and nuclear factor-κB inhibitor (IκB)–nuclear factor-κB (NFκB) activation in rat muscle, in the absence of mitochondrial dysfunction. *Diabetologia, 55*(3), 773–782. doi:10.1007/s00125-011-2396-x

21. Chow, L., From, A., & Seaquist, E. (2010). Skeletal muscle insulin resistance: the interplay of local lipid excess and mitochondrial dysfunction. *Metabolism, 59*(1), 70–85. doi:10.1016/j.metabol.2009.07.009

22. Boden, G. (2006). Fatty acid—induced inflammation and insulin resistance in skeletal muscle and liver. *Current Diabetes Reports, 6*(3), 177–181. doi:10.1007/s11892-006-0031-x

23. Kahn, S. E., Hull, R. L., & Utzschneider, K. M. (2006). Mechanisms linking obesity to insulin resistance and type 2 diabetes. *Nature, 444*(7121), 840–846. doi:10.1038/nature05482

24. Phielix, E., Meex, R., Ouwens, D. M., Sparks, L., Hoeks, J., Schaart, G., et al. (2012). High Oxidative Capacity Due to Chronic Exercise Training Attenuates Lipid-Induced Insulin Resistance. *Diabetes.* doi:10.2337/db11-1832

25. Dela, F., & Helge, J. W. (2013). Insulin resistance and mitochondrial function in skeletal muscle. *The International Journal of Biochemistry & Cell Biology, 45*(1), 11–15. doi:10.1016/j.biocel.2012.09.019 (Insulin resistance 30% decrease in ATP)

26. Petersen, K. F., Dufour, S., Befroy, D., Garcia, R., & Shulman, G. I. (2004). Impaired mitochondrial activity in the insulin-resistant offspring of patients with type 2 diabetes. *New England Journal of Medicine, 350*(7), 664–671. doi:10.1056/NEJMoa031314

27. Befroy, D. E., Petersen, K. F., Dufour, S., Mason, G. F., de Graaf, R. A., Rothman, D. L., & Shulman, G. I. (2007). Impaired Mitochondrial Substrate Oxidation in Muscle of Insulin-Resistant Offspring of Type 2 Diabetic Patients. *Diabetes, 56*(5), 1376–1381. doi:10.2337/db06-0783

28. Brumbaugh, D. E., Crume, T. L., Nadeau, K., Scherzinger, A., & Dabelea, D. (2012). Intramyocellular Lipid Is Associated with Visceral Adiposity, Markers of Insulin Resistance, and Cardiovascular Risk in Prepubertal Children: The EPOCH Study. *Journal of Clinical Endocrinology & Metabolism, 97*(7), E1099–E1105. doi:10.1210/jc.2011-3243

29. Bäckhed, F., Ding, H., Wang, T., Hooper, L. V., Koh, G. Y., Nagy, A., et al. (2004). The gut microbiota as an environmental factor that regulates fat storage. *Proceedings of the National Academy of Sciences of the United States of America, 101*(44), 15718–15715723. doi:10.1073/pnas.0407076101

30. Bäckhed, F. (2011). Programming of host metabolism by the gut microbiota. *Annals of nutrition & metabolism, 58 Suppl 2*, 44–52. doi:10.1159/000328042

31. Delzenne, N. M., Neyrinck, A. M., Bäckhed, F., & Cani, P. D. (2011). Targeting gut microbiota in obesity: effects of prebiotics and probiotics. *Nature Reviews | Endocrinology,* 1–8. doi:10.1038/nrendo.2011.126

32. Mandard, S., Zandbergen, F., van Straten, E., Wahli, W., Kuipers, F., Müller, M., & Kersten, S. (2006). The fasting-induced adipose factor/angiopoietin-like protein 4 is physically associated with lipoproteins and governs plasma lipid levels and adiposity. *The Journal of Biological Chemistry, 281*(2), 934–944. doi:10.1074/jbc.M506519200

33. Lichtenstein, L., & Kersten, S. (2010). Modulation of plasma TG lipolysis by Angiopoietin-like proteins and GPIHBP1. *Biochimica et Biophysica Acta, 1801*(4), 415–420. doi:10.1016/j.bbalip.2009.12.015

34. Xie, W., Gu, D., Li, J., Cui, K., & Zhang, Y. (2011). Effects and Action Mechanisms of Berberine and Rhizoma coptidis on Gut Microbes and Obesity in High-Fat Diet-Fed C57BL/6J Mice. *PLoS ONE, 6*(9), e24520. doi:10.1371/journal.pone.0024520.t003

35. Yin, J., Xing, H., & Ye, J. (2008). Efficacy of berberine in patients with type 2 diabetes mellitus. *Metabolism, 57*(5), 712–717. doi:10.1016/j.metabol.2008.01.013

36. Gruzman, A., Babai, G., & Sasson, S. (2009). Adenosine monophosphate-activated protein kinase (AMPK) as a new target for antidiabetic drugs: a review on metabolic, pharmacological and chemical considerations. *The review of diabetic studies: RDS, 6*(1), 13.

37. Handschin, C., & Spiegelman, B. M. (2008). The role of exercise and PGC-1alpha in inflammation and chronic disease. *Nature, 454*(7203), 463–469. doi:10.1038/nature07206

38. Lin, J., Handschin, C., & Spiegelman, B. M. (2005). Metabolic control through the PGC-1 family of transcription coactivators. *Cell Metabolism, 1*(6), 361–370. doi:10.1016/j.cmet.2005.05.004

39. Reznick, R. M., & Shulman, G. I. (2006). The role of AMP-activated protein kinase in mitochondrial biogenesis. *The Journal of Physiology, 574*(Pt 1), 33–39. doi:10.1113/jphysiol.2006.109512

40. Narkar, V. A., Downes, M., Yu, R. T., Embler, E., Wang, Y.-X., Banayo, E., et al. (2008). AMPK and PPARδ Agonists Are Exercise Mimetics. *Cell, 134*(3), 405–415. doi:10.1016/j.cell.2008.06.051

41. Treebak, J. T., & Wojtaszewski, J. (2008). Role of 5′ AMP-activated protein kinase in skeletal muscle. *International Journal of Obesity, 32,* S13–S17.

42. Long, Y. C., & Zierath, J. R. (2006). AMP-activated protein kinase signaling in metabolic regulation. *Journal of Clinical Investigation, 116*(7), 1776–1783.

43. Layne, A. S., Nasrallah, S., South, M. A., Howell, M. E. A., McCurry, M. P., Ramsey, M. W., et al. (2011). Impaired Muscle AMPK Activation in the Metabolic Syndrome May Attenuate Improved Insulin Action after Exercise Training. *Journal of Clinical Endocrinology & Metabolism, 96*(6), 1815–1826. doi:10.1210/jc.2010-2532

44. Befroy, D. E., Petersen, K. F., Dufour, S., Mason, G. F., Rothman, D. L., & Shulman, G. I. (2008). Increased substrate oxidation and mitochondrial uncoupling in skeletal muscle of endurance-trained individuals. *Proceedings of the National Academy of Sciences*, *105*(43), 16409–16410. doi:10.1073/iti4308105

45. Bäckhed, F., Manchester, J. K., Semenkovich, C. F., & Gordon, J. I. (2007). Mechanisms underlying the resistance to diet-induced obesity in germ-free mice. *Proceedings of the National Academy of Sciences of the United States of America*, *104*(3), 979–984.

46. Boyle, J. G., Logan, P. J., Jones, G. C., Small, M., Sattar, N., Connell, J., et al. (2011). AMP-activated protein kinase is activated in adipose tissue of individuals with type 2 diabetes treated with metformin: a randomised glycaemia-controlled crossover study. *Diabetologia*, *54*(7), 1799–1809.

47. Musi, N., Hirshman, M. F., Nygren, J., Svanfeldt, M., Bavenholm, P., Rooyackers, O., et al. (2002). Metformin Increases AMP-Activated Protein Kinase Activity in Skeletal Muscle of Subjects With Type 2 Diabetes. *Diabetes*, *51*(7), 2074–2081. doi:10.2337/diabetes.51.7.2074

48. Wilson, A. J., Prapavessis, H., Jung, M. E., Cramp, A. G., Vascotto, J., Lenhardt, L., et al. (2009). Lifestyle modification and metformin as long-term treatment options for obese adolescents: study protocol. *BMC Public Health*, *9*(1), 434. doi:10.1186/1471-2458-9-434

49. Baur, D. M., Klotsche, J., Hamnvik, O.-P. R., Sievers, C., Pieper, L., Wittchen, H.-U., et al. (2011). Type 2 diabetes mellitus and medications for type 2 diabetes mellitus are associated with risk for and mortality from cancer in a German primary care cohort. *Metabolism*, *60*(10), 1363–1371. doi:10.1016/j.metabol.2010.09.012

50. Rayalam, S., Della-Fera, M. A., & Baile, C. A. (2008). Phytochemicals and regulation of the adipocyte life cycle. *The Journal of Nutritional Biochemistry*, *19*(11), 717–726. doi:10.1016/j.jnutbio.2007.12.007

51. Aggarwal, B. B. (2010). Targeting inflammation-induced obesity and metabolic diseases by curcumin and other nutraceuticals. *Annual Review of Nutrition*, *30*, 173–199. doi:10.1146/annurev.nutr.012809.104755

52. Carbonelli, M. G., Di Renzo, L., Bigioni, M., Di Daniele, N., De Lorenzo, A., & Fusco, M. A. (2010). Alpha-lipoic acid supplementation: a tool for obesity therapy? *Current Pharmaceutical Design*, *16*(7), 840–846.

53. Koh, E. H., Lee, W. J., Lee, S. A., Kim, E. H., Cho, E. H., Jeong, E., et al. (2011). Effects of Alpha-Lipoic Acid on Body Weight in Obese Subjects. *AJM*, *124*(1), 85.e1–85.e8. doi:10.1016/j.amjmed.2010.08.005

54. Lee, H. J., Lee, Y.-H., Park, S. K., Kang, E. S., Kim, H.-J., Lee, Y. C., et al. (2009). Korean red ginseng (Panax ginseng) improves insulin sensitivity and attenuates the development of diabetes in Otsuka Long-Evans Tokushima fatty rats. *Metabolism*, *58*(8), 1170–1177. doi:10.1016/j.metabol.2009.03.015

55. Kim, T., Davis, J., Zhang, A. J., He, X., & Mathews, S. T. (2009). Biochemical and Biophysical Research Communications. *Biochemical and Biophysical Research Communications, 388*(2), 377–382. doi:10.1016/j. bbrc.2009.08.018

56. Berings, M., Wehlou, C., Verrijken, A., Deschepper, E., Mertens, I., Kaufman, J.-M., et al. (2012). Glucose Intolerance and the Amount of Visceral Adipose Tissue Contribute to an Increase in Circulating Triglyceride Concentrations in Caucasian Obese Females. *PLoS ONE, 7*(9), e45145. doi:10.1371/journal.pone.0045145.s001

57. Chen, D., Pamu, S., Cui, Q., Chan, T. H., & Dou, Q. P. (2012). Novel epigallocatechin gallate (EGCG) analogs activate AMP-activated protein kinase pathway and target cancer stem cells. *Bioorganic & Medicinal Chemistry, 20*(9), 3031–3037. doi:10.1016/j.bmc.2012.03.002

58. Collins, Q. F., Liu, H. Y., Pi, J., Liu, Z., Quon, M. J., & Cao, W. (2007). Epigallocatechin-3-gallate (EGCG), A Green Tea Polyphenol, Suppresses Hepatic Gluconeogenesis through 5'-AMP-activated Protein Kinase. *Journal of Biological Chemistry, 282*(41), 30143–30149. doi:10.1074/jbc. M702390200

59. Hwang, J.-T., Park, I.-J., Shin, J.-I., Lee, Y. K., Lee, S. K., Baik, H. W., et al. (2005). Genistein, EGCG, and capsaicin inhibit adipocyte differentiation process via activating AMP-activated protein kinase. *Biochemical and Biophysical Research Communications, 338*(2), 694–699. doi:10.1016/j. bbrc.2005.09.195

60. Ahn, J., Lee, H., Kim, S., Park, J., & Ha, T. (2008). The anti-obesity effect of quercetin is mediated by the AMPK and MAPK signaling pathways. *Biochemical and Biophysical Research Communications, 373*(4), 545–549. doi:10.1016/j.bbrc.2008.06.077

61. Sell, H., Habich, C., & Eckel, J. (2012). Adaptive immunity in obesity and insulin resistance. *Nature Reviews | Endocrinology, 8*(12), 709–716. doi:10.1038/nrendo.2012.114

62,. Ye, J. (2008). Emerging role of adipose tissue hypoxia in obesity and insulin resistance. *International Journal of Obesity, 33*(1), 54–66. doi:10.1038/ ijo.2008.229

63. Semenza, G. L. (2011). Oxygen sensing, homeostasis, and disease. *N Engl J Med, 365*(6), 537–547.

64. Schwartz, R. S., Eltzschig, H. K., & Carmeliet, P. (2011). Hypoxia and inflammation. *N Engl J Med, 364*(7), 656–665.

65. Shi, L. Z., Wang, R., Huang, G., Vogel, P., Neale, G., Green, D. R., & Chi, H. (2011). HIF1 -dependent glycolytic pathway orchestrates a metabolic checkpoint for the differentiation of TH17 and Treg cells. *Journal of Experimental Medicine, 208*(7), 1367–1376. doi:10.1146/annurev- immunol-030409-101212

66. Biswas, S. K., & Mantovani, A. (2012). Orchestration of Metabolism by Macrophages. *Cell Metab.*, *15*(4), 432–437. doi:10.1016/j.cmet.2011.11.013

67. Fox, C. J., Hammerman, P. S., & Thompson, C. B. (2005). Fuel feeds function: energy metabolism and the T-cell response. *Nature Reviews Immunology*, *5*(11), 844–852. doi:10.1038/nri1710

68. Rathmell, J. C. (2012). Metabolism and autophagy in the immune system: immunometabolism comes of age. *Immunological Reviews*, *249*(1), 5–13. doi:10.1111/j.1600-065X.2012.01158.x

69. Barbi, J., Pardoll, D., & Pan, F. (2013). Metabolic control of the Treg/Th17 axis. *Immunological Reviews*, *252*(1), 52–77. doi:10.1111/imr.12029

70. Verbist, K. C., Wang, R., & Green, D. R. (2012). T cell metabolism and the immune response. *Seminars in Immunology*, *24*(6), 399–404. doi:10.1016/j.smim.2012.12.006

71. Collier, B., Dossett, L. A., May, A. K., & Diaz, J. J. (2006). Glucose Control and the Inflammatory Response. *Nutrition in Clinical Practice*, *23*(1), 3–15. doi:10.1177/011542650802300103

72. Neels, J. G., & Olefsky, J. M. (2006). Inflamed fat: what starts the fire? *Journal of Clinical Investigation*, *116*(1), 33–35.

73. Cildir, G., Akıncılar, S. C., & Tergaonkar, V. (2013). Chronic adipose tissue inflammation: all immune cells on the stage. *Trends in Molecular Medicine*, *19*(8), 487–500. doi:10.1016/j.molmed.2013.05.001

74. Blagih, J., & Jones, R. G. (2012). Polarizing Macrophages through Reprogramming of Glucose Metabolism. *Cell Metab.*, *15*(6), 793–795. doi:10.1016/j.cmet.2012.05.008

75. MacIver, N. J., Jacobs, S. R., Wieman, H. L., Wofford, J. A., Coloff, J. L., & Rathmell, J. C. (2008). Glucose metabolism in lymphocytes is a regulated process with significant effects on immune cell function and survival. *Journal of Leukocyte Biology*, *84*(4), 949–957. doi:10.1189/jlb.0108024

76. Biswas, S. K., Chittezhath, M., Shalova, I. N., & Lim, J.-Y. (2012). Macrophage polarization and plasticity in health and disease. *Immunologic Research*. doi:10.1007/s12026-012-8291-9

77. Viardot, A., Heilbronn, L. K., Samocha-Bonet, D., Mackay, F., Campbell, L. V., & Samaras, K. (2012). Obesity is associated with activated and insulin resistant immune cells. *Diabetes/Metabolism Research and Reviews*, n/a–n/a. doi:10.1002/dmrr.2302

78. Wang, R., & Green, D. R. (2012). The immune diet: meeting the metabolic demands of lymphocyte activation. *F1000 biology reports*, *4*, 9. doi:10.3410/B4-9

79. Ahima, R. S., Saper, C. B., Flier, J. S., & Elmquist, J. K. (2000). Leptin Regulation of Neuroendocrine Systems. *Frontiers in Neuroendocrinology*, *21*(3), 263–307. doi:10.1006/frne.2000.0197

80. Zhang, Y., & Proenca, R. (1994). Positional cloning of the mouse *obese* gene and its human homologue. *Nature, 372,* 425–432. doi:10.1038/372425a0

81. Coleman, D. L. (2010). *A historical perspective on leptin. Nature medicine* (Vol. 16, pp. 1097–1099). doi:10.1038/nm1010-1097

82. Mattsson, C. (2007). Estrogens and Glucocorticoid Hormones in Adipose Tissue Metabolism. *Current Medicinal Chemistry, 14*(27), 2918–2924.

83. Shah, N. R., & Braverman, E. R. (2012). Measuring Adiposity in Patients: The Utility of Body Mass Index (BMI), Percent Body Fat, and Leptin. *PLoS ONE, 7*(4), e33308. doi:10.1371/journal.pone.0033308.t004

84. Cella, F., Giordano, G., & Cordera, R. (2000). Serum leptin concentrations during the menstrual cycle in normal-weight women: effects of an oral triphasic estrogen-progestin medication. *European journal of endocrinology / European Federation of Endocrine Societies, 142*(2), 174–178.

85. de Lartigue, G., Barbier de la Serre, C., Espero, E., Lee, J., & Raybould, H. E. (2012). Leptin Resistance in Vagal Afferent Neurons Inhibits Cholecystokinin Signaling and Satiation in Diet Induced Obese Rats. *PLoS ONE, 7*(3), e32967. doi:10.1371/journal.pone.0032967.g006

86. Spiegel, K., Leproult, R., L'hermite-Balériaux, M., Copinschi, G., Penev, P. D., & Van Cauter, E. (2004). Leptin levels are dependent on sleep duration: relationships with sympathovagal balance, carbohydrate regulation, cortisol, and thyrotropin. *Journal of Clinical Endocrinology & Metabolism, 89*(11), 5762–5771. doi:10.1210/jc.2004-1003

87. Rocha, V. Z., & Folco, E. J. (2011). Inflammatory concepts of obesity. *International Journal of Inflammation, 2011,* 529061. doi:10.4061/2011/529061

88. Temporal Patterns of Circulating Leptin Levels in Lean and Obese Adolescents: Relationships to Insulin, Growth Hormone, and Free Fatty Acids Rhythmicity*. (2001). Temporal Patterns of Circulating Leptin Levels in Lean and Obese Adolescents: Relationships to Insulin, Growth Hormone, and Free Fatty Acids Rhythmicity*, 1–7.

89. Cani, P. D., Osto, M., Geurts, L., & Everard, A. (2012). Involvement of gut microbiota in the development of low-grade inflammation and type 2 diabetes associated with obesity. *Gut Microbes, 3*(4), 279–288. doi:10.4161/gmic.19625

90. Lago, R., Gómez, R., Lago, F., Gómez-Reino, J., & Gualillo, O. (2008). Leptin beyond body weight regulation—Current concepts concerning its role in immune function and inflammation. *Cellular Immunology, 252*(1-2), 139–145. doi:10.1016/j.cellimm.2007.09.004

91. Matarese, G., Procaccini, C., De Rosa, V., Horvath, T. L., & La Cava, A. (2010). Regulatory T cells in obesity: the leptin connection. *Trends in Molecular Medicine, 16*(6), 247–256. doi:10.1016/j.molmed.2010.04.002

92. Duffaut, C., Galitzky, J., Lafontan, M., & Bouloumié, A. (2009). Unexpected trafficking of immune cells within the adipose tissue during the onset of obesity. *Biochemical and Biophysical Research Communications, 384*(4), 482–485. doi:10.1016/j.bbrc.2009.05.002

93. Chatzigeorgiou, A., Karalis, K. P., Bornstein, S. R., & Chavakis, T. (2012). Lymphocytes in obesity-related adipose tissue inflammation. *Diabetologia, 55*(10), 2583–2592. doi:10.1007/s00125-012-2607-0

94. Kalupahana, N. S., Moustaid-Moussa, N., & Claycombe, K. J. (2012). Immunity as a link between obesity and insulin resistance. *Journal of Molecular Aspects of Medicine, 33*(1), 26–34. doi:10.1016/j.mam.2011.10.011

95. Hanson, L. A., Padyukov, L., Strandvik, B., & Wrammer, L. (2000). The immune system of the hunter-gatherer meets poverty and excess. *Lakartidningen, 97*(15), 1823–1825.

96. Lord, G. M., Matarese, G., Howard, J. K., Baker, R. J., Bloom, S. R., & Lechler, R. I. (1998). Leptin modulates the T-cell immune response and reverses starvation-induced immunosuppression. *Nature, 394*(6696), 897–901.

97. Faggioni, R., Feingold, K. R., & Grunfeld, C. (2001). Leptin regulation of the immune response and the immunodeficiency of malnutrition. *The FASEB Journal, 15*(14), 2565–2571. doi:10.1096/fj.01-0431rev

98. Procaccini, C., Jirillo, E., & Matarese, G. (2011). Leptin as an immunomodulator. *Journal of Molecular Aspects of Medicine*, 1–11. doi:10.1016/j.mam.2011.10.012

99. Fantuzzi, G., & Faggioni, R. (2000). Leptin in the regulation of immunity, inflammation, and hematopoiesis. *Journal of Leukocyte Biology, 68*(4), 437–446.

100. Mattioli, B., Straface, E., Quaranta, M. G., Giordani, L., & Viora, M. (2005). Leptin promotes differentiation and survival of human dendritic cells and licenses them for Th1 priming. *J Immunol, 174*(11), 6820–6828.

101. Silha, J. V., Krsek, M., Skrha, J. V., Sucharda, P., Nyomba, B. L. G., & Murphy, L. J. (2003). Plasma resistin, adiponectin and leptin levels in lean and obese subjects: correlations with insulin resistance. *European journal of endocrinology / European Federation of Endocrine Societies, 149*(4), 331–335.

102. Zimmet, P. Z., Collins, V. R., de Courten, M. P., Hodge, A. M., Collier, G. R., Dowse, G. K., et al. (1998). Is there a relationship between leptin and insulin sensitivity independent of obesity? A population-based study in the Indian Ocean nation of Mauritius. *International Journal of Obesity, 22*(2), 171–177. doi:10.1038/sj.ijo.0800559

103. Harris, R. B. S. (2000). Leptin-much more than a satiety signal. *Annual Review of Nutrition, 20*(1), 45–75. doi:10.1146/annurev.nutr.20.1.45

104. Huang, K.-C., Lin, R. C. Y., Kormas, N., Lee, L.-T., Chen, C.-Y., Gill, T. P., & Caterson, I. D. (2004). Plasma leptin is associated with insulin resistance independent of age, body mass index, fat mass, lipids, and pubertal development in nondiabetic adolescents. *International Journal of Obesity*, *28*(4), 470–475. doi:10.1038/sj.ijo.0802531

105. Zimmet, P., Hodge, A., Nicolson, M., Staten, M., De Courten, M., Moore, J., et al. (1996). Serum leptin concentration, obesity, and insulin resistance in Western Samoans: cross sectional study. *BMJ, 313*(7063), 965–969.

106. Kim-Motoyama, H., Yamaguchi, T., Katakura, T., Miura, M., Ohashi, Y., Yazaki, Y., & Kadawaki, T. (1997). Serum Leptin Levels Are Associated with Hyperinsulinemia Independent of Body Mass Index but Not with Visceral Obesity. *Biochemical and Biophysical Research Communications*, *239*(1), 340–344. doi:10.1006/bbrc.1997.7329

107. Franks, P. W., Brage, S., Luan, J., Ekelund, U., Rahman, M., Farooqi, I. S., et al. (2005). Leptin predicts a worsening of the features of the metabolic syndrome independently of obesity. *Obesity research, 13*(8), 1476–1484. doi:10.1038/oby.2005.178

108. Patel, S. B., Reams, G. P., Spear, R. M., Freeman, R. H., & Villarreal, D. (n.d.). Leptin: Linking obesity, the metabolic syndrome, and cardiovascular disease. *Current Hypertension Reports, 10*(2), 131–137. doi:10.1007/s11906-008-0025-y

109. Cojocaru, M., Cojocaru, I. M., Siloşi, I., & Rogoz, S. (2013). Role of leptin in autoimmune diseases. *Mædica, 8*(1), 68–74.

110. Matarese, G., La Cava, A., Sanna, V., Lord, G. M., Lechler, R. I., Fontana, S., & Zappacosta, S. (2002). Balancing susceptibility to infection and autoimmunity: a role for leptin? *TRENDS in Immunology, 23*(4), 182–187.

111. Moore, S. E., Morgan, G., Collinson, A. C., Swain, J. A., O'Connell, M. A., & Prentice, A. M. (2002). Leptin, malnutrition, and immune response in rural Gambian children. *Archives of Disease in Childhood, 87*, 192–197.

112. Dumond, H. L. N., Presle, N., Terlain, B., Mainard, D., Loeuille, D., Netter, P., & Pottie, P. (2003). Evidence for a key role of leptin in osteoarthritis. *Arthritis and Rheumatism, 48*(11), 3118–3129. doi:10.1002/art.11303

113. Yusuf, E., Nelissen, R. G., Ioan-Facsinay, A., Stojanovic-Susulic, V., DeGroot, J., van Osch, G., et al. (2010). Association between weight or body mass index and hand osteoarthritis: a systematic review. *Annals of the Rheumatic Diseases, 69*(4), 761–765. doi:10.1136/ard.2008.106930

114. Sowers, M. R., & Karvonen-Gutierrez, C. A. (2010). The evolving role of obesity in knee osteoarthritis. *Current Opinion in Rheumatology, 22*(5), 533–537. doi:10.1097/BOR.0b013e32833b4682

115. Simopoulou, T., Malizos, K. N., Iliopoulos, D., Stefanou, N., Papatheodorou, L., Ioannou, M., & Tsezou, A. (2007). Differential expression of leptin and leptin's receptor isoform (Ob-Rb) mRNA between advanced and minimally affected osteoarthritic cartilage; effect on cartilage metabolism. *Osteoarthritis and Cartilage*, *15*(8), 872–883. doi:10.1016/j.joca.2007.01.018

116. Nelson, F., Zvirbulis, R., Zonca, B., Pasierb, M., Wilton, P., Martinez-Puig, D., & Wu, W. (2013). An oral preparation containing hylauronic acid (ORALVISC) can reduce osteoarthritis knee pain and serum and synovial fluid bradykinin. *Osteoarthritis and Cartilage*, *21*(S), S150. doi:10.1016/j.joca.2013.02.320

117. Shehzad, A., Ha, T., Subhan, F., & Lee, Y. S. (2011). New mechanisms and the anti-inflammatory role of curcumin in obesity and obesity-related metabolic diseases. *European Journal of Nutrition*, *50*(3), 151–161. doi:10.1007/s00394-011-0188-1

118. Flachs, P., Rossmeisl, M., Bryhn, M., & Kopecky, J. (2009). Cellular and molecular effects of n–3 polyunsaturated fatty acids on adipose tissue biology and metabolism. *Clinical Science*, *116*(1), 1. doi:10.1042/CS20070456

119. Titos, E., Rius, B., Gonzalez-Periz, A., Lopez-Vicario, C., Moran-Salvador, E., Martinez-Clemente, M., et al. (2011). Resolvin D1 and Its Precursor Docosahexaenoic Acid Promote Resolution of Adipose Tissue Inflammation by Eliciting Macrophage Polarization toward an M2-Like Phenotype. *The Journal of Immunology*, *187*(10), 5408–5418. doi:10.4049/jimmunol.1100225

120. Olefsky, J. M., & Glass, C. K. (2010). Macrophages, Inflammation, and Insulin Resistance. *Annual Review of Physiology*, *72*(1), 219–246. doi:10.1146/annurev-physiol-021909-135846

121. Spencer, M., Finlin, B. S., Unal, R., Zhu, B., Morris, A. J., Shipp, L. R., et al. (2013). Omega-3 Fatty Acids Reduce Adipose Tissue Macrophages in Human Subjects With Insulin Resistance. *Diabetes*, *62*(5), 1709–1717.

122. Lundström, S. L., Yang, J., Brannan, J. D., Haeggström, J. Z., Hammock, B. D., Nair, P., et al. (2013). Lipid mediator serum profiles in asthmatics significantly shift following dietary supplementation with omega-3 fatty acids. *Molecular Nutrition & Food Research*, *57*(8), 1378–1389. doi:10.1002/mnfr.201200827

123. Spite, M., Clària, J., & Serhan, C. N. (2013). Resolvins, Specialized Proresolving Lipid Mediators, and Their Potential Roles in Metabolic Diseases. *Cell Metab.*, 1–16. doi:10.1016/j.cmet.2013.10.006

124. Serhan, C. N., Hong, S., Gronert, K., Colgan, S. P., Devchand, P. R., Mirick, G., & Moussignac, R. L. (2002). Resolvins: A Family of Bioactive Products of Omega-3 Fatty Acid Transformation Circuits Initiated by Aspirin Treatment that Counter Proinflammation Signals. *Journal of Experimental Medicine*, *196*(8), 1025–1037. doi:10.1084/jem.20020760

125. Serhan, C. N., Chiang, N., & Van Dyke, T. E. (2008). Resolving inflammation: dual anti-inflammatory and pro-resolution lipid mediators. *Nature Reviews Immunology, 8*(5), 349–361. doi:10.1038/nri2294

126. Mas, E., Croft, K. D., Zahra, P., Barden, A., & Mori, T. A. (2012). Resolvins D1, D2, and Other Mediators of Self-Limited Resolution of Inflammation in Human Blood following n-3 Fatty Acid Supplementation. *Clinical Chemistry, 58*(10), 1476–1484. doi:10.1373/clinchem.2012.190199

127. Lee, B.-C., & Lee, J. (2013). Cellular and molecular players in adipose tissue inflammation in the development of obesity-induced insulin resistance. *Biochimica et Biophysica Acta.* doi:10.1016/j.bbadis.2013.05.017

128. Kopecky, J., Rossmeisl, M., Flachs, P., Kuda, O., Brauner, P., Jilkova, Z., et al. (2009). n-3 PUFA: bioavailability and modulation of adipose tissue function. *Proceedings of the Nutrition Society, 68*(04), 361. doi:10.1017/S0029665109990231

129. Kalupahana, N. S., Claycombe, K. J., & Moustaid-Moussa, N. (2011). (n-3) Fatty acids alleviate adipose tissue inflammation and insulin resistance: mechanistic insights. *Adv Nutr, 2*(4), 304–316. doi:10.3945/an.111.000505

130. Hill, A. M., Buckley, J. D., Murphy, K. J., & Howe, P. R. C. (2007). Combining fish-oil supplements with regular aerobic exercise improves body composition and cardiovascular disease risk factors. *Am J Clin Nutr, 85*(5), 1267–1274.

131. Kelley, D. S., Adkins, Y., Woodhouse, L. R., Swislocki, A., Mackey, B. E., & Siegel, D. (2012). Docosahexaenoic Acid Supplementation Improved Lipocentric but Not Glucocentric Markers of Insulin Sensitivity in Hypertriglyceridemic Men. *Metabolic Syndrome and Related Disorders, 10*(1), 32–38. doi:10.1089/met.2011.0081

132. Doughman, S. D., Ryan, A. S., Krupanidhi, S., Sanjeevi, C. B., & Mohan, V. (2013). High DHA dosage from algae oil improves postprandial hypertriglyceridemia and is safe for type-2 diabetics. *International Journal of Diabetes in Developing Countries, 33*(2), 75–82. doi:10.1007/s13410-013-0125-3

133. Oelrich, B., Dewell, A., & Gardner, C. D. (2011). Effect of fish oil supplementation on serum triglycerides, LDL cholesterol and LDL subfractions in hypertriglyceridemic adults. *Nutrition, Metabolism and Cardiovascular Diseases,* 1–8. doi:10.1016/j.numecd.2011.06.003

134. Vargas, M. L., Almario, R. U., Buchan, W., Kim, K., & Karakas, S. E. (2011). Metabolic and endocrine effects of long-chain versus essential omega-3 polyunsaturated fatty acids in polycystic ovary syndrome. *Metabolism, 60*(12), 1711–1718. doi:10.1016/j.metabol.2011.04.007

135. Nettleton, J., & Katz, R. (2005). n-3 long-chain polyunsaturated fatty acids in type 2 diabetes: A review. *Journal of the American Dietetic Association, 105*(3), 428–440. doi:10.1016/j.jada.2004.11.029

136. Belluzzi, A., Brignola, C., Campieri, M., Pera, A., Boschi, S., & Miglioli, M. (1996). Effect of an enteric-coated fish-oil preparation on relapses in Crohn's disease. *N Engl J Med*, *334*(24), 1557–1560.

137. Schneider, I., Schuchardt, J. P., Meyer, H., & Hahn, A. (2011). Effect of gastric acid resistant coating of fish oil capsules on intestinal uptake of eicosapentaenoic acid and docosahexaenoic acid. *Journal of Functional Foods*, *3*(2), 129–133. doi:10.1016/j.jff.2011.03.001

138. Davidson, M. H., Johnson, J., Rooney, M. W., Kyle, M. L., & Kling, D. F. (2012). A novel omega-3 free fatty acid formulation has dramatically improved bioavailability duringa low-fat diet compared with omega-3-acid ethyl esters: The Eclipse (Epanova. *Journal of Clinical Lipidology*, *6*(6), 573–584. doi:10.1016/j.jacl.2012.01.002

139. Schacky, von, C. (2010). Omega-3 Index and Sudden Cardiac Death. *Nutrients*, *2*(3), 375–388. doi:10.3390/nu2030375

140. Aarsetoey, H., Aarsetoey, R., Lindner, T., Staines, H., Harris, W. S., & Nilsen, D. W. T. (2011). Low Levels of the Omega-3 Index are Associated with Sudden Cardiac Arrest and Remain Stable in Survivors in the Subacute Phase. *Lipids*, *46*(2), 151–161. doi:10.1007/s11745-010-3511-3

CHAPTERS 5: YOUR GUT AT WORK

1. Drucker, D. J. (2006). The biology of incretin hormones. *Cell Metabolism*, *3*(3), 153–165. doi:10.1016/j.cmet.2006.01.004

2. Tilg, H., Moschen, A. R., & Kaser, A. (2009). Obesity and the Microbiota. *YGAST*, *136*(5), 1476–1483. doi:10.1053/j.gastro.2009.03.030

3. Reis, B. S., & Mucida, D. (2012). The Role of the Intestinal Context in the Generation of Tolerance and Inflammation. *Clinical and Developmental Immunology*, *2012*, 1–6. doi:10.1155/2012/157948

4. Cummings, J. H., Antoine, J.-M., Azpiroz, F., Bourdet-Sicard, R., Brandtzaeg, P., Calder, P. C., et al. (2004). PASSCLAIM--gut health and immunity. *European Journal of Nutrition*, *43 Suppl 2*, II118–II173. doi:10.1007/s00394-004-1205-4

5. Relman, D. A. (2012). Microbiology: Learning about who we are. *Nature*, *486*(7402), 194–195. doi:doi:10.1038/486194a

6. Zoetendal, E. G., Vaughan, E. E., & de Vos, W. M. (2006). A microbial world within us. *Molecular Microbiology*, *59*(6), 1639–1650. doi:10.1111/j.1365-2958.2006.05056.x

7. Neish, A. S. (2009). Microbes in gastrointestinal health and disease. *Gastroenterology*, *136*(1), 65–80. doi:10.1053/j.gastro.2008.10.080

8. Engelstoft, M. S., Egerod, K. L., Holst, B., & Schwartz, T. W. (2008). A Gut Feeling for Obesity: 7TM Sensors on Enteroendocrine Cells. *Cell Metab.*, *8*(6), 447–449. doi:10.1016/j.cmet.2008.11.004

9. Badman, M. K., & Flier, J. S. (2005). The gut and energy balance: visceral allies in the obesity wars. *Science Magazine, 307*(5717), 1909–1914. doi:10.1126/science.1104815

10. Larder, R., & O'Rahilly, S. (2012). Guts over glory—why diets fail. *Nature Medicine, 18*(5), 666–667. doi:10.1038/nm.2747

11. Mandel, A. L., & Breslin, P. A. S. (2012). High Endogenous Salivary Amylase Activity Is Associated with Improved Glycemic Homeostasis following Starch Ingestion in Adults. *Journal of Nutrition, first published online April 4, 2012*. doi:10.3945/jn.111.156984

12. Berthoud, H.-R., Shin, A. C., & Zheng, H. (2011). Obesity surgery and gut–brain communication. *Physiology and Behavior, 105*(1), 106–119. doi:10.1016/j.physbeh.2011.01.023

13. Janssen, S., & Depoortere, I. (2012). Nutrient sensing in the gut: new roadsto therapeutics? *Trends in Endocrinology & Metabolism*, 1–9. doi:10.1016/j.tem.2012.11.006

14. Hage, M. P., Safadi, B., Salti, I., & Nasrallah, M. (2012). Role of Gut-Related Peptides and Other Hormones in the Amelioration of Type 2 Diabetes after Roux-en-Y Gastric Bypass Surgery. *ISRN Endocrinology, 2012*, 1–13. doi:10.5402/2012/504756

15. Howard-McNatt, M., Simon, T., Wang, Y., & Fink, A. S. (2002). Insulin Inhibits Secretin-Induced Pancreatic Bicarbonate Output Via Cholinergic Mechanisms. *Pancreas, 24*(4), 380.

16. Dockray, G. J. (2009). Cholecystokinin and gut–brain signalling. *Regulatory Peptides, 155*(1-3), 6–10. doi:10.1016/j.regpep.2009.03.015

17. de Aguiar Vallim, T. Q., Tarling, E. J., & Edwards, P. A. (2013). Pleiotropic Roles of Bile Acids in Metabolism. *Cell Metab.*, 1–13. doi:10.1016/j.cmet.2013.03.013

18. Camilleri, M., Madsen, K., Spiller, R., Van Meerveld, B. G., & Verne, G. N. (2012). Intestinal barrier function in health and gastrointestinal disease. *Neurogastroenterology & Motility, 24*(6), 503–512. doi:10.1111/j.1365-2982.2012.01921.x

19. Geurts, L., Neyrinck, A. M., Delzenne, N. M., Knauf, C., & Cani, P. D. (2013). Gut microbiota controls adipose tissue expansion, gut barrier and glucose metabolism: novel insights into molecular targets and interventions using prebiotics. *Beneficial Microbes, 1*(-1), 1–15. doi:10.3920/BM2012.0065

20. Vanormelingen, C., Tack, J., & Andrews, C. N. (2013). Diabetic gastroparesis. *British medical bulletin, 105*, 213–230. doi:10.1093/bmb/ldt003

21. Scott, W. R., & Batterham, R. L. (2011). Roux-en-Y gastric bypass and laparoscopic sleeve gastrectomy: understanding weight loss and improvements in type 2 diabetes after bariatric surgery. *AJP: Regulatory, Integrative and Comparative Physiology, 301*(1), R15–R27. doi:10.1152/ajpregu.00038.2011

22. Manabe, N., Wong, B. S., Camilleri, M., Burton, D., Mckinzie, S., & Zinsmeister, A. R. (2010). Lower functional gastrointestinal disorders: evidence of abnormal colonic transit in a 287 patient cohort. *Neurogastroenterol Motil, 22*(3), 293–e82. doi:10.1111/j.1365-2982.2009.01442.x

23. Bener, A., Ghuloum, S., Al-Hamaq, A. O., & Dafeeah, E. E. (2012). Association between psychological distress and gastrointestinal symptoms in diabetes mellitus. *World Journal of Diabetes, 3*(6), 123–129. doi:10.4239/wjd.v3.i6.123

24. Merrouche, M., Sabate, J.-M., Jouet, P., Harnois, F., Scaringi, S., Coffin, B., & Msika, S. (2013). Gastro-esophageal reflux and esophageal motility disorders in morbidly obese patients before and after bariatric surgery. *Obesity Surgery, 17*(7), 894–900.

25. Murray, L., Johnston, B., Lane, A., Harvey, I., Donovan, J., Nair, P., & Harvey, R. (2003). Relationship between body mass and gastro-oesophageal reflux symptoms: The Bristol Helicobacter Project. *International Journal of Epidemiology, 32*(4), 645–650.

26. Ayazi, S., Hagen, J. A., Chan, L. S., DeMeester, S. R., Lin, M. W., Ayazi, A., et al. (2009). Obesity and gastroesophageal reflux: quantifying the association between body mass index, esophageal acid exposure, and lower esophageal sphincter status in a large series of patients with reflux symptoms. *Journal of Gastrointestinal Surgery, 13*(8), 1440–1447. doi:10.1093/ije/dyg108

27. Jackson, S. J., Leahy, F. E., McGowan, A. A., Bluck, L. J. C., Coward, W. A., & Jebb, S. A. (2004). Delayed gastric emptying in the obese: an assessment using the non-invasive 13C-octanoic acid breath test. *Diabetes, Obesity and Metabolism, 6*(4), 264–270. doi:10.1111/j.1462-8902.2004.0344.x

28. Friedenberg, F. K., Xanthopoulos, M., Foster, G. D., & Richter, J. E. (2008). The association between gastroesophageal reflux disease and obesity. *Am J Gastroenterol., 103*(8), 2111–2122. doi:10.1111/j.1572-0241.2008.01946.x

29. Bagyánszki, M., & Bódi, N. (2012). Diabetes-related alterations in the enteric nervous system and its microenvironment. *World Journal of Diabetes, 3*(5), 80–93. doi:10.4239/wjd.v3.i5.80

30. Bäckhed, F. (2011). Programming of host metabolism by the gut microbiota. *Annals of nutrition & metabolism, 58 Suppl 2*, 44–52. doi:10.1159/000328042

31. Miller, B. F. (2003). Miller-Keane Encyclopedia and Dictionary of Medicine, Nursing, and Allied Health Volume 1 of Encyclopedia and Dictionary of Medicine, Nursing, and Allied Health (7 ed.). W. B. Saunders. ISBN: 9780721697918

32. Stainier, D. Y. R. (2005). No Organ Left Behind: Tales of Gut Development and Evolution. *Science, 307*(5717), 1902–1904. doi:10.1126/science.1108709

33. Abu-Shanab, A., & Quigley, E. M. M. (2010). The role of the gut microbiota in nonalcoholic fatty liver disease. *Nature Reviews Gastroenterology and Hepatology*, *7*(12), 691–701. doi:doi:10.1038/nrgastro.2010.172

34. Cesaro, C., Tiso, A., Del Prete, A., Cariello, R., Tuccillo, C., Cotticelli, G., et al. (2011). Gut microbiota and probiotics in chronic liver diseases. *Digestive and Liver Disease*, *43*(6), 431–438. doi:10.1016/j.dld.2010.10.015

35. Marchesini, G., Bugianesi, E., Forlani, G., Cerrelli, F., Lenzi, M., Manini, R., et al. (2003). Nonalcoholic fatty liver, steatohepatitis, and the metabolic syndrome. *Hepatology*, *37*(4), 917–923. doi:10.1053/jhep.2003.50161

36. Völzke, H. (2012). Multicausality in fatty liver disease: Is there a rationale to distinguish between alcoholic and non-alcoholic origin? *World Journal of Gastroenterology*, *18*(27), 3492. doi:10.3748/wjg.v18.i27.3492

37. Ludwig, J., Viggiano, T. R., & McGill, D. B. (1980). Nonalcoholic steatohepatitis: Mayo Clinic experiences with a hitherto unnamed disease. *Mayo Clinic Proceedings*, *55*(7), 434–438.

38. Ford, E. S., Schulze, M. B., Bergmann, M. M., Thamer, C., Joost, H. G., & Boeing, H. (2008). Liver Enzymes and Incident Diabetes: Findings from the European Prospective Investigation Into Cancer and Nutrition (EPIC)-Potsdam Study. *Diabetes Care*, *31*(6), 1138–1143. doi:10.2337/dc07-2159

39. Kwon, O. W., Jun, D. W., Lee, S. M., Lee, K. N., Lee, H. L., Lee, O. Y., et al. (2012). Carbohydrate but not fat is associated with elevated aminotransferases. *Alimentary Pharmacology & Therapeutics*, n/a–n/a. doi:10.1111/j.1365-2036.2012.05061.x

40. Ren, J., Pang, Z. C., Gao, W. G., Nan, H. R., Wang, S. J., Zhang, L., & Qiao, Q. (2010). C-Reactive Protein and Gamma-Glutamyltransferase Concentrations in Relation to the Prevalence of Type 2 Diabetes Diagnosed by Glucose or HbA1c Criteria in Chinese Adults in Qingdao, China. *Experimental Diabetes Research*, *2010*(3), 1–8. doi:10.1111/j.1464-5491.2010.02943.x

41. Balkau, B., Lange, C., Vol, S., Fumeron, F., Bonnet, F., Group Study D.E.S.I.R. (2010). Nine-year incident diabetes is predicted by fatty liver indices: the French D.E.S.I.R. study. *BMC gastroenterology*, *10*, 56. doi:10.1186/1471-230X-10-56

42. Ryoo, J. H., Oh, C. M., Kim, H. S., Park, S. K., & Choi, J. M. (2013). Clinical association between serum γ-glutamyltransferase levels and the development of insulin resistance in Korean men: a 5-year follow-up study. *Diabetic Medicine*, n/a–n/a. doi:10.1111/dme.12315

43. Lee, D. H., Steffes, M. W., & Jacobs, D. R. (2008). Can persistent organic pollutants explain the association between serum gamma-glutamyltransferase and type 2 diabetes? *Diabetologia*, *51*(3), 402–407. doi:10.1007/s00125-007-0896-5

44. Lee, D.-H., Blomhoff, R., & Jacobs, D. R. (2004). Review Is Serum Gamma Glutamyltransferase a Marker of Oxidative Stress? *Free Radical Research*, *38*(6), 535–539. doi:10.1080/10715760410001694026

45. Cacciatore, I., Cornacchia, C., Pinnen, F., Mollica, A., & Di Stefano, A. (2010). Prodrug Approach for Increasing Cellular Glutathione Levels. *Molecules*, *15*(3), 1242–1264. doi:10.3390/molecules15031242

46. Ballatori, N., Krance, S. M., Notenboom, S., Shi, S., Tieu, K., & Hammond, C. L. (2009). Glutathione dysregulation and the etiology and progression of human diseases. *Biological Chemistry*, *390*(3), 191–214. doi:10.1515/BC.2009.033

47. Raza, H. (2011). Dual localization of glutathione S-transferase in the cytosol and mitochondria: implications in oxidative stress, toxicity and disease. *The FEBS journal*, *278*(22), 4243–4251. doi:10.1111/j.1742-4658.2011.08358.x

48. Lee, D.-H., Blomhoff, R., & Jacobs, D. R. (2004). Review Is Serum Gamma Glutamyltransferase a Marker of Oxidative Stress? *Free Radical Research*, *38*(6), 535–539. doi:10.1080/10715760410001694026

49. Fraser, A., Sattar, N., Ebrahim, S., & Lawlor, D. A. (2008). Is Serum-Glutamylatransferase a Biomarker of Xenobiotics Which Are Conjugated by Glutathione? *Arteriosclerosis, Thrombosis, and Vascular Biology*, *28*(4), e29–e29. doi:10.1161/ATVBAHA.107.161299

50. Edlinger, M., Nagel, G., Hilbe, W., Diem, G., Concin, H., Strasak, A. M., & Ulmer, H. (2011). Associations of serum uric acid and gamma-glutamyltransferase with cancer in the Vorarlberg Health Monitoring and Promotion Programme (VHM&PP) – a short review. *memo - Magazine of European Medical Oncology*, *4*(1), 50–54. doi:10.1007/s12254-011-0249-4

51. Nakanishi, N., Suzuki, K., & Tatara, K. (2004). Serum gamma-glutamyltransferase and risk of metabolic syndrome and type 2 diabetes in middle-aged Japanese men. *Diabetes Care*, *27*(6), 1427–1432.

52. Lee, D. S., Evans, J. C., Robins, S. J., Wilson, P. W., Albano, I., Fox, C. S., et al. (2007). Gamma Glutamyl Transferase and Metabolic Syndrome, Cardiovascular Disease, and Mortality Risk: The Framingham Heart Study. *Arteriosclerosis, Thrombosis, and Vascular Biology*, *27*(1), 127–133. doi:10.1161/01.ATV.0000251993.20372.40

53. Yamada, J., Tomiyama, H., Yambe, M., Koji, Y., Motobe, K., Shiina, K., et al. (2006). Elevated serum levels of alanine aminotransferase and gamma glutamyltransferase are markers of inflammation and oxidative stress independent of the metabolic syndrome. *Atherosclerosis*, *189*(1), 198–205. doi:10.1016/j.atherosclerosis.2005.11.036

54. Onata, A., Hergençc, G., Karabulutd, A., Türkmene, S., Doğanf, Y., Uyareld, H., et al. (n.d.). Serum gamma glutamyltransferase as a marker of metabolic syndrome and coronary disease likelihood in nondiabetic middle-aged and elderly adults. *Preventive Medicine*, *43*(2), 136–139.

55. Andre, P., Balkau, B., Vol, S., Charles, M. A., Eschwege, E., on behalf of the DESIR Study Group. (2007). -Glutamyltransferase Activity and Development of the Metabolic Syndrome (International Diabetes Federation Definition) in Middle-Aged Men and Women: Data From the Epidemiological Study on the Insulin Resistance Syndrome (DESIR) cohort. *Diabetes Care, 30*(9), 2355–2361. doi:10.2337/dc07-0440

56. Kim, D. J., Noh, J. H., Cho, N. H., Lee, B. W., Choi, Y. H., Jung, J. H., et al. (2005). Serum gamma-glutamyltransferase within its normal concentration range is related to the presence of diabetes and cardiovascular risk factors. *Diabetic Medicine, 22*(9), 1134–1140. doi:10.1111/j.1464-5491.2005.01581.x

57. Casals-Casas, C., & Desvergne, B. (2011). Endocrine Disruptors: From Endocrine to Metabolic Disruption. *Annual Review of Physiology, 73*(1), 135–162. doi:10.1146/annurev-physiol-012110-142200

58. Vandenberg, L. N., Colborn, T., Hayes, T. B., Heindel, J. J., Jacobs, D. R., Lee, D. H., et al. (2012). Hormones and Endocrine-Disrupting Chemicals: Low-Dose Effects and Nonmonotonic Dose Responses. *Endocrine Reviews, 33*(3), 378–455. doi:10.1210/er.2011-1050

59. Guillette, L. J., & Iguchi, T. (2012). Life in a Contaminated World. *Science, 337*(6102), 1614–1615. doi:10.1126/science.1226985

60. Grun, F., & Blumberg, B. (2009). Minireview: The Case for Obesogens. *Molecular Endocrinology, 23*(8), 1127–1134. doi:10.1210/me.2008-0485

61. Holtcamp, W. (2012, February). Obesogens: an environmental link to obesity. *Environmental Health Perspectives*, pp. a62–8. doi:10.1289/ehp.120-a62

62. Faerch, K., Hojlund, K., Vind, B. F., Vaag, A., Dalgard, C., Nielsen, F., & Grandjean, P. (2012). Increased Serum Concentrations of Persistent Organic Pollutants among Prediabetic Individuals: Potential Role of Altered Substrate Oxidation Patterns. *Journal of Clinical Endocrinology & Metabolism.* doi:10.1210/jc.2012-1342

63. Forgacs, I., & Loganayagam, A. (2008). Overprescribing proton pump inhibitors. *BMJ, 336*(7634), 2–3. doi:10.1136/bmj.39406.449456.BE

64. Lewis, S. J., Franco, S., Young, G., & O'Keefe, S. J. (1996). Altered bowel function and duodenal bacterial overgrowth in patients treated with omeprazole. *Alimentary Pharmacology & Therapeutics, 10*(4), 557–561. doi:10.1046/j.1365-2036.1996.d01-506.x

65. Bajaj, J. S., Zadvornova, Y., Heuman, D. M., Hafeezullah, M., Hoffmann, R. G., Sanyal, A. J., & Saeian, K. (2009). Association of Proton Pump Inhibitor Therapy With Spontaneous Bacterial Peritonitis in Cirrhotic Patients With Ascites. *Am J Gastroenterol., 104*(5), 1130–1134. doi:10.1038/ajg.2009.80

66. Kanno, T., Matsuki, T., Oka, M., Utsunomiya, H., Inada, K., Magari, H., et al. (2009). Gastric acid reduction leads to an alteration in lower intestinal microflora. *Biochemical and Biophysical Research Communications*, *381*(4), 666–670. doi:10.1016/j.bbrc.2009.02.109

67. Tennant, S. M. S., Hartland, E. L. E., Phumoonna, T. T., Lyras, D. D., Rood, J. I. J., Robins-Browne, R. M. R., & van Driel, I. R. I. (2008). Influence of gastric acid on susceptibility to infection with ingested bacterial pathogens. *Infection and Immunity*, *76*(2), 639–645. doi:10.1128/IAI.01138-07

68. Bavishi, C., & DuPont, H. L. (2011). Systematic review: the use of proton pump inhibitors and increased susceptibility to enteric infection. *Alimentary Pharmacology & Therapeutics*, *34*(11-12), 1269–1281. doi:10.1111/j.1365-2036.2011.04874.x

69. Ramírez, E., Cabañas, R., Laserna, L. S., Fiandor, A., Tong, H., Prior, N., et al. (2013). Proton pump inhibitors are associated with hypersensitivity reactions to drugs in hospitalized patients: a nested case-control in a retrospective cohort study. *Clinical & Experimental Allergy*, *43*(3), 344–352. doi:10.1111/cea.12034

70. Pali-Schöll, I., Herzog, R., Wallmann, J., Szalai, K., Brunner, R., Lukschal, A., et al. (2010). Antacids and dietary supplements with an influence on the gastric pH increase the risk for food sensitization. *Clinical & Experimental Allergy*, *40*(7), 1091–1098. doi:10.1111/j.1365-2222.2010.03468.x

71. Biswas, S. S., Benedict, S. H. S., Lynch, S. G. S., & LeVine, S. M. S. (2012). Potential immunological consequences of pharmacological suppression of gastric acid production in patients with multiple sclerosis. *BMC Medicine*, *10*, 57–57. doi:10.1186/1741-7015-10-57

72. Saltzman, J. R., Kowdley, K. V., Pedrosa, M. C., Sepe, T., Golner, B., Perrone, G., & Russell, R. M. (1994). Bacterial overgrowth without clinical malabsorption in elderly hypochlorhydric subjects. *YGAST*, *106*(3), 615–623.

73. Stabler, S. P. S. (2013). Clinical practice. Vitamin B12 deficiency. *N Engl J Med*, *368*(2), 149–160. doi:10.1056/NEJMcp1113996

74. Watari, I., Oka, S., Tanaka, S., Aoyama, T., Imagawa, H., Shishido, T., et al. (2013). Effectiveness of polaprezinc for low-dose aspirin-induced small-bowel mucosal injuries as evaluated by capsule endoscopy: a pilot randomized controlled study. *BMC gastroenterology*, *13*, 108–108. doi:10.1186/1471-230X-13-108

75. Mahmood, A., FitzGerald, A. J., Marchbank, T., Ntatsaki, E., Murray, D., Ghosh, S., & Playford, R. J. (2007). Zinc carnosine, a health food supplement that stabilises small bowel integrity and stimulates gut repair processes. *Gut*, *56*(2), 168–175. doi:10.1136/gut.2006.099929

76. Houten, S. M., Watanabe, M., & Auwerx, J. (2006). Endocrine functions of bile acids. *The EMBO Journal*, *25*(7), 1419–1425. doi:10.1038/sj.emboj.7601049

77. Wu, T., Bound, M. J., Standfield, S. D., Jones, K. L., Horowitz, M., & Rayner, C. K. (2013). Effects of Taurocholic Acid on Glycemic, Glucagon-like Peptide-1, and Insulin Responses to Small Intestinal Glucose Infusion in Healthy Humans. *Journal of Clinical Endocrinology & Metabolism*, *98*(4), E718–E722. doi:10.1210/jc.2012-3961

78. Watanabe, M., Houten, S. M., Mataki, C., Christoffolete, M. A., Kim, B. W., Sato, H., et al. (2006). Bile acids induce energy expenditure by promoting intracellular thyroid hormone activation. *Nature*, *439*(7075), 484–489. doi:10.1038/nature04330

79. Swann, J. R., Want, E. J., Geier, F. M., Spagou, K., Wilson, I. D., Sidaway, J. E., et al. (2011). Systemic gut microbial modulation of bile acid metabolism in host tissue compartments. *PNAS*, *108*(1), 4523–4530.

80. Thomas, C., Gioiello, A., Noriega, L., Strehle, A., Oury, J., Rizzo, G., et al. (2009). TGR5-Mediated Bile Acid Sensing Controls Glucose Homeostasis. *Cell Metabolism*, *10*(3), 167–177. doi:10.1016/j.cmet.2009.08.001

81. Ockenga, J., Valentini, L., Schuetz, T., Wohlgemuth, F., Glaeser, S., Omar, A., et al. (2012). Plasma Bile Acids Are Associated with Energy Expenditure and Thyroid Function in Humans. *Journal of Clinical Endocrinology & Metabolism*, *97*(2), 535–542. doi:10.1210/jc.2011-2329

82. Musso, G., Gambino, R., & Cassader, M. (2011). Interactions Between Gut Microbiota and Host Metabolism Predisposing to Obesity and Diabetes. *Annual Review of Medicine*, *62*(1), 361–380. doi:10.1146/annurev-med-012510-175505

83. Begley, M. I., Gahan, C. G. M., & Hill, C. (2005). The interaction between bacteria and bile. *FEMS Microbiology Reviews*, *29*(4), 625–651. doi:10.1016/j.femsre.2004.09.003

84. Vacca, M., Degirolamo, C., Mariani-Costantini, R., Palasciano, G., & Moschetta, A. (2011). Lipid-sensing nuclear receptors in the pathophysiology and treatment of the metabolic syndrome. *Wiley Interdisciplinary Reviews: Systems Biology and Medicine*, *3*(5), 562–587. doi:10.1002/wsbm.137

85. Ahmad, N. N., Pfalzer, A., & Kaplan, L. M. (2013). Roux-en-Y gastric bypass normalizes the blunted postprandial bile acid excursion associated with obesity. *International Journal of Obesity*, –. doi:10.1038/ijo.2013.38

86. Steinert, R. E., Peterli, R., Keller, S., Meyer-Gerspach, A. C., Drewe, J., Peters, T., & Beglinger, C. (2013). Bile acids and gut peptide secretion after bariatric surgery: A 1-year prospective randomized pilot trial. *Obesity*, *21*(12), E660–E668. doi:10.1002/oby.20522

87. Kohli, R., Setchell, K. D., Kirby, M., Myronovych, A., Ryan, K. K., Ibrahim, S. H., et al. (2013). A Surgical Model in Male Obese Rats Uncovers Protective Effects of Bile Acids Post-Bariatric Surgery. *Endocrinology*. doi:10.1210/en.2012-2069

88. Glicksman, C., Pournaras, D. J., Wright, M., Roberts, R., Mahon, D., Welbourn, R., et al. (2010). Postprandial plasma bile acid responses in normal weight and obese subjects. *Annals of Clinical Biochemistry, 47*(5), 482–484. doi:10.1258/acb.2010.010040

89. Werling, M., Vincent, R. P., Cross, G. F., Marschall, H.-U., Fändriks, L., Lönroth, H., et al. (2013). Enhanced fasting and post-prandial plasma bile acid responses after Roux-en-Y gastric bypass surgery. *Scandinavian Journal of Gastroenterology, 48*(11), 1257–1264. doi:10.3109/00365521.2013.8336 47

90. Roberts, R. E., Glicksman, C., Alaghband-Zadeh, J., Sherwood, R. A., Akuji, N., & le Roux, C. W. (2010). The relationship between postprandial bile acid concentration, GLP-1, PYY and ghrelin. *Clinical Endocrinology, 74*(1), 67–72. doi:10.1111/j.1365-2265.2010.03886.x

91. Sayin, S. I., Wahlström, A., Felin, J., Jäntti, S., Marschall, H.-U., Bamberg, K., et al. (2013). Gut Microbiota Regulates Bile Acid Metabolism by Reducing the Levels of Tauro-beta-muricholic Acid, a Naturally Occurring FXR Antagonist. *Cell Metabolism, 17*(2), 225–235. doi:10.1016/j. cmet.2013.01.003

92. Murphy, K. G., & Bloom, S. R. (2006). Gut hormones and the regulation of energy homeostasis. *Nature, 444*(7121), 854–859. doi:10.1038/ nature05484

93. Toft-Nielsen, M. B., Damholt, M. B., Madsbad, S., Hilsted, L. M., Hughes, T. E., Michelsen, B. K., & Holst, J. J. (2001). Determinants of the impaired secretion of glucagon-like peptide-1 in type 2 diabetic patients. *Journal of Clinical Endocrinology & Metabolism, 86*(8), 3717–3723.

94. Vilsbøll, T., Krarup, T., Deacon, C. F., Madsbad, S., & Holst, J. J. (2001). Reduced postprandial concentrations of intact biologically active glucagon-like peptide 1 in type 2 diabetic patients. *Diabetes, 50*(3), 609–613.

95. Mudaliar, S., & Henry, R. R. (2012). The incretin hormones: from scientific discovery to practical therapeutics. *Diabetologia, 55*(7), 1865–1868. doi:10.1007/s00125-012-2561-x

96. Meier, J. J., & Nauck, M. A. (2008). Is secretion of glucagon-like peptide-1 reduced in type 2 diabetes mellitus? *Nature clinical practice. Endocrinology & metabolism, 4*(11), 606–607. doi:10.1038/ncpendmet0946

97. Sumithran, P., Prendergast, L. A., Delbridge, E., Purcell, K., Shulkes, A., Kriketos, A., & Proietto, J. (2011). Long-term persistence of hormonal adaptations to weight loss. *N Engl J Med, 365*(17), 1597–1604. doi:10.1056/NEJMoa1105816

98. Anagnostis, P., Athyros, V. G., Adamidou, F., Panagiotou, A., Kita, M., Karagiannis, A., & Mikhailidis, D. P. (2011). Glucagon-like peptide-1-based therapies and cardiovascular disease: looking beyond glycaemic control. *Diabetes, Obesity and Metabolism, 13*(4), 302–312. doi:10.1111/ j.1463-1326.2010.01345.x

99. Makdissi, A., Ghanim, H., Vora, M., Green, K., Abuaysheh, S., Chaudhuri, A., et al. (2012). Sitagliptin Exerts an Antinflammatory Action. *Journal of Clinical Endocrinology & Metabolism, 97*(9), 3333–3341. doi:10.1210/jc.2012-1544

100. Chaudhuri, A., Ghanim, H., Vora, M., Sia, C. L., Korzeniewski, K., Dhindsa, S., et al. (2012). Exenatide Exerts a Potent Antiinflammatory Effect. *Journal of Clinical Endocrinology & Metabolism, 97*(1), 198–207. doi:10.1210/jc.2011-1508

101. Lee, Y. S., Park, M. S., Choung, J. S., Kim, S. S., Oh, H. H., Choi, C. S., et al. (2012). Glucagon-like peptide-1 inhibits adipose tissue macrophage infiltration and inflammation in an obese mouse model of diabetes. *Diabetologia, 55*(9), 2456–2468. doi:10.1007/s00125-012-2592-3

102. Ben-Shlomo, S., Zvibel, I., Varol, C., Spektor, L., Shlomai, A., Santo, E. M., et al. (2013). Role of glucose-dependent insulinotropic polypeptide in adipose tissue inflammation of dipeptidylpeptidase 4-deficient rats. *Obesity*, n/a–n/a. doi:10.1002/oby.20340

103. Lee, K. S., Kim, D. H., Jang, J. S., Nam, G. E., Shin, Y. N., Bok, A. R., et al. (2012). Eating rate is associated with cardiometabolic risk factors in Korean adults. *Nutrition, Metabolism and Cardiovascular Diseases*, 1–7. doi:10.1016/j.numecd.2012.02.003

104. McKay, A. B., & Wall, D. (2008). Overprescribing PPIs: An old problem. *BMJ, 336*(7636), 109. doi:10.1136/bmj.39458.462338.3A

105. Swithers, S. E., Laboy, A. F., Clark, K., Cooper, S., & Davidson, T. L. (2012). Experience with the high-intensity sweetener saccharin impairs glucose homeostasis and GLP-1 release in rats. *Behavioural Brain Research, 233*(1), 1–14. doi:10.1016/j.bbr.2012.04.024

106. Pepino, M. Y., Tiemann, C. D., Patterson, B. W., Wice, B. M., & Klein, S. (2013). Sucralose Affects Glycemic and Hormonal Responses to an Oral Glucose Load. *Diabetes Care, 36*(9), 2530–2535. doi:10.2337/dc12-2221

107. Di Bartolomeo, F., Startek, J. B., & Van den Ende, W. (2013). Prebiotics to fight diseases: reality or fiction? *Phytotherapy research : PTR, 27*(10), 1457–1473. doi:10.1002/ptr.4901

108. Everard, A., Lazarevic, V., Derrien, M., Girard, M., Muccioli, G. G., Muccioli, G. M., et al. (2011). Responses of gut microbiota and glucose and lipid metabolism to prebiotics in genetic obese and diet-induced leptin-resistant mice. *Diabetes, 60*(11), 2775–2786. doi:10.2337/db11-0227

109. Delzenne, N., Cani, P., & Neyrinck, A. (2007). Modulation of Glucagon-like Peptide 1 and Energy Metabolism by Inulin and Oligofructose: Experimental Data. *Journal of Nutrition*, (137:), 2547S–2551S.

110. Cani, P. D., Lecourt, E., Dewulf, E. M., Sohet, F. M., Pachikian, B. D., Naslain, D., et al. (2009). Gut microbiota fermentation of prebiotics increases satietogenic and incretin gut peptide production with consequences for appetite sensation and glucose response after a meal. *American Journal of Clinical Nutrition, 90*(5), 1236–1243. doi:10.3945/ajcn.2009.28095

111. Russo, F., Linsalata, M., Clemente, C., Chiloiro, M., Orlando, A., Marconi, E., et al. (2012). Inulin-enriched pasta improves intestinal permeability and modifies the circulating levels of zonulin and glucagon-like peptide 2 in healthy young volunteers. *Nutrition Research, 32*(12), 940–946. doi:10.1016/j.nutres.2012.09.010

112. Ramirez-Farias, C., Slezak, K., Fuller, Z., Duncan, A., Holtrop, G., & Louis, P. (2008). Effect of inulin on the human gut microbiota: stimulation of Bifidobacterium adolescentis and Faecalibacterium prausnitzii. *British Journal of Nutrition, 101*(04), 533. doi:10.1017/S0007114508019880

113. Costabile, A., Kolida, S., Klinder, A., Gietl, E., Bäuerlein, M., Frohberg, C., et al. (2010). A double-blind, placebo-controlled, cross-over study to establish the bifidogenic effect of a very-long-chain inulin extracted from globe artichoke (Cynara scolymus) in healthy human subjects. *British Journal of Nutrition, 104*(07), 1007–1017. doi:10.1017/S0007114510001571

114. Moran-Ramos, S., Tovar, A. R., & Torres, N. (2012). Diet: friend or foe of enteroendocrine cells--how it interacts with enteroendocrine cells. *Adv Nutr, 3*(1), 8–20. doi:10.3945/an.111.000976

115. Nilsson, A., Johansson, E., Ekström, L., & Björck, I. (2013). Effects of a Brown Beans Evening Meal on Metabolic Risk Markers and Appetite Regulating Hormones at a Subsequent Standardized Breakfast: A Randomized Cross-Over Study. *PLoS ONE, 8*(4), e59985. doi:10.1371/journal.pone.0059985.s002

116. Al-masri, I. M., Mohammad, M. K., & Tahaa, M. O. (2009). Inhibition of dipeptidyl peptidase IV (DPP IV) is one of the mechanisms explaining the hypoglycemic effect of berberine. *Journal of Enzyme Inhibition and Medicinal Chemistry, 24*(5), 1061–1066.

117. Yu, Y., Liu, L., Wang, X., Liu, X., Liu, X., Xie, L., & Wang, G. (2010). Modulation of glucagon-like peptide-1 release by berberine: In vivo and in vitro studies. *Biochemical Pharmacology, 79*(7), 1000–1006. doi:10.1016/j.bcp.2009.11.017

118. Dao, T.-M. A., Waget, A., Klopp, P., Serino, M., Vachoux, C., Pechere, L., et al. (2011). Resveratrol Increases Glucose Induced GLP-1 Secretion in Mice: A Mechanism which Contributes to the Glycemic Control. *PLoS ONE, 6*(6), e20700. doi:10.1371/journal.pone.0020700.t001

119. Geraedts, M. C. P., Troost, F. J., Tinnemans, R., Söderholm, J. D., Brummer, R.-J., & Saris, W. H. M. (2010). Release of satiety hormones in response to specific dietary proteins is different between human and murine small intestinal mucosa. *Annals of nutrition & metabolism*, *56*(4), 308–313. doi:10.1159/000312664

120. Geraedts, M. C. P., Troost, F. J., Munsters, M. J. M., Stegen, J. H. C. H., de Ridder, R. J., Conchillo, J. M., et al. (2011). Intraduodenal Administration of Intact Pea Protein Effectively Reduces Food Intake in Both Lean and Obese Male Subjects. *PLoS ONE*, *6*(9), e24878. doi:10.1371/journal. pone.0024878.t001

121. Geraedts, M. C. P., Troost, F. J., & Saris, W. H. M. (2012). Addition of sucralose enhances the release of satiety hormones in combination with pea protein. *Molecular Nutrition & Food Research*, *56*(3), 417–424. doi:10.1002/mnfr.201100297

122. Pols, T. W. H., Noriega, L. G., Nomura, M., Auwerx, J., & Schoonjans, K. (2011). The bile acid membrane receptor TGR5 as an emerging target in metabolism and inflammation. *Journal of Hepatology*, *54*(6), 1263–1272. doi:10.1016/j.jhep.2010.12.004

CHAPTER 6: A CHANGING VIEW OF THE GUT

1. Liou, A. P., Paziuk, M., Luevano, J. M., Machineni, S., Turnbaugh, P. J., & Kaplan, L. M. (2013). Conserved Shifts in the Gut Microbiota Due to Gastric Bypass Reduce Host Weight and Adiposity. *Science Translational Medicine*, *5*(178), 178ra41–178ra41. doi:10.1126/scitranslmed.3005687

2. Holmes, E., Kinross, J., Gibson, G. R., Burcelin, R., Jia, W., Pettersson, S., & Nicholson, J. K. (2012). Therapeutic Modulation of Microbiota-Host Metabolic Interactions. *Science Translational Medicine*, *4*(137), 137rv6–137rv6. doi:10.1126/scitranslmed.3004244

3. Delzenne, N. M., Neyrinck, A. M., & Cani, P. D. (2011). Modulation of the gut microbiota by nutrients with prebiotic properties: consequences for host health in the context of obesity and metabolic syndrome. *Microbial Cell Factories*, *10*(Suppl 1), S10. doi:10.1186/1475-2859-10-S1-S10

4. Million, M., & Raoult, D. (2013). The role of the manipulation of the gut microbiota in obesity. *Current infectious disease reports*, *15*(1), 25–30. doi:10.1007/s11908-012-0301-5

5. Pimentel, G. D., Micheletti, T. O., Pace, F., Rosa, J. C., Santos, R. V., & Lira, F. S. (2012). Gut-central nervous system axis is a target for nutritional therapies. *Nutrition Journal*, *11*(1), 1–23. doi:10.1186/1475-2891-11-22

6. Pimentel, G. D., Micheletti, T. O., & Pace, F. (2013). Nutritional Targets for Modulation of the Microbiota in Obesity. *Drug Development Research*, *74*(6), 393–402. doi:10.1002/ddr.21092

7.   Vrieze, A., Van Nood, E., Holleman, F., Salojärvi, J., Kootte, R. S.,
     Bartelsman, J. F. W. M., et al. (2012). Transfer of Intestinal Microbiota
     From Lean Donors Increases Insulin Sensitivity in Individuals With
     Metabolic Syndrome. *Gastroenterology*, *143*(4), 913–916.e7. doi:10.1053/j.
     gastro.2012.06.031

8.   Ridaura, V. K., Faith, J. J., Rey, F. E., Cheng, J., Duncan, A. E., Kau, A. L., et
     al. (2013). Gut Microbiota from Twins Discordant for Obesity Modulate
     Metabolism in Mice. *Science*, *341*(6150), 1241214–1241214. doi:10.1126/
     science.1241214

9.   Angelakis, E., Armougom, F., Million, M., & Raoult, D. (2012). The
     relationship between gut microbiota and weight gain in humans. *Future
     Microbiology*, *7*(1), 91–109. doi:10.2217/fmb.11.142

10. Payne, A. N., Chassard, C., Zimmermann, M., Müller, P., Stinca, S., &
     Lacroix, C. (2011). The metabolic activity of gut microbiota in obese
     children is increased compared with normal-weight children and exhibits
     more exhaustive substrate utilization. *Nutrition and Diabetes*, *1*(7), e12–8.
     doi:10.1038/nutd.2011.8

11. Hegde, V., & Dhurandhar, N. V. (2013). Microbes and obesity--
     interrelationship between infection, adipose tissue and the immune system.
     *Clinical microbiology and infection : the official publication of the European
     Society of Clinical Microbiology and Infectious Diseases*, *19*(4), 314–320.
     doi:10.1111/1469-0691.12157

12. Qin, J., Li, Y., Cai, Z., Li, S., Zhu, J., Zhang, F., et al. (2012). A
     metagenome-wide association study of gut microbiota in type 2 diabetes.
     Nature, *490*(7418), 55–60. doi:10.1038/nature11450

13. Shen, J., Obin, M. S., & Zhao, L. (2013). The gut microbiota, obesity and
     insulin resistance. Journal of Molecular Aspects of Medicine, *34*(1), 39–58.
     doi:10.1016/j.mam.2012.11.001

14. Brown, K., DeCoffe, D., Molcan, E., & Gibson, D. L. (2012). Diet-Induced
     Dysbiosis of the Intestinal Microbiota and the Effects on Immunity and
     Disease. *Nutrients*, *4*(12), 1095–1119. doi:10.3390/nu4081095

15. Bengmark, S. (2013). Processed Foods, Dysbiosis, Systemic Inflammation,
     and Poor Health. *Current Nutrition & Food Science*, *9*(2), 113–143.

16. Martins dos Santos, V., Müller, M., & de Vos, W. M. (2010). Systems biology
     of the gut: the interplay of food, microbiota and host at the mucosal
     interface. *Current Opinion in Biotechnology*, *21*(4), 539–550. doi:10.1016/j.
     copbio.2010.08.003

17. Reis, B. S., & Mucida, D. (2012). The Role of the Intestinal Context in the
     Generation of Tolerance and Inflammation. *Clinical and Developmental
     Immunology*, *2012*, 1–6. doi:10.1155/2012/157948

18. Ulluwishewa, D., Anderson, R. C., McNabb, W. C., Moughan, P. J., Wells,
     J. M., & Roy, N. C. (2011). Regulation of Tight Junction Permeability by
     Intestinal Bacteria and Dietary Components. *Journal of Nutrition*, *141*(5),
     769–776. doi:10.3945/jn.110.135657

19. Garg, A., Chren, M.-M., Sands, L. P., Matsui, M. S., Marenus, K. D., Feingold, K. R., & Elias, P. M. (2001). Psychological stress perturbs epidermal permeability barrier homeostasis: implications for the pathogenesis of stress-associated skin disorders. *Archives of Dermatology*, *137*(1), 53.

20. Li, X., Kan, E. M., Lu, J., Cao, Y., Wong, R. K., Keshavarzian, A., & Wilder-Smith, C. H. (2013). Combat-training increases intestinal permeability, immune activation and gastrointestinal symptoms in soldiers. *Alimentary Pharmacology & Therapeutics*, *37*(8), 799–809. doi:10.1111/apt.12269

21. Moreira, A. P. B., Texeira, T. F. S., Ferreira, A. B., do Carmo Gouveia Peluzio, M., & de Cássia Gonçalves Alfenas, R. (2012). Influence of a high-fat diet on gut microbiota, intestinal permeability and metabolic endotoxaemia. *British Journal of Nutrition*, *108*(05), 801–809. doi:10.1017/S0007114512001213

22. Miele, L., Valenza, V., La Torre, G., Montalto, M., Cammarota, G., Ricci, R., et al. (2009). Increased intestinal permeability and tight junction alterations in nonalcoholic fatty liver disease. *Hepatology*, *49*(6), 1877–1887. doi:10.1002/hep.22848

23. Harte, A. L., Varma, M. C., Tripathi, G., McGee, K. C., Al-Daghri, N. M., Al-Attas, O. S., et al. (2012). High Fat Intake Leads to Acute Postprandial Exposure to Circulating Endotoxin in Type 2 Diabetic Subjects. *Diabetes Care*, *35*(2), 375–382. doi:10.2337/dc11-1593

24. Esteve, E., Ricart, W., & Fernández-Real, J.-M. (2011). Gut microbiota interactions with obesity, insulin resistance and type 2 diabetes: did gut microbiote co-evolve with insulin resistance? *Current Opinion in Clinical Nutrition and Metabolic Care*, 1. doi:10.1097/MCO.0b013e328348c06d

25. Stehle, J. R., Leng, X., Kitzman, D. W., Nicklas, B. J., Kritchevsky, S. B., & High, K. P. (2012). Lipopolysaccharide-binding protein, a surrogate marker of microbial translocation, is associated with physical function in healthy older adults. *The Journals of Gerontology Series A: Biological Sciences and Medical Sciences*, *67*(11), 1212–1218. doi:10.1093/gerona/gls178

26. Mehta, N. N., McGillicuddy, F. C., Anderson, P. D., Hinkle, C. C., Shah, R., Pruscino, L., et al. (2009). Experimental endotoxemia induces adipose inflammation and insulin resistance in humans. *Diabetes*, *59*(1), 172–181. doi:10.2337/db09-0367

27. Teixeira, T. F. S., Souza, N. C. S., Chiarello, P. G., Franceschini, S. C. C., Bressan, J., Ferreira, C. L. L. F., & do Carmo G Peluzio, M. (2012). Intestinal permeability parameters in obese patients are correlated with metabolic syndrome risk factors. *Clinical Nutrition*, *31*(5), 735–740. doi:10.1016/j.clnu.2012.02.009

28. Moreno-Navarrete, J. M., Sabater, M., Ortega, F., Ricart, W., & Fernández-Real, J.-M. (2012). Circulating Zonulin, a Marker of Intestinal Permeability, Is Increased in Association with Obesity-Associated Insulin Resistance. *PLoS ONE*, *7*(5), e37160. doi:10.1371/journal.pone.0037160.t003

29. Gummesson, A., Carlsson, L. M. S., Storlien, L. H., Bäckhed, F., Lundin, P., Löfgren, L., et al. (2011). Intestinal Permeability Is Associated With Visceral Adiposity in Healthy Women. *Obesity*, 1–3. doi:10.1038/oby.2011.251

30. Żak-Gołąb, A., Kocełak, P., Aptekorz, M., Zientara, M., Juszczyk, Ł., Martirosian, G., et al. (2012). Gut microbiota, microinflammation, metabolic profile and zonulin concentration in obese and normal weight subjects. *Cardiovascular Diabetology*, *11*(1), 116. doi:10.1038/oby.2009.319

31. Pop, M. (2012). We are what we eat: how the diet of infants affects their gut microbiome. *Genome Biology*, *13*(4), 152–152. doi:10.1186/gb-2012-13-4-152

32. Lee, K. S., Kim, D. H., Jang, J. S., Nam, G. E., Shin, Y. N., Bok, A. R., et al. (2012). Eating rate is associated with cardiometabolic risk factors in Korean adults. *Nutrition, Metabolism and Cardiovascular Diseases*, 1–7. doi:10.1016/j.numecd.2012.02.003

33. Otsuka, R., Tamakoshi, K., Yatsuya, H., Murata, C., Sekiya, A., Wada, K., et al. (2006). Eating Fast Leads to Obesity: Findings Based on Self-administered Questionnaires among Middle-aged Japanese Men and Women. *Journal of Epidemiology*, *16*(3), 117–124. doi:10.2188/jea.16.117

34. Ohkuma, T., Fujii, H., Iwase, M., Kikuchi, Y., Ogata, S., Idewaki, Y., et al. (2013). Impact of eating rate on obesity and cardiovascular risk factors according to glucose tolerance status: the Fukuoka Diabetes Registry and the Hisayama Study. *Diabetologia*, *56*(1), 70–77. doi:10.1007/s00125-012-2746-3

35. Li, J., Zhang, N., Hu, L., Li, Z., Li, R., Li, C., & Wang, S. (2011). Improvement in chewing activity reduces energy intake in one meal and modulates plasma gut hormone concentrations in obese and lean young Chinese men. *American Journal of Clinical Nutrition*, *94*(3), 709–716. doi:10.3945/ajcn.111.015164

36. Zhu, Y., Hsu, W. H., & Hollis, J. H. (2012). Increasing the number of masticatory cycles is associated with reduced appetite and altered postprandial plasma concentrations of gut hormones, insulin and glucose. *British Journal of Nutrition*, 1–7. doi:10.1017/S0007114512005053

37. Andrade, A. M., Greene, G. W., & Melanson, K. J. (2008). Eating Slowly Led to Decreases in Energy Intake within Meals in Healthy Women. *Journal of the American Dietetic Association*, *108*(7), 1186–1191. doi:10.1016/j.jada.2008.04.026

38. Helman, C. A. (1998). Chewing gum is as effective as food in stimulating cephalic phase gastric secretion. *Am J Gastroenterol.*, *83*(6), 640–642.

39. Lunding, J. A., Nordström, L. M., Haukelid, A.-O., Gilja, O. H., Berstad, A., & Hausken, T. (2008). Vagal activation by sham feeding improves gastric motility in functional dyspepsia. *Neurogastroenterology and motility : the official journal of the European Gastrointestinal Motility Society*, *20*(6), 618–624. doi:10.1111/j.1365-2982.2007.01076.x

40. Reutrakul, S., Hood, M. M., Crowley, S. J., Morgan, M. K., Teodori, M., & Knutson, K. L. (2013). The Relationship Between Breakfast Skipping, Chronotype, and Glycemic Control in Type 2 Diabetes. *Chronobiology International*, 1–8. doi:10.3109/07420528.2013.821614

41. Nurul-Fadhilah, A., Teo, P. S., Huybrechts, I., & Foo, L. H. (2013). Infrequent Breakfast Consumption Is Associated with Higher Body Adiposity and Abdominal Obesity in Malaysian School-Aged Adolescents. *PLoS ONE*, *8*(3), e59297. doi:10.1371/journal.pone.0059297.t003

42. Jakubowicz, D., Barnea, M., Wainstein, J., & Froy, O. (2013). High Caloric intake at breakfast vs. dinner differentially influences weight loss of overweight and obese women. *Obesity*, *21*(12), 2504–2512. doi:10.1002/oby.20460

43. Garaulet, M., Gómez-Abellán, P., Alburquerque-Béjar, J. J., Lee, Y.-C., Ordovas, J. M., & Scheer, F. A. J. L. (2013). Timing of food intake predicts weight loss effectiveness. *International Journal of Obesity*, *37*(4), 604–611. doi:10.1038/ijo.2012.229

44. Astbury, N. M., Taylor, M. A., & Macdonald, I. A. (2011). Breakfast consumption affects appetite, energy intake, and the metabolic and endocrine responses to foods consumed later in the day in male habitual breakfast eaters. *Journal of Nutrition*, *141*(7), 1381–1389. doi:10.3945/jn.110.128645

45. Farshchi, H. R., Taylor, M. A., & Macdonald, I. A. (2005). Deleterious effects of omitting breakfast on insulin sensitivity and fasting lipid profiles in healthy lean women. *Am J Clin Nutr*, *81*(2), 388–396.

46. Jakubowicz, D. D., Froy, O. O., Wainstein, J. J., & Boaz, M. M. (2012). Meal timing and composition influence ghrelin levels, appetite scores and weight loss maintenance in overweight and obese adults. Steroids, *77*(4), 323–331. doi:10.1016/j.steroids.2011.12.006

47. Pavlov, V. A., & Tracey, K. J. (2012). The vagus nerve and the inflammatory reflex—linking immunity and metabolism. *Nature Reviews | Endocrinology*, *8*(12), 743–754. doi:10.1038/nrendo.2012.189

48. Vinik, A. I., Erbas, T., & Casellini, C. M. (2013). Diabetic cardiac autonomic neuropathy, inflammation and cardiovascular disease. *Journal of Diabetes Investigation*, *4*(1), 4–18. doi:10.1111/jdi.12042

49. Mizock, B. A. (2001). Alterations in fuel metabolism in critical illness: hyperglycaemia. *Best Practice & Research Clinical Endocrinology & Metabolism*, *15*(4), 533–551. doi:10.1053/beem.2001.0168

50. Cancello, R., Zulian, A., Maestrini, S., Mencarelli, M., Barba, Della, A., Invitti, C., et al. (2012). The nicotinic acetylcholine receptor α7 in subcutaneous mature adipocytes: downregulation in human obesity and modulation by diet-induced weight loss. *International Journal of Obesity*, *36*(12), 1552–1557. doi:10.1038/ijo.2011.275

51. Mayer, E. A. (2011). Gut feelings: the emerging biology of gut–brain communication. *Nature Reviews Neuroscience*, *12*(8), 453–466. doi:10.1038/nrn3071

52. Kennedy, P. J., Clarke, G., Quigley, E. M. M., Groeger, J. A., Dinan, T. G., & Cryan, J. F. (2011). Gut memories: Towards a cognitive neurobiology of irritable bowel syndrome. *Neuroscience and Biobehavioral Reviews*, *36*(1), 310–340. doi:10.1016/j.neubiorev.2011.07.001

53. de Lartigue, G., La Serre, de, C. B., & Raybould, H. E. (2011). Vagal afferent neurons in high fat diet-induced obesity; intestinal microflora, gut inflammation and cholecystokinin. *Physiology and Behavior*, *105*(1), 100–105. doi:10.1016/j.physbeh.2011.02.040

54. Gershon, M. (1999). *The Second Brain: A Groundbreaking New Understanding of Nervous Disorders of the Stomach and Intestine.* HarperCollins. 336 pages. ISBN: 9780060930721

55. Grenham, S., Clarke, G., Cryan, J. F., & Dinan, T. G. (2011). Brain-gut-microbe communication in health and disease. *Frontiers in Physiology*, *2*, 94–94. doi:10.3389/fphys.2011.00094

56. Hussain, S. S., & Bloom, S. R. (2012). The regulation of food intake by the gut-brain axis: implications for obesity. *International Journal of Obesity*, *37*(5), 625–633. doi:10.1038/ijo.2012.93

57 .Phillips, L. K., & Prins, J. B. (2012). Update on incretin hormones. *Annals of the New York Academy of Sciences*, *1243*(1), E55–E74. doi:10.1111/j.1749-6632.2012.06491.x

58. Elsenbruch, S., Holtmann, G., Oezcan, D., Lysson, A., Janssen, O., Goebel, M. U., & Schedlowski, M. (2004). Are There Alterations of Neuroendocrine and Cellular Immune Responses to Nutrients in Women with Irritable Bowel Syndrome? *The American Journal of Gastroenterology*, *99*(4), 703–710. doi:10.1111/j.1572-0241.2004.04138.x

59. Huston, J. M., & Tracey, K. J. (2011). The pulse of inflammation: heart rate variability, the cholinergic anti-inflammatory pathway and implications for therapy. *Journal of Internal Medicine*, *269*(1), 45–53. doi:10.1111/j.1365-2796.2010.02321.x

60. Lujan, H. L., & DiCarlo, S. E. (2013). Physical activity, by enhancing parasympathetic tone and activating the cholinergic anti-inflammatory pathway, is a therapeutic strategy to restrain chronic inflammation and prevent many chronic diseases. *Medical Hypotheses*, *80*(5), 548–552. doi:10.1016/j.mehy.2013.01.014

61. Swarbrick, M. M. (2011). Putting Out Fat's Fire with the Cholinergic Antiinflammatory Pathway. *Endocrinology*, *152*(3), 748–750. doi:10.1210/en.2011-0041

62. Wang, X., Yang, Z., Xue, B., & Shi, H. (2011). Activation of the Cholinergic Antiinflammatory Pathway Ameliorates Obesity-Induced Inflammation and Insulin Resistance. *Endocrinology*, *152*(3), 836–846. doi:10.1210/en.2010-0855

63. Borovikova, L. V., Ivanova, S., Zhang, M., Yang, H., Botchkina, G. I., Watkins, L. R., et al. (2000). Vagus nerve stimulation attenuates the systemic inflammatory response to endotoxin. *Nature, 405*(6785), 458–462. doi:10.1038/35013070

64. Thayer, J. F., & Sternberg, E. (2006). Beyond Heart Rate Variability: Vagal Regulation of Allostatic Systems. *Annals of the New York Academy of Sciences, 1088*(1), 361–372. doi:10.1196/annals.1366.014

65. Haarala, A., Kähönen, M., Eklund, C., Jylhävä, J., Koskinen, T., Taittonen, L., et al. (2011). Heart rate variability is independently associated with C-reactive protein but not with Serum amyloid A. The Cardiovascular Risk in Young Finns Study. *European Journal of Clinical Investigation, 41*(9), 951–957. doi:10.1111/j.1365-2362.2011.02485.x

66. Thayer, J. F., & Fischer, J. E. (2009). Heart rate variability, overnight urinary norepinephrine and C-reactive protein: evidence for the cholinergic anti-inflammatory pathway in healthy human adults. *Journal of Internal Medicine, 265*(4), 439–447. doi:10.1111/j.1365-2796.2008.02023.x

67. Thayer, J. F., Yamamoto, S. S., & Brosschot, J. F. (2010). The relationship of autonomic imbalance, heart rate variability and cardiovascular disease risk factors. *International Journal of Cardiology, 141*(2), 122–131. doi:10.1016/j.ijcard.2009.09.543

68. Soares-Miranda, L., Sandercock, G., Vale, S., Santos, R., Abreu, S., Moreira, C., & Mota, J. (2012). Metabolic syndrome, physical activity and cardiac autonomic function. *Diabetes/Metabolism Research and Reviews, 28*(4), 363–369. doi:10.1002/dmrr.2281

CHAPTER 7: EXERCISE TO LOSE BELLY FAT

1. Nisoli, E., & Carruba, M. O. (2006). Nitric oxide and mitochondrial biogenesis. *Journal of Cell Science, 119*, 2855–2862.

2. Canto, C., Jiang, L. Q., Deshmukh, A. S., Mataki, C., Coste, A., Lagouge, M., et al. (2010). Interdependence of AMPK and SIRT1 for metabolic adaptation to fasting and exercise in skeletal muscle. *Cell Metabolism, 11*(3), 213–219. doi:10.1016/j.cmet.2010.02.006

3. Wenz, T. (2013). Regulation of mitochondrial biogenesis and PGC-1α under cellular stress. *Mitochondrion, 13*(2), 134–142. doi:10.1016/j.mito.2013.01.006

4. Reznick, R. M., & Shulman, G. I. (2006). The role of AMP-activated protein kinase in mitochondrial biogenesis. *The Journal of Physiology, 574*(Pt 1), 33–39. doi:10.1113/jphysiol.2006.109512

5. Misra, P. (2008). AMP activated protein kinase: a next generation target for total metabolic control. *Expert Opinion on Therapeutic Targets, 12*(1), 91–100.

6. Bäckhed, F., Manchester, J. K., Semenkovich, C. F., & Gordon, J. I. (2007). Mechanisms underlying the resistance to diet-induced obesity in germ-free mice. *Proceedings of the National Academy of Sciences of the United States of America*, *104*(3), 979–984.

7. Gauthier, M.-S., O'Brien, E. L., Bigornia, S., Mott, M., Cacicedo, J. M., Xu, X. J., et al. (2011). Decreased AMP-activated protein kinase activity is associated with increased inflammation in visceral adipose tissue and with whole-body insulin resistance in morbidly obese humans. *Biochemical and Biophysical Research Communications*, *404*(1), 382–387. doi:10.1016/j. bbrc.2010.11.127

8. Kahn, B. B., Alquier, T., Carling, D., & Hardie, D. G. (2005). AMP-activated protein kinase: Ancient energy gauge provides clues to modern understanding of metabolism. *Cell Metabolism*, *1*(1), 15–25. doi:10.1016/j. cmet.2004.12.003

9. Li, Y., Xu, S., Mihaylova, M. M., Bin Zheng, Hou, X., Jiang, B., et al. (2011). AMPK Phosphorylates and Inhibits SREBP Activity to Attenuate Hepatic Steatosis and Atherosclerosis in Diet-Induced Insulin-Resistant Mice. *Cell Metabolism*, *13*(4), 376–388. doi:10.1016/j.cmet.2011.03.009

10. Richter, E. A., & Ruderman, N. B. (2009). AMPK and the biochemistry of exercise: implications for human health and disease. *The Biochemical journal*, *418*(2), 261–275. doi:10.1042/BJ20082055

11. Little, J. P., Safdar, A., Wilkin, G. P., Tarnopolsky, M. A., & Gibala, M. J. (2010). A practical model of low-volume high-intensity interval training induces mitochondrial biogenesis in human skeletal muscle: potential mechanisms. *The Journal of Physiology*, *588*(6), 1011–1022. doi:10.1113/ jphysiol.2009.181743

12. Civitarese, A. E., Carling, S., Heilbronn, L. K., Hulver, M. H., Ukropcova, B., Deutsch, W. A., et al. (2007). Calorie restriction increases muscle mitochondrial biogenesis in healthy humans. *PLOS Medicine*, *4*(3), e76. doi:10.1371/journal.pmed.0040076

13. Lindholm, C. R., Ertel, R. L., Bauwens, J. D., Schmuck, E. G., Mulligan, J. D., & Saupe, K. W. (2012). A high-fat diet decreases AMPK activity in multiple tissues in the absence of hyperglycemia or systemic inflammation in rats. *Journal of Physiology and Biochemistry*, *69*(2), 165–175. doi:10.1007/s13105-012-0199-2

14. Steinberg, G. R. (2007). Inflammation in obesity is the common link between defects in fatty acid metabolism and insulin resistance. *Cell cycle (Georgetown, Tex.)*, *6*(8), 888–894.

15. Kola, B., Christ-Crain, M., Lolli, F., Arnaldi, G., Giacchetti, G., Boscaro, M., et al. (2008). Changes in Adenosine 5"-Monophosphate-Activated Protein Kinase as a Mechanism of Visceral Obesity in Cushing"s Syndrome. *Journal of Clinical Endocrinology & Metabolism*, *93*(12), 4969–4973. doi:10.1210/ jc.2008-1297

16. Salminen, A., Hyttinen, J. M. T., & Kaarniranta, K. (2011). AMP-activated protein kinase inhibits NF-κβ signaling and inflammation: impact on healthspan and lifespan. *Journal of Molecular Medicine, 89*(7), 667–676. doi:10.1007/s00109-011-0748-0

17. Cacicedo, J. M., Yagihashi, N., Keaney, J. F., Jr., Ruderman, N. B., & Ido, Y. (2004). AMPK inhibits fatty acid-induced increases in NF-κβ transactivation in cultured human umbilical vein endothelial cells. *Biochemical and Biophysical Research Communications, 324*(4), 1204–1209. doi:10.1016/j.bbrc.2004.09.177

18. Green, C. J., Pedersen, M., Pedersen, B. K., & Scheele, C. (2011). Elevated NF-κβ Activation Is Conserved in Human Myocytes Cultured From Obese Type 2 Diabetic Patients and Attenuated by AMP-Activated Protein Kinase. *Diabetes, 60*(11), 2810–2819. doi:10.2337/db11-0263

19. Hundal, H., Green, C., Macrae, K., Fogarty, S., Hardie, D., & Sakamoto, K. (2011). Counter modulation of fatty acid-induced proinflammatory NFkB signalling in rat skeletal muscle cells by AMPK. *Biochemical Journal Immediate Publication, 35*(2), 463–474.

20. Bijland, S., Mancini, S. J., & Salt, I. P. (2013). Role of AMP-activated protein kinase in adipose tissue metabolism and inflammation. *Clinical Science, 124*(8), 491–507. doi:10.1210/jc.2008-1297

21. Little, J. P., Safdar, A., Bishop, D., Tarnopolsky, M. A., & Gibala, M. J. (2011). An acute bout of high-intensity interval training increases the nuclear abundance of PGC-1α and activates mitochondrial biogenesis in human skeletal muscle. *AJP: Regulatory, Integrative and Comparative Physiology, 300*(6), R1303–10. doi:10.1152/ajpregu.00538.2010

22. Kitada, M., Kume, S., Takeda-Watanabe, A., Tsuda, S.-I., Kanasaki, K., & Koya, D. (2013). Calorie restriction in overweight males ameliorates obesity-related metabolic alterations and cellular adaptations through anti-aging effects, possibly including AMPK and SIRT1 activation. *Biochimica et Biophysica Acta, 1830*(10), 4820–4827. doi:10.1016/j.bbagen.2013.06.014

23. Finley, L. W., Lee, J., Souza, A., Desquiret-Dumas, V., Bullock, K., Rowe, G. C., et al. (2012). Skeletal muscle transcriptional coactivator PGC-1α mediates mitochondrial, but not metabolic, changes during calorie restriction. *Proceedings of the National Academy of Sciences of the United States of America, 109*(8), 2931–2936. doi:10.1073/pnas.1115813109/-/DCSupplemental

24. Huffman, K. M., Redman, L. M., Landerman, L. R., Pieper, C. F., Stevens, R. D., Muehlbauer, M. J., et al. (2012). Caloric Restriction Alters the Metabolic Response to a Mixed-Meal: Results from a Randomized, Controlled Trial. *PLoS ONE, 7*(4), e28190. doi:10.1371/journal.pone.0028190.s002

25. Burns Kraft, T. F., Dey, M., Rogers, R. B., Ribnicky, D. M., Gipp, D. M., Cefalu, W. T., et al. (2008). Phytochemical Composition and Metabolic Performance-Enhancing Activity of Dietary Berries Traditionally Used by Native North Americans. *Journal of Agricultural and Food Chemistry, 56*(3), 654–660. doi:10.1021/jf071999d

26. Philp, A. (2011). Should Willy Wonka have been a sports nutritionist? *The Journal of Physiology, 589*(19), 4643–4643. doi:10.1113/jphysiol.2011.218438

27. Liu, J., Shen, W., Zhao, B., Wang, Y., Wertz, K., Weber, P., & Zhang, P. (2009). Targeting mitochondrial biogenesis for preventing and treating insulin resistance in diabetes and obesity: Hope from natural mitochondrial nutrients. *Advanced Drug Delivery Reviews, 61*(14), 1343–1352. doi:10.1016/j.addr.2009.06.007

28. Nunn, A. V., Guy, G. W., Brodie, J. S., & Bell, J. D. (2010). Inflammatory modulation of exercise salience: using hormesis to return to a healthy lifestyle. *Nutrition & Metabolism, 7*(1), 87. doi:10.1186/1743-7075-7-87

29. Mattson, M. P., & Calabrese, E. J. (2010). *Hormesis: A Revolution in Biology, Toxicology and Medicine.* Springer. ISBN: 1607614952

30. Calabrese, E., Iavicoli, I., & Calabrese, V. (2013). Hormesis: Its impact on medicine and health. *Human & Experimental Toxicology, 32*(2), 120–152. doi:10.1177/0960327112455069

31. Gurd, B. (2011). Deacetylation of PGC-1α by SIRT1: importance for skeletal muscle function and exercise-induced mitochondrial biogenesis. *Applied Physiology, Nutrition, and Metabolism, 36*(5), 589–597.

32. Dumke, C. L., Mark Davis, J., Angela Murphy, E., Nieman, D. C., Carmichael, M. D., Quindry, J. C., et al. (2009). Successive bouts of cycling stimulates genes associated with mitochondrial biogenesis. *European Journal of Applied Physiology, 107*(4), 419–427. doi:10.1007/s00421-009-1143-1

33. Fadini, G. P., Ceolotto, G., Pagnin, E., De Kreutzenberg, S., & Avogaro, A. (2010). At the crossroads of longevity and metabolism: the metabolic syndrome and lifespan determinant pathways. *Aging Cell, 10*(1), 10–17. doi:10.1111/j.1474-9726.2010.00642.x

34. Wang, Y., Liang, Y., & Vanhoutte, P. M. (2011). SIRT1 and AMPK in regulating mammalian senescence: A critical review and a working model. *FEBS Letters, 585*(7), 986–994. doi:10.1016/j.febslet.2010.11.047

35. Tiainen, A.-M., Männistö, S., Blomstedt, P. A., Moltchanova, E., Perälä, M.-M., Kaartinen, N. E., et al. (2012). Leukocyte telomere length and its relation to food and nutrient intake in an elderly population. *European Journal of Clinical Nutrition, 66*(12), 1290–1294. doi:10.1038/ejcn.2012.143

36. Buxton, J. L., Walters, R. G., Visvikis-Siest, S., Meyre, D., Froguel, P., & Blakemore, A. I. F. (2011). Childhood Obesity Is Associated with Shorter Leukocyte Telomere Length. *Journal of Clinical Endocrinology & Metabolism*, *96*(5), 1500–1505. doi:10.1210/jc.2010-2924

37. Rodenhiser, D., & Mann, M. (2006). Epigenetics and human disease: translating basic biology into clinical applications. *Canadian Medical Association Journal*, *174*(3), 341–348. doi:10.1503/cmaj.050774

38. Cencioni, C., Spallotta, F., Martelli, F., Valente, S., Mai, A., Zeiher, A., & Gaetano, C. (2013). Oxidative Stress and Epigenetic Regulation in Ageing and Age-Related Diseases. *International Journal of Molecular Sciences*, *14*(9), 17643–17663. doi:10.3390/ijms140917643

39. Bencko, V. (1977). Carcinogenic, teratogenic, and mutagenic effects of arsenic. *Environmental Health Perspectives*, *19*, 179.

40. Anand, P., Kunnumakara, A. B., Sundaram, C., Harikumar, K. B., Tharakan, S. T., Lai, O. S., et al. (2008). Cancer is a preventable disease that requires major lifestyle changes. *Pharmaceutical research*, *25*(9), 2097–2116.

41. Kwon, H.-S., & Ott, M. (2008). The ups and downs of SIRT1. *Trends in Biochemical Sciences*, *33*(11), 517–525. doi:10.1016/j.tibs.2008.08.001

42. Houtkooper, R. H., Pirinen, E., & Auwerx, J. (2012). Sirtuins as regulators of metabolism and healthspan. *Nature Publishing Group*, *13*(4), 225–238. doi:10.1038/nrm3293

43. Dashwood, R. H., & Ho, E. (2007). Dietary histone deacetylase inhibitors: from cells to mice to man, *17*(5), 363–369. doi:10.1016/j.semcancer.2007.04.001

44. Dolinoy, D. C., Weidman, J. R., & Jirtle, R. L. (2007). Epigenetic gene regulation: linking early developmental environment to adult disease. *Reproductive toxicology (Elmsford, N.Y.)*, *23*(3), 297–307. doi:10.1016/j.reprotox.2006.08.012

45. Mai, A., & Altucci, L. (2009). Epi-drugs to fight cancer: From chemistry to cancer treatment, the road ahead. *The International Journal of Biochemistry & Cell Biology*, *41*(1), 199–213. doi:10.1016/j.biocel.2008.08.020

46. Das, P. M., & Singal, R. (2004). DNA methylation and cancer. *Journal of Clinical Oncology*, *22*(22), 4632–4642. doi:10.1200/JCO.2004.07.151

47. Milagro, F. I., Mansego, M. L., De Miguel, C., & Martínez, J. A. (2012). Dietary factors, epigenetic modifications and obesity outcomes: Progresses and perspectives. *Journal of Molecular Aspects of Medicine*, 1–31. doi:10.1016/j.mam.2012.06.010

48. Obeid, R., & Herrmann, W. (2009). Homocysteine and lipids: S-Adenosyl methionine as a key intermediate. *FEBS Letters*, *583*(8), 1215–1225. doi:10.1016/j.febslet.2009.03.038

49. James, S. J., Cutler, P., Melnyk, S., Jernigan, S., Janak, L., Gaylor, D. W., & Neubrander, J. A. (2004). Metabolic biomarkers of increased oxidative stress and impaired methylation capacity in children with autism. *Am J Clin Nutr*, *80*(6), 1611–1617.

50. Yang, H., Yang, T., Baur, J. A., Perez, E., Matsui, T., Carmona, J. J., et al. (2007). Nutrient-Sensitive Mitochondrial NAD+ Levels Dictate Cell Survival. *Cell, 130*(6), 1095–1107. doi:10.1016/j.cell.2007.07.035

51. Finkel, T., Deng, C.-X., & Mostoslavsky, R. (2009). Recent progress in the biology and physiology of sirtuins. *Nature, 460*(7255), 587–591.

52. Brooks, C. L., & Gu, W. (2008). How does SIRT1 affect metabolism, senescence and cancer? *Nature Reviews Cancer, 9*(2), 123–128. doi:10.1038/nrc2562

53. Chalkiadaki, A., & Guarente, L. (2012). Sirtuins mediate mammalian metabolic responses to nutrient availability. *Nature Reviews | Endocrinology*, 1–10. doi:10.1038/nrendo.2011.225

54. Chang, H.-C., & Guarente, L. (2013). SIRT1 Mediates Central Circadian Control in the SCN by a Mechanism that Decays with Aging. *Cell, 153*(7), 1448–1460.

55. O'Callaghan, N., Parletta, N., Milte, C. M., & Benassi-Evans, B. (2013). Telomere shortening in elderly people with mild cognitive impairment may be attenuated with omega-3 fatty acid supplementation: A randomised controlled pilot study. *Nutrition.* doi:10.1016/j.nut.2013.09.013

56. Blackburn, E. H. (2005). Telomeres and telomerase: their mechanisms of action and the effects of altering their functions. *FEBS Letters, 579*(4), 859–862. doi:10.1016/j.febslet.2004.11.036

57. Zannolli, R., Mohn, A., Buoni, S., Pietrobelli, A., Messina, M., Chiarelli, F., & Miracco, C. (2008). Telomere length and obesity. *Acta Paediatrica, 97*(7), 952–954. doi:10.1111/j.1651-2227.2008.00783.x

58. Lee, M., Martin, H., Firpo, M. A., & Demerath, E. W. (2010). Inverse association between adiposity and telomere length: The fels longitudinal study. *American Journal of Human Biology, 23*(1), 100–106. doi:10.1002/ajhb.21109

59. Zee, R. Y., Castonguay, A. J., Barton, N. S., Germer, S., & Martin, M. (2010). Mean leukocyte telomere length shortening and type 2 diabetes mellitus: a case-control study. *Translational Research, 155*(4), 166–169.

60. Harte, A. L., da Silva, N. F., Miller, M. A., Cappuccio, F. P., Kelly, A., O'Hare, J. P., et al. (2012). Telomere Length Attrition, a Marker of Biological Senescence, Is Inversely Correlated with Triglycerides and Cholesterol in South Asian Males with Type 2 Diabetes Mellitus. *Experimental Diabetes Research, 2012*(24), 1–7. doi:10.1185/03007995.2010.490468

61. Kong, C. M., Lee, X. W., & Wang, X. (2013). Telomere shortening in human diseases. *FEBS Journal, 280*(14), 3180–3193. doi:10.1111/febs.12326

62. Wang, Y.-Y., Chen, A.-F., Wang, H.-Z., Xie, L.-Y., Sui, K.-X., & Zhang, Q.-Y. (2011). Association of shorter mean telomere length with large artery stiffness in patients with coronary heart disease. *The Aging Male, 14*(1), 27–32. doi:10.3109/13685538.2010.529196

63. Diaz, V. A., Mainous, A. G., Player, M. S., & Everett, C. J. (2009). Telomere length and adiposity in a racially diverse sample. *International Journal of Obesity*, *34*(2), 261–265. doi:10.1038/ijo.2009.198

64. Njajou, O. T., Cawthon, R. M., Blackburn, E. H., Harris, T. B., Li, R., Sanders, J. L., et al. (2011). Shorter telomeres are associated with obesity and weight gain in the elderly. *International Journal of Obesity*, *36*(9), 1176–1179. doi:10.1038/ijo.2011.196

65. Müezzinler, A., Zaineddin, A. K., & Brenner, H. (2013). Body mass index and leukocyte telomere length in adults: a systematic review and meta-analysis. *Obesity Reviews*, n/a–n/a. doi:10.1111/obr.12126

66. Gardner, J. P., Li, S., Srinivasan, S. R., Chen, W., Kimura, M., Lu, X., et al. (2005). Rise in insulin resistance is associated with escalated telomere attrition. *Circulation*, *111*(17), 2171–2177.

67. Masi, S., Nightingale, C. M., Day, I. N. M., Guthrie, P., Rumley, A., Lowe, G. D. O., et al. (2012). Inflammation and Not Cardiovascular Risk Factors Is Associated With Short Leukocyte Telomere Length in 13- to 16-Year-Old Adolescents. *Arteriosclerosis, Thrombosis, and Vascular Biology*, *32*, 2029–2034.

68. Steffens, J. P., Masi, S., D'Aiuto, F., & Spolidorio, L. C. (2013). Telomere length and its relationship with chronic diseases – New perspectives for periodontal research. *Archives of Oral Biology*, *58*(2), 111–117. doi:10.1016/j.archoralbio.2012.09.009

69. Qu, S., Wen, W., Shu, X. O., Chow, W. H., Xiang, Y. B., Wu, J., et al. (2013). Association of Leukocyte Telomere Length With Breast Cancer Risk: Nested Case-Control Findings From the Shanghai Women's Health Study. *American Journal of Epidemiology*, *177*(7), 617–624. doi:10.1093/aje/kws291

70. Tzanetakou, I. P., Katsilambros, N. L., Benetos, A., Mikhailidis, D. P., & Perrea, D. N. (2011). "Is obesity linked to aging?" Adipose tissue and the role of telomeres. *Ageing Research Reviews*, 1–40. doi:10.1016/j.arr.2011.12.003

71. Monickaraj, F., Aravind, S., Gokulakrishnan, K., Sathishkumar, C., Prabu, P., Prabu, D., et al. (2012). Accelerated aging as evidenced by increased telomere shortening and mitochondrial DNA depletion in patients with type 2 diabetes. *Molecular and Cellular Biochemistry*, *365*(1-2), 343–350. doi:10.1007/s11010-012-1276-0

72. Ludlow,, A. T., Zimmerman, J. B., Witkowski, S., Hearn, J. W., Hatfiield, B. D., & Roth, S. M. (2008). Relationship between Physical Activity Level, Telomere Length, and Telomerase Activity. *Medicine & Science in Sports & Exercise*, *40*(10), 1764–1771. doi:10.1249/MSS.0b013e31817c92aa

73. Aviv, A. (2009). Leukocyte telomere length: the telomere tale continues. *American Journal of Clinical Nutrition*, *89*(6), 1721–1722. doi:10.3945/ajcn.2009.27807

74. Marcon, F., Siniscalchi, E., Crebelli, R., Saieva, C., Sera, F., Fortini, P., et al. (2011). Diet-related telomere shortening and chromosome stability. *Mutagenesis*, *27*(1), 49–57. doi:10.1093/mutage/ger056

75. Mikus, C. R., Oberlin, D. J., Libla, J., Boyle, L. J., & Thyfault, J. P. (2012). Glycaemic control is improved by 7 days of aerobic exercise training in patients with type 2 diabetes. *Diabetologia*, *55*(5), 1417–1423. doi:10.1007/s00125-012-2490-8

76. Lira, V. A., Benton, C. R., Yan, Z., & Bonen, A. (2010). PGC-1alpha regulation by exercise training and its influences on muscle function and insulin sensitivity. *AJP: Endocrinology and Metabolism*, *299*(2), E145–61. doi:10.1152/ajpendo.00755.2009

77. Giannopoulou, I., Ploutz-Snyder, L. L., Carhart, R., Weinstock, R. S., Fernhall, B., Goulopoulou, S., & Kanaley, J. A. (2005). Exercise is required for visceral fat loss in postmenopausal women with type 2 diabetes. *Journal of Clinical Endocrinology & Metabolism*, *90*(3), 1511–1518. doi:10.1210/jc.2004-1782

78. Vissers, D., Hens, W., Taeymans, J., Baeyens, J.-P., Poortmans, J., & Van Gaal, L. (2013). The Effect of Exercise on Visceral Adipose Tissue in Overweight Adults: A Systematic Review and Meta-Analysis. *PLoS ONE*, *8*(2), e56415. doi:10.1371/journal.pone.0056415.s002

79. Cuff, D. J., Meneilly, G. S., Martin, A., Ignaszewski, A., Tildesley, H. D., & Frohlich, J. J. (2003). Effective exercise modality to reduce insulin resistance in women with type 2 diabetes. *Diabetes Care*, *26*(11), 2977–2982.

80. Ross, R., & Bradshaw, A. J. (2009). The future of obesity reduction: beyond weight loss. *Nature Reviews | Endocrinology*, *5*(6), 319–326. doi:10.1038/nrendo.2009.78

81. Sigal, R. J., Kenny, G. P., Boulé, N. G., Wells, G. A., Prud'homme, D., Fortier, M., et al. (2007). Effects of Aerobic Training, Resistance Training, or Both on Glycemic Control in Type 2 DiabetesA Randomized Trial. *Annals of Internal Medicine*, *147*(6), 357–369.

82. Church, T. S., Blair, S. N., Cocreham, S., Johannsen, N., Johnson, W., Kramer, K., et al. (2010). Effects of Aerobic and Resistance Training on Hemoglobin A 1cLevels in Patients With Type 2 Diabetes. *JAMA: The Journal of the American Medical Association*, *304*(20), 2253. doi:10.1001/jama.2010.1710

83. Poehlman, E. T., Dvorak, R. V., DeNino, W. F., Brochu, M., & Ades, P. A. (2000). Effects of resistance training and endurance training on insulin sensitivity in nonobese, young women: a controlled randomized trial. *Journal of Clinical Endocrinology & Metabolism*, *85*(7), 2463–2468.

84. Tokmakidis, S., Zois, C., Volaklis, K., Kotsa, K., & Touvra, A.-M. (2004). The effects of a combined strength and aerobic exercise program on glucose control and insulin action in women with type 2 diabetes. *European Journal of Applied Physiology*, *92*(4-5), 437–442. doi:10.1007/s00421-004-1174-6

85. Poehlman, E. T., Denino, W. F., Beckett, T., Kinaman, K. A., Dionne, I. J., Dvorak, R., & Ades, P. A. (2002). Effects of endurance and resistance training on total daily energy expenditure in young women: a controlled randomized trial. *Journal of Clinical Endocrinology & Metabolism, 87*(3), 1004–1009.

86. Suh, S., Jeong, I.-K., Kim, M. Y., Kim, Y. S., Shin, S., Kim, S. S., & Kim, J. H. (2011). Effects of Resistance Training and Aerobic Exercise on Insulin Sensitivity in Overweight Korean Adolescents: A Controlled Randomized Trial. *Diabetes & Metabolism Journal, 35*(4), 418. doi:10.4093/dmj.2011.35.4.418

87. Davidson, L. E., Hudson, R., Kilpatrick, K., Kuk, J. L., McMillan, K., Janiszewski, P. M., et al. (2009). Effects of Exercise Modality on Insulin Resistance and Functional Limitation in Older AdultsA Randomized Controlled Trial. *Arch Intern Med, 169*(2), 122–131. doi:10.1001/archinternmed.2008.558

88. Willis, L. H., Slentz, C. A., Bateman, L. A., Shields, A. T., Piner, L. W., Bales, C. W., et al. (2012). Effects of aerobic and/or resistance training on body mass and fat mass in overweight or obese adults. *Journal of Applied Physiology, 113*(12), 1831–1837. doi:10.1152/japplphysiol.01370.2011

89. Grøntved, A., Rimm, E. B., Willett, W. C., Andersen, L. B., & Hu, F. B. (2012). A Prospective Study of Weight Training and Risk of Type 2 Diabetes Mellitus in MenWeight Training and Risk of Type 2 Diabetes. *Arch Intern Med, 172*(17), 1306–1312. doi:10.1001/archinternmed.2012.3138

90. Perez-Gomez, J., Vicente-Rodríguez, G., Ara Royo, I., Martínez-Redondo, D., Puzo Foncillas, J., Moreno, L. A., et al. (2013). Effect of endurance and resistance training on regional fat mass and lipid profile. *Nutrición hospitalaria, 28*(2), 340–346. doi:10.3305/nh.2013.28.2.6200

91. Slentz, C. A., Aiken, L. B., Houmard, J. A., Bales, C. W., Johnson, J. L., Tanner, C. J., et al. (2005). Inactivity, exercise, and visceral fat. Strride: a randomized, controlled study of exercise intensity and amount. *J Appl Physiol, 99*(4), 1613–1618. doi:10.1152/japplphysiol.00124.2005

92. Slentz, C. A., Houmard, J. A., Johnson, J. L., Bateman, L. A., Tanner, C. J., McCartney, J. S., et al. (2007). Inactivity, exercise training and detraining, and plasma lipoproteins. Strride: a randomized, controlled study of exercise intensity and amount. *Journal of Applied Physiology, 103*(2), 432–442. doi:10.1152/japplphysiol.01314.2006

93. Abbenhardt, C., McTiernan, A., Alfano, C. M., Wener, M. H., Campbell, K. L., Duggan, C., et al. (2013). Effects of individual and combined dietary weight loss and exercise interventions in postmenopausal women on adiponectin and leptin levels. *Journal of Internal Medicine*, n/a–n/a. doi:10.1111/joim.12062

94. Laursen, P. B., & Jenkins, D. G. (2002). The scientific basis for high-intensity interval training: optimising training programmes and maximising performance in highly trained endurance athletes. *Sports medicine (Auckland, N.Z.), 32*(1), 53–73.

95. Gibala, M. J., & McGee, S. L. (2008). Metabolic adaptations to short-term high-intensity interval training: a little pain for a lot of gain? *Exercise and sport sciences reviews, 36*(2), 58–63. doi:10.1097/JES.0b013e318168ec1f

96. Gibala, M. J., McGee, S. L., Garnham, A. P., Howlett, K. F., Snow, R. J., & Hargreaves, M. (2009). Brief intense interval exercise activates AMPK and p38 MAPK signaling and increases the expression of PGC-1alpha in human skeletal muscle. *J Appl Physiol, 106*(3), 929–934. doi:10.1152/japplphysiol.90880.2008

97. Boutcher, S. H. (2011). High-Intensity Intermittent Exercise and Fat Loss. *Journal of Obesity, 2011*(4), 1–10. doi:10.1038/sj.ijo.0802846

98. Heydari, M., Freund, J., & Boutcher, S. H. (2012). The Effect of High-Intensity Intermittent Exercise on Body Composition of Overweight Young Males. *Journal of Obesity, 2012*(12), 1–8. doi:10.2478/v10036-009-0014-5

99. Talanian, J. L., Galloway, S. D. R., Heigenhauser, G. J. F., Bonen, A., & Spriet, L. L. (2007). Two weeks of high-intensity aerobic interval training increases the capacity for fat oxidation during exercise in women. *Journal of Applied Physiology, 102*(4), 1439–1447. doi:10.1152/japplphysiol.01098.2006

100. Crisp, N. A., Fournier, P. A., Licari, M. K., Braham, R., & Guelfi, K. J. (2012a). Adding sprints to continuous exercise at the intensity that maximises fat oxidation: Implications for acute energy balance and enjoyment. *Metabolism, 61*(9), 1280–1288. doi:10.1016/j.metabol.2012.02.009

101. Crisp, N. A., Fournier, P. A., Licari, M. K., Braham, R., & Guelfi, K. J. (2012b). Optimising sprint interval exercise to maximise energy expenditure and enjoyment in overweight boys. *Applied Physiology, Nutrition, and Metabolism, 37*(6), 1222–1231. doi:10.1139/h2012-111

102. Johnson, J. L., Slentz, C. A., Houmard, J. A., Samsa, G. P., Duscha, B. D., Aiken, L. B., et al. (2007). Exercise training amount and intensity effects on metabolic syndrome (from Studies of a Targeted Risk Reduction Intervention through Defined Exercise). *AJC, 100*(12), 1759–1766.

103. Aoi, W., Naito, Y., & Yoshikawa, T. (2011). Dietary Exercise as a Novel Strategy for the Prevention and Treatment of Metabolic Syndrome: Effects on Skeletal Muscle Function. *Journal of Nutrition and Metabolism, 2011*, 1–11. doi:10.1155/2011/676208

104. Pedersen, B. K., & Febbraio, M. A. (2012). Muscles, exercise and obesity: skeletal muscle as a secretory organ. *Nature Reviews | Endocrinology, 8*(8), 457–465. doi:10.1038/nrendo.2012.49

105. Perandini, L. A., de Sá-Pinto, A. L., Roschel, H., Benatti, F. B., Lima, F. R., Bonfá, E., & Gualano, B. (2012). Exercise as a therapeutic tool to counteract inflammation and clinical symptoms in autoimmune rheumatic diseases. *Autoimmunity Reviews*, *12*(2), 218–224. doi:10.1016/j.autrev.2012.06.007

106. Scott, J. M., Koelwyn, G. J., Hornsby, W. E., Khouri, M., Peppercorn, J., Douglas, P. S., & Jones, L. W. (2013). Exercise Therapy as Treatment for Cardiovascular and Oncologic Disease After a Diagnosis of Early-Stage Cancer. *Seminars in Oncology*, *40*(2), 218–228. doi:10.1053/j.seminoncol.2013.01.001

107. Fink, L. N., Oberbach, A., Costford, S. R., Chan, K. L., Sams, A., Blüher, M., & Klip, A. (2013). Expression of anti-inflammatory macrophage genes within skeletal muscle correlates with insulin sensitivity in human obesity and type 2 diabetes. *Diabetologia*, *56*(7), 1623–1628. doi:10.1007/s00125-013-2897-x

108. Wernbom, M., Augustsson, J., & Thomeé, R. (2007). The influence of frequency, intensity, volume and mode of strength training on whole muscle cross-sectional area in humans. *Sports medicine (Auckland, N.Z.)*, *37*(3), 225–264.

109. Gonzalez, J. T., & Stevenson, E. J. (2011). New perspectives on nutritional interventions to augment lipid utilisation during exercise. *British Journal of Nutrition*, *107*(03), 339–349. doi:10.1017/S0007114511006684

110. Álvares, T. S., Meirelles, C. M., Bhambhani, Y. N., Paschoalin, V. M. F., & Gomes, P. P. S. C. (2011). L-Arginine as a Potential Ergogenic Aid in Healthy Subjects. *Sports medicine (Auckland, N.Z.)*, *41*(3), 233–248. doi:10.2165/11538590-000000000-00000

111. Cooke, M. B., Rybalka, E., Williams, A. D., Cribb, P. J., & Hayes, A. (2009). Creatine supplementation enhances muscle force recovery after eccentrically-induced muscle damage in healthy individuals. *Journal of the International Society of Sports Nutrition*, *6*(1), 13. doi:10.1186/1550-2783-6-13

112. Álvares, T. S., Meirelles, C. M., Bhambhani, Y. N., Paschoalin, V. M. F., & Gomes, P. P. S. C. (2011). L-Arginine as a Potential Ergogenic Aid in Healthy Subjects. *Sports Medicine (Auckland, N.Z.)*, *41*(3), 233–248. doi:10.2165/11538590-000000000-00000

113. Bloomer, R. J., Farney, T. M., Trepanowski, J. F., McCarthy, C. G., Canale, R. E., & Schilling, B. K. (2010). Comparison of pre-workout nitric oxide stimulating dietary supplements on skeletal muscle oxygen saturation, blood nitrate/nitrite, lipid peroxidation, and upper body exercise performance in resistance trained men. *Journal of the International Society of Sports Nutrition*, *7*(1), 16. doi:10.1186/1550-2783-7-16

114. Cooke, M. B., Rybalka, E., Williams, A. D., Cribb, P. J., & Hayes, A. (2009). Creatine supplementation enhances muscle force recovery after eccentrically-induced muscle damage in healthy individuals. *Journal of the International Society of Sports Nutrition*, *6*(1), 13. doi:10.1186/1550-2783-6-13

115. Derave, W., Ozdemir, M. S., Harris, R. C., Pottier, A., Reyngoudt, H., Koppo, K., et al. (2007). beta-Alanine supplementation augments muscle carnosine content and attenuates fatigue during repeated isokinetic contraction bouts in trained sprinters. *Journal of Applied Physiology*, *103*(5), 1736–1743. doi:10.1152/japplphysiol.00397.2007

116. Gonzalez, J. T., & Stevenson, E. J. (2011). New perspectives on nutritional interventions to augment lipid utilisation during exercise. *British Journal of Nutrition*, *107*(03), 339–349. doi:10.1017/S0007114511006684

117. Smith, A. E., Walter, A. A., Graef, J. L., Kendall, K. L., Moon, J. R., Lockwood, C. M., et al. (2009). Effects of β-alanine supplementation and high-intensity interval training on endurance performance and body composition in men; a double-blind trial. *Journal of the International Society of Sports Nutrition*, *6*(1), 5. doi:10.1186/1550-2783-6-5

118. Volek, J. S., Kraemer, W. J., Rubin, M. R., Gómez, A. L., Ratamess, N. A., & Gaynor, P. (2002). L-Carnitine L-tartrate supplementation favorably affects markers of recovery from exercise stress. *Am J Physiol Endocrinol Metab*, *282*(2), E474–82. doi:10.1152/ajpendo.00277.2001

119. Zoeller, R. F., Stout, J. R., O'Kroy, J. A., Torok, D. J., & Mielke, M. (2006). Effects of 28 days of beta-alanine and creatine monohydrate supplementation on aerobic power, ventilatory and lactate thresholds, and time to exhaustion. *Amino Acids*, *33*(3), 505–510. doi:10.1007/s00726-006-0399-6

120. Chromiak, J. A., Smedley, B., Carpenter, W., Brown, R., Koh, Y. S., Lamberth, J. G., et al. (2004). Effect of a 10-Week strength training program and recovery drink on body composition, muscular strength and endurance, and anaerobic power and capacity. *Nutrition*, *20*(5), 420–427. doi:10.1016/j.nut.2004.01.005

121. Hulmi, J. J., Tannerstedt, J., Selanne, H., Kainulainen, H., Kovanen, V., & Mero, A. A. (2009). Resistance exercise with whey protein ingestion affects mTOR signaling pathway and myostatin in men. *Journal of Applied Physiology*, *106*(5), 1720–1729. doi:10.1152/japplphysiol.00087.2009

122. Smith, A. E., Fukuda, D. H., Kendall, K. L., & Stout, J. R. (2010). The effects of a pre-workout supplement containing caffeine, creatine, and amino acids during three weeks of high-intensity exercise on aerobic and anaerobic performance. *Journal of the International Society of Sports Nutrition*, *7*(1), 10. doi:10.1186/1550-2783-7-10

123. Tipton, K. D., Elliott, T. A., Cree, M. G., Aarsland, A. A., Sanford, A. P., & Wolfe, R. R. (2006). Stimulation of net muscle protein synthesis by whey protein ingestion before and after exercise. *AJP: Endocrinology and Metabolism*, *292*(1), E71–E76. doi:10.1152/ajpendo.00166.2006

124. Hayes, L. D., Bickerstaff, G. F., & Baker, J. S. (2010). Interactions of cortisol, testosterone, and resistance training: influence of circadian rhythms. *Chronobiology International, 27*(4), 675–705. doi:10.3109/07420521003778773

125. Handschin, C., & Spiegelman, B. M. (2008). The role of exercise and PGC-1alpha in inflammation and chronic disease. *Nature, 454*(7203), 463–469. doi:10.1038/nature07206

126. Yates, T., Khunti, K., Wilmot, E. G., Brady, E., Webb, D., Srinivasan, B., et al. (2012). Self-Reported Sitting Time and Markers of Inflammation, Insulin Resistance, and Adiposity. *American Journal of Preventive Medicine, 42*(1), 1–7. doi:10.1016/j.amepre.2011.09.022

127. Hamilton, M. T., Hamilton, D. G., & Zderic, T. W. (2007). Role of low energy expenditure and sitting in obesity, metabolic syndrome, type 2 diabetes, and cardiovascular disease. *Diabetes, 56*(11), 2655–2667. doi:10.2337/db07-0882

128. Healy, G. N., Dunstan, D. W., Salmon, J., Cerin, E., Shaw, J. E., Zimmet, P. Z., & Owen, N. (2008). Breaks in sedentary time: beneficial associations with metabolic risk. *Diabetes Care, 31*(4), 661–666. doi:10.2337/dc07-2046

129. Rutten, G. M., Savelberg, H. H., Biddle, S. J. H., & Kremers, S. P. J. (2013). Interrupting long periods of sitting: good STUFF. *The international journal of behavioral nutrition and physical activity, 10*(1), 1–1. doi:10.1186/1479-5868-10-1

130. Ando, T., Usui, C., Ohkawara, K., Miyake, R., Miyashita, M., Park, J., et al. (2013). Effects of Intermittent Physical Activity on Fat Utilization over a Whole Day. *Medicine & Science in Sports & Exercise, 1.* doi:10.1249/MSS.0b013e3182885e4b

CHAPTER 8: SLEEP MORE, WEIGH LESS

1. Hanlon, E. C., & Van Cauter, E. (2011). Colloquium Paper: Quantification of sleep behavior and of its impact on the cross-talk between the brain and peripheral metabolism. *Proceedings of the National Academy of Sciences, 108*(Supplement_3), 15609–15616. doi:10.1073/pnas.1101338108

2. Kilkus, J. M., Booth, J. N., Bromley, L. E., Darukhanavala, A. P., Imperial, J. G., & Penev, P. D. (2009). Sleep and Eating Behavior in adults at Risk for Type 2 Diabetes. *Obesity, 20*(1), 112–117. doi:10.1038/oby.2011.319

3. Knutson, K. L., Spiegel, K., Penev, P., & Van Cauter E. (2007). The metabolic consequences of sleep deprivation. *Sleep Med Rev, 11*(3), 163-168.

4. Fonken, L. K., Aubrecht, T. G., Meléndez-Fernández, O. H., Weil, Z. M., & Nelson, R. J. (2013). Dim light at night disrupts molecular circadian rhythms and increases body weight. *Journal of Biological Rhythms, 28*(4), 262–271. doi:10.1177/0748730413493862

5. Santana, A. A., Pimentel, G. D., Romualdo, M., Oyama, L. M., Santos, R. V. T., Pinho, R. A., et al. (2012). Sleep duration in elderly obese patients correlated negatively with intake fatty. *Lipids in Health and Disease*, *11*(1), 99. doi:10.1186/1476-511X-11-99

6. Silva, C. M., Sato, S., & Margolis, R. N. (2010). No time to lose: workshop on circadian rhythms and metabolic disease. (Vol. 24, pp. 1456–1464). Presented at the Genes & development. doi:10.1101/gad.1948310

7. Hayes, L. D., Bickerstaff, G. F., & Baker, J. S. (2010). Interactions of cortisol, testosterone, and resistance training: influence of circadian rhythms. *Chronobiology International*, *27*(4), 675–705. doi:10.3109/07420521003778773

8. Spiegel, K., Leproult, R., L'hermite-Balériaux, M., Copinschi, G., Penev, P. D., & Van Cauter, E. (2004). Leptin levels are dependent on sleep duration: relationships with sympathovagal balance, carbohydrate regulation, cortisol, and thyrotropin. *Journal of Clinical Endocrinology & Metabolism*, *89*(11), 5762–5771. doi:10.1210/jc.2004-1003

9. Reynolds, A. C., Dorrian, J., Liu, P. Y., Van Dongen, H. P. A., Wittert, G. A., Harmer, L. J., & Banks, S. (2012). Impact of Five Nights of Sleep Restriction on Glucose Metabolism, Leptin and Testosterone in Young Adult Men. *PLoS ONE*, *7*(7), e41218. doi:10.1371/journal.pone.0041218. t001

10. Vollmers, C., Gill, S., DiTacchio, L., Pulivarthy, S. R., Le, H. D., & Panda, S. (2009). Time of feeding and the intrinsic circadian clock drive rhythms in hepatic gene expression. *Proceedings of the National Academy of Sciences*, *106*(50), 21453–21458. doi:10.1073/pnas.0909591106

11. Froy, O. (2010). Metabolism and circadian rhythms--implications for obesity. *Endocrine Reviews*, *31*(1), 1–24. doi:10.1210/er.2009-0014

12. Ekmekcioglu, C., & Touitou, Y. (2010). Chronobiological aspects of food intake and metabolism and their relevance on energy balance and weight regulation. *Obesity Reviews*, *12*(1), 14–25. doi:10.1111/j.1467-789X.2010.00716.x

13. Manfredini, R., Fabbian, F., Manfredini, F., Salmi, R., Gallerani, M., & Bossone, E. (2013). Chronobiology in aortic diseases - "is this really a random phenomenon?". *Progress in Cardiovascular Diseases*, *56*(1), 116–124. doi:10.1016/j.pcad.2013.04.001

14. Boivin, D. B., Tremblay, G. M., & James, F. O. (2007). Working on atypical schedules. *Sleep Medicine*, *8*(6), 578–589. doi:10.1016/j.sleep.2007.03.015

15. Bray, M. S., & Young, M. E. (2012). Chronobiological Effects on Obesity. *Current Obesity Reports*, *1*(1), 9–15. doi:10.1007/s13679-011-0005-4

16. Reddy, A. B., & O'Neill, J. S. (2010). Healthy clocks, healthy body, healthy mind. *Trends in Cell Biology*, *20*(1), 36–44. doi:10.1016/j.tcb.2009.10.005

17. Gouin, J.-P., Connors, J., Kiecolt-Glaser, J. K., Glaser, R., Malarkey, W. B., Atkinson, C., et al. (2010). Altered expression of circadian rhythm genes among individuals with a history of depression. *Journal of Affective Disorders*, *126*(1-2), 161–166. doi:10.1016/j.jad.2010.04.002

18. Nojkov, B., Rubenstein, J. H., Chey, W. D., & Hoogerwerf, W. A. (2010). The impact of rotating shift work on the prevalence of irritable bowel syndrome in nurses. *Am J Gastroenterol.*, *105*(4), 842–847. doi:10.1038/ajg.2010.48

19. Partonen, T. (2012). Clock gene variants in mood and anxiety disorders. *Journal of Neural Transmission*, *119*(10), 1133–1145. doi:10.1007/s00702-012-0810-2

20. Lévi, F. (2006). Chronotherapeutics: The Relevance of Timing in Cancer Therapy. *Cancer Causes and Control*, *17*(4), 611–621. doi:10.1007/s10552-005-9004-7

21. Innominato, P. F., Lévi, F. A., & Bjarnason, G. A. (2010). Chronotherapy and the molecular clock: clinical implications in oncology. *Adv Drug Deliv Rev*, *62*(9-10), 979–1001. doi:10.1016/j.addr.2010.06.002

22. Eckel-Mahan, K., & Sassone-Corsi, P. (2013). Metabolism and the Circadian Clock Converge. *Physiological Reviews*, *93*(1), 107–135. doi:10.1152/physrev.00016.2012

23. Dibner, C., Schibler, U., & Albrecht, U. (2010). The mammalian circadian timing system: organization and coordination of central and peripheral clocks. *Annual Review of Physiology*, *72*, 517–549. doi:10.1146/annurev-physiol-021909-135821

24. Wijnen, H., & Young, M. W. (2006). Interplay of Circadian Clocks and Metabolic Rhythms. *Annual Review of Genetics*, *40*(1), 409–448. doi:10.1146/annurev.genet.40.110405.090603

25. Buijs, R. M., Van Eden, C. G., Goncharuk, V. D., & Kalsbeek, A. (2003). The biological clock tunes the organs of the body: timing by hormones and the autonomic nervous system. *Journal of Endocrinology*, *177*(1), 17–26. doi:10.1677/joe.0.1770017

26. Garaulet, M., & Madrid, J. A. (2010). Chronobiological aspects of nutrition, metabolic syndrome and obesity. *Advanced Drug Delivery Reviews*, *62*(9-10), 967–978. doi:10.1016/j.addr.2010.05.005

27. Cagampang, F. R., & Bruce, K. D. (2012). The role of the circadian clock system in nutrition and metabolism. *British Journal of Nutrition*, *108*(3), 381–392. doi:10.1017/S0007114512002139

28. Hashiramoto, A., Yamane, T., Tsumiyama, K., Yoshida, K., Komai, K., Yamada, H., et al. (2010). Mammalian Clock Gene Cryptochrome Regulates Arthritis via Proinflammatory Cytokine TNF-α. *The Journal of Immunology*, *184*(3), 1560–1565. doi:10.4049/jimmunol.0903284

29. Straub, R. H., & Cutolo, M. (2007). Circadian rhythms in rheumatoid arthritis: implications for pathophysiology and therapeutic management. *Arthritis and Rheumatism*.

30. Do, Y. K., Shin, E., Bautista, M. A., & Foo, K. (2013). The associations between self-reported sleep duration and adolescent health outcomes: what is the role of time spent on Internet use? *Sleep Medicine, 14*(2), 195–200. doi:10.1016/j.sleep.2012.09.004

31. Asterholm, I. W., & Scherer, P. E. (2012). Metabolic jet lag when the fat clock is out of sync. *Nature Medicine, 18*(12), 1738–1740. doi:10.1038/nm.3010

32. Ramsey, K. M., & Bass, J. (2009). Obeying the clock yields benefits for metabolism. *Proceedings of the National Academy of Sciences, 106*(11), 4069–4070. doi:10.1073/pnas.0901304106

33. Richards, J., & Gumz, M. L. (2012). Advances in understanding the peripheral circadian clocks. *FASEB J, 26*(9), 3602–3613. doi:10.1096/fj.12-203554

34. Ptitsyn, A. A., Zvonic, S., Conrad, S. A., Scott, L. K., Mynatt, R. L., & Gimble, J. M. (2006). Circadian Clocks Are Resounding in Peripheral Tissues. *PLoS Computational Biology, 2*(3), e16. doi:10.1371/journal.pcbi.0020016

35. Prasai, M. J., Mughal, R. S., Wheatcroft, S. B., Kearney, M. T., Grant, P. J., & Scott, E. M. (2013). Diurnal Variation in Vascular and Metabolic Function in Diet-Induced Obesity. *Diabetes, 62*(6), 1981–1989.

36. Scheiermann, C., Kunisaki, Y., Lucas, D., Chow, A., Jang, J. E., Zhang, D., et al. (2012). Adrenergic nerves govern circadian leukocyte recruitment to tissues. *Immunity, 37*(2), 290-301. doi:10.1016/j.immuni.2012.05.02

37. Scheiermann, C., Kunisaki, Y., & Frenette, P. S. (2013). Circadian control of the immune system. *Nature Reviews Immunology, 13*(3), 190–198. doi:10.1038/nri3386

38. Castanon-Cervantes, O., Wu, M., Ehlen, J. C., Paul, K., Gamble, K. L., Johnson, R. L., et al. (2010). Dysregulation of inflammatory responses by chronic circadian disruption. *The Journal of Immunology, 185*(10), 5796–5805. doi:10.4049/jimmunol.1001026

39. Keller, M., Mazuch, J., Abraham, U., Eom, G. D., Herzog, E. D., Volk, H.-D., et al. (2009). A circadian clock in macrophages controls inflammatory immune responses. *Proceedings of the National Academy of Sciences, 106*(50), 21407–21412. doi:10.1073/pnas.0906361106

40. Sahar, S., & Sassone-Corsi, P. (2011). Regulation of metabolism: thecircadian clock dictates the time. *Trends in Endocrinology & Metabolism, 23*(1), 1–8. doi:10.1016/j.tem.2011.10.005

41. Hastings, M. H., Maywood, E. S., & Reddy, A. B. (2008). Two Decades of Circadian Time. *Journal of Neuroendocrinology, 20*(6), 812–819. doi:10.1111/j.1365-2826.2008.01715.x

42. Kovac, J., Husse, J., & Oster, H. (2009). A time to fast, a time to feast: The crosstalk between metabolism and the circadian clock. *Molecules and Cells, 28*(2), 75–80. doi:10.1007/s10059-009-0113-0

43. Kreier, F., Yilmaz, A., Kalsbeek, A., Romijn, J. A., Sauerwein, H. P., Fliers, E., & Buijs, R. M. (2003). Hypothesis: shifting the equilibrium from activity to food leads to autonomic unbalance and the metabolic syndrome. *Diabetes, 52*(11), 2652–2656.

44. Champaneri, S., Xu, X., Carnethon, M. R., Bertoni, A. G., Seeman, T., Roux, A. D., & Golden, S. H. (2012). Diurnal salivary cortisol and urinary catecholamines are associated with diabetes mellitus: the Multi-Ethnic Study of Atherosclerosis. *Metabolism, 61*(7), 986–995. doi:10.1016/j.metabol.2011.11.006

45. Garaulet, M., s, J. M. O. A., & Madrid, J. A. (2010). The chronobiology, etiology and pathophysiology of obesity. *International Journal of Obesity, 34*(12), 1667–1683. doi:10.1038/ijo.2010.118

46. Spiegel, K., Knutson, K., Leproult, R., Tasali, E., & Van Cauter, E. (2005). Sleep loss: a novel risk factor for insulin resistance and Type 2 diabetes. *J Appl Physiol, 99*(5), 2008–2019. doi:10.1152/japplphysiol.00660.2005

47. Spiegel, K., Tasali, E., Penev, P., & Van Cauter, E. (2004). Brief communication: sleep curtailment in healthy young men is associated with decreased leptin levels, elevated ghrelin levels, and increased hunger and appetite. *Annals of Internal Medicine, 141*(11), 846–850.

48. Boden, G., Chen, X., & Polansky, M. (1999). Disruption of circadian insulin secretion is associated with reduced glucose uptake in first-degree relatives of patients with type 2 diabetes. *Diabetes, 48*(11), 2182–2188.

49. Huang, W., Ramsey, K. M., Marcheva, B., & Bass, J. (2011). Circadian rhythms, sleep, and metabolism. *The Journal of Clinical Investigation, 121*(6), 2133–2141. doi:10.1172/JCI46043

50. Almoosawi, S., Prynne, C. J., Hardy, R., & Stephen, A. M. (2013). Time-of-day and nutrient composition of eating occasions: prospective association with the metabolic syndrome in the 1946 British birth cohort. *International Journal of Obesity, 37*(5), 725–731. doi:10.1038/ijo.2012.103

51. Hayes, L. D., Bickerstaff, G. F., & Baker, J. S. (2010). Interactions of cortisol, testosterone, and resistance training: influence of circadian rhythms. *Chronobiology International, 27*(4), 675–705. doi:10.3109/07420521003778773

52. Zhang, X., Dube, T. J., & Esser, K. A. (2009). Working around the clock: circadian rhythms and skeletal muscle. *Journal of Applied Physiology, 107*(5), 1647–1654. doi:10.1152/japplphysiol.00725.2009

53. Tahara, Y., & Shibata, S. (2013). Chronobiology and nutrition. *Neuroscience, 253*, 78–88. doi:10.1016/j.neuroscience.2013.08.049

54. Enck, P., Kaiser, C., Felber, M., Riepl, R. L., Klauser, A., Klosterhalfen, S., & Otto, B. (2009). Circadian variation of rectal sensitivity and gastrointestinal peptides in healthy volunteers. *Neurogastroenterol Motil, 21*(1), 52–58. doi:10.1111/j.1365-2982.2008.01182.x

55. Arasaradnam, M., Morgan, L., Wright, J., & Gama, R. (2002). Diurnal variation in lipoprotein lipase activity. *Ann Clin Biochem, 39*(2), 136–139. doi:10.1258/0004563021901883

56. Gimble, J. M., & Floyd, Z. E. (2009). Fat circadian biology. *J Appl Physiol, 107*(5), 1629–1637. doi:10.1152/japplphysiol.00090.2009

57. Bass, J., & Takahashi, J. S. (2010). Circadian integration of metabolism and energetics. *Science, 330*(6009), 1349–1354. doi:10.1126/science.1195027

58. Munford, R. S. (2005). Detoxifying endotoxin: time, place and person. *J Endotoxin Res, 11*(2), 69–84. doi:10.1177/09680519050110020201

59. Summa, K. C., Voigt, R. M., Forsyth, C. B., Shaikh, M., Cavanaugh, K., Tang, Y., et al. (2013). Disruption of the Circadian Clock in Mice Increases Intestinal Permeability and Promotes Alcohol-Induced Hepatic Pathology and Inflammation. *PLoS ONE, 8*(6), e67102. doi:10.1371/journal.pone.0067102.g011

60. Shi, S.-Q., Ansari, T. S., McGuinness, O. P., Wasserman, D. H., & Johnson, C. H. (2013). Circadian disruption leads to insulin resistance and obesity. *Current biology : CB, 23*(5), 372–381. doi:10.1016/j.cub.2013.01.048

61. Zanquetta, M. M., Corrêa-Giannella, M., Monteiro, M., & Villares, S. M. (2010). Body weight, metabolism and clock genes. *Diabetology & Metabolic Syndrome, 2*(1), 53. doi:10.1186/1758-5996-2-53

62. Zmrzljak, U. P., & Rozman, D. (2012). Circadian regulation of the hepatic endobiotic and xenobiotic detoxification pathways: the time matters. *Chemical Research in Toxicology, 25*(4), 811–824. doi:10.1021/tx200538r

63. Claudel, T., Cretenet, G., Saumet, A., & Gachon, F. (2007). Crosstalk between xenobiotics metabolism and circadian clock. *FEBS Lett, 581*(19), 3626–3633. doi:10.1016/j.febslet.2007.04.009

64. Peek, C. B., Affinati, A. H., Ramsey, K. M., Kuo, H. Y., Yu, W., Sena, L. A., et al. (2013). Circadian clock NAD+ cycle drives mitochondrial oxidative metabolism in mice. *Science, 342*(6158), 1243417. doi:10.1126/science.1243417

65. Rey, G., & Reddy, A. B. (2013). Physiology. Rhythmic respiration. *Science, 342*(6158), 570–571. doi:10.1126/science.1246658

66. Dyar, K. A., Ciciliot, S., Wright, L. E., Biensø, R. S., Tagliazucchi, G. M., Patel, V. R., et al. (2013). Muscle insulin sensitivity and glucose metabolism are controlled by the intrinsic muscle clock. *Mol Metab*, 1–13. [in press]

67. Lin, Y. C., & Chen, P. C. (2012). Persistent rotating shift work exposure is a tough second hit contributing to abnormal liver function among on-site workers having sonographic fatty liver. *Asia Pac J Public Health*. doi:10.1177/1010539512469248

68. Bechtold, D. A., Gibbs, J. E., & Loudon, A. S. I. (2010). Circadian dysfunction in disease. *Trends in Pharmacological Sciences, 31*(5), 191–198. doi:10.1016/j.tips.2010.01.002

69. Haus, E. (2007). Chronobiology in the endocrine system. *Advanced Drug Delivery Reviews*, *59*(9-10), 985–1014. doi:10.1016/j.addr.2007.01.001

70. Besedovsky, L., Lange, T., & Born, J. (2011). Sleep and immune function. *Pflügers Archiv - European Journal of Physiology*, *463*(1), 121–137. doi:10.1007/s00424-011-1044-0

71. Cutolo, M., & Straub, R. H. (2008). Circadian rhythms in arthritis: Hormonal effects on the immune/inflammatory reaction. *Autoimmunity Reviews*, *7*(3), 223–228. doi:10.1016/j.autrev.2007.11.019

72. White, W. B. (2003). Matching the circadian rhythms of hypertension with pharmacotherapy. *Clinical Cardiology*, *26*(S4), 10–15.

73. Möller-Levet, C. S., Archer, S. N., Bucca, G., Laing, E. E., Slak, A., Kabiljo, R., et al. (2013). Effects of insufficient sleep on circadian rhythmicity and expression amplitude of the human blood transcriptome. *Proceedings of the National Academy of Sciences of the United States of America*, *110*(12), E1132–E1141. doi:10.1073/pnas.1217154110/-/DCSupplemental

74. Wu, X., Xie, H., Yu, G., Hebert, T., Goh, B. C., Smith, S. R., & Gimble, J. M. (2009). Expression profile of mRNAs encoding core circadian regulatory proteins in human subcutaneous adipose tissue: correlation with age and body mass index. *International Journal of Obesity*, *33*(9), 971–977. doi:10.1038/ijo.2009.137

75. Markwald, R. R., Melanson, E. L., Smith, M. R., Higgins, J., Perreault, L., Eckel, R. H., & Wright, K. P. (2013). Impact of insufficient sleep on total daily energy expenditure, food intake, and weight gain. *Proceedings of the National Academy of Sciences*, *110*(14), 5695–5700. doi:10.1073/pnas.1216951110

76. Kilkus, J. M., Booth, J. N., Bromley, L. E., Darukhanavala, A. P., Imperial, J. G., & Penev, P. D. (2009). Sleep and eating behavior in adults at risk for type 2 diabetes. *Obesity*, *20*(1), 112–117. doi:10.1038/oby.2011.319

77. Ford, E. S., Li, C., Wheaton, A. G., Chapman, D. P., Perry, G. S., & Croft, J. B. (2013). Sleep duration and body mass index and waist circumference among Us adults. *Obesity*, n/a–n/a. doi:10.1002/oby.20558

78. Reutrakul, S., Hood, M. M., Crowley, S. J., Morgan, M. K., Teodori, M., Knutson, K. L., & Van Cauter, E. (2013). Chronotype is independently associated with glycemic control in type 2 diabetes. *Diabetes Care, 36*(9), 2523–2529. doi:10.2337/dc12-2697

79. Baron, K. G., Reid, K. J., Kern, A. S., & Zee, P. C. (2009). Role of sleep timing in caloric intake and BMI. *Obesity*, *19*(7), 1374–1381. doi:10.1038/oby.2011.100

80. Verhoef, S. P., Camps, S. G., Gonnissen, H. K., Westerterp, K. R., & Westerterp-Plantenga, M. S. (2013). Concomitant changes in sleep duration and body weight and body composition during weight loss and 3-mo weight maintenance. *Am J Clin Nutr, 98*(1), 25–31. doi:10.3945/ajcn.112.054650

81. Chaput, J.-P., McNeil, J., Després, J.-P., Bouchard, C., & Tremblay, A. (2013). Short sleep duration as a risk factor for the development of the metabolic syndrome in adults. *Preventive Medicine*, 1–6. doi:10.1016/j.ypmed.2013.09.022

82. Tuñón, M. J., González, P., López, P., Salido, G.M., & Madrid, J.A. (1992). Circadian rhythms in glutathione and glutathione-S transferase activity of rat liver. *Arch Int Physiol Biochim Biophys*, 100(1), 83–87.

83. Merikanto, I., Lahti, T., Puolijoki, H., Vanhala, M., Peltonen, M., Laatikainen, T., et al. (2013). Associations of Chronotype and Sleep With Cardiovascular Diseases and Type 2 Diabetes. *Chronobiology International*, 30(4), 470–477. doi:10.3109/07420528.2012.741171

84. Atkinson, G., Jones, H., & Ainslie, P. N. (2009). Circadian variation in the circulatory responses to exercise: relevance to the morning peaks in strokes and cardiac events. *European Journal of Applied Physiology*, 108(1), 15–29. doi:10.1007/s00421-009-1243-y

85. Bridges, E. J., & Woods, S. L. (2001). Cardiovascular chronobiology: do you know what time it is? *Progress in cardiovascular nursing*, 16(2), 65–79.

86. Gómez-Abellán, P., Madrid, J. A., Ordovás, J. M., & Garaulet, M. (2012). Chronobiological aspects of obesity and metabolic syndrome. *Endocrinol Nutr.*, 59(1), 50–61. doi:10.1016/j.endoen.2011.08.002

87. Ju, S.-Y., & Choi, W.-S. (2013). Sleep duration and metabolic syndrome in adult populations: a meta-analysis of observational studies. *Nutrition and Diabetes*, 3(5), e65–9. doi:10.1038/nutd.2013.8

88. Katano, S., Nakamura, Y., Nakamura, A., Murakami, Y., Tanaka, T., Takebayashi, T., et al. (2011). Relationship between sleep duration and clustering of metabolic syndrome diagnostic components. *Diabetes Metab Syndr Obes*, 4, 119-125. doi:10.2147/DMSO.S16147

89. Erren, T. C., & Reiter, R. J. (2009). Light Hygiene: Time to make preventive use of insights--old and new--into the nexus of the drug light, melatonin, clocks, chronodisruption and public health. *Medical Hypotheses*, 73(4), 537–541. doi:10.1016/j.mehy.2009.06.003

90. Reiter, R. J., Tan, D. X., Korkmaz, A., Erren, T. C., Piekarski, C., Tamura, H., & Manchester, L. C. (2007). Light at Night, Chronodisruption, Melatonin Suppression, and Cancer Risk: A Review. *Crit Rev Oncog*, 13(4), 303–328. doi:10.1615/CritRevOncog.v13.i4.30

91. Korkmaz, A., Topal, T., Tan, D. X., & Reiter, R. J. (2009). Role of melatonin in metabolic regulation. *Rev Endoc Metab Disord*, 10(4), 261–270. doi:10.1007/s11154-009-9117-5

92. Roenneberg, T., Allebrandt, K. V., Merrow, M., & Vetter, C. (2012). Social jetlag and obesity. *Curr Biol*, 22(10), 939–943. doi:10.1016/j.cub.2012.03.038

93. Kantermann, T. (2013). Circadian biology: sleep-styles shaped by light-styles. *Curr Biol*, 23(16), R689–R690. doi:10.1016/j.cub.2013.06.065

94. Skene, D. J. (2003). Optimization of light and melatonin to phase-shift human circadian rhythms. *J Neuroendocrinol, 15*(4), 438–441.

95. Hack, L. M., Lockley, S. W., Arendt, J., & Skene, D. J. (2003). The effects of low-dose 0.5-mg melatonin on the free-running circadian rhythms of blind subjects. *J Biol Rhythms, 18*(5), 420–429. doi:10.1177/0748730403256796

96. Skene, D. J., & Arendt, J. (2007). Circadian rhythm sleep disorders in the blind and their treatment with melatonin. *Sleep Med, 8*(6), 651–655. doi:10.1016/j.sleep.2006.11.013

97. Lowden, A., Åkerstedt, T., & Wibom, R. (2004). Suppression of sleepiness and melatonin by bright light exposure during breaks in night work. *J Sleep Res, 13*(1), 37–43.

98. Crowley, S. J., Lee, C., Tseng, C. Y., Fogg, L. F., & Eastman, C. I. (2003). Combinations of bright light, scheduled dark, sunglasses, and melatonin to facilitate circadian entrainment to night shift work. *J Biol Rhythms, 18*(6), 513–523. doi:10.1177/0748730403258422

99. Tan, D. X., Manchester, L. C., Fuentes-Broto, L., Paredes, S. D., & Reiter, R. J. (2011). Significance and application of melatonin in the regulation of brown adipose tissue metabolism: relation to human obesity. *Obes Rev, 12*(3), 167–188. doi:10.1111/j.1467-789X.2010.00756.x

100. Schroeder, A. M., & Colwell, C. S. (2013). How to fix a broken clock. *Trends Pharmacol Sci, 34*(11), 605-19. doi:10.1016/j.tips.2013.09.002

101. Koziróg, M., Poliwczak, A. R., Duchnowicz, P., Koter-Michalak, M., Sikora, J., & Broncel, M. (2011). Melatonin treatment improves blood pressure, lipid profile, and parameters of oxidative stress in patients with metabolic syndrome. *J Pineal Res, 50*(3), 261–266. doi:10.1111/j.1600-079X.2010.00835.x

102. Gonciarz, M., Gonciarz, Z., Bielanski, W., Mularczyk, A., Konturek, P. C., Brzozowski, T., & Konturek, S. J. (2012). The effects of long-term melatonin treatment on plasma liver enzymes levels and plasma concentrations of lipids and melatonin in patients with nonalcoholic steatohepatitis: a pilot study. *J Physiol Pharmacol, 63*(1), 35–40.

103. Gonciarz, M., Bielański, W., Partyka, R., Brzozowski, T., Konturek, P. C., Eszyk, J., et al. (2013). Plasma insulin, leptin, adiponectin, resistin, ghrelin, and melatonin in nonalcoholic steatohepatitis patients treated with melatonin. *J Pineal Res, 54*(2), 154–161. doi:10.1111/j.1600-079X.2012.01023.x

104. Danilenko, K., & Ragino, Y. (2013). Melatonin and its use in atherosclerosis and dyslipidemia. *ChronoPhysiol Ther, 3*, 15-20. doi:10.2147/CPT.S40209

105. Scheer, F. A., Van Montfrans, G. A., van Someren, E. J., Mairuhu, G., & Buijs, R. M. (2004). Daily nighttime melatonin reduces blood pressure in male patients with essential hypertension. *Hypertension, 43*(2), 192–197.

106. Ochoa, J. J., Díaz-Castro, J., Kajarabille, N., García, C., Guisado, I. M., De Teresa, C., & Guisado, R. (2011). Melatonin supplementation ameliorates oxidative stress and inflammatory signaling induced by strenuous exercise in adult human males. *J Pineal Res, 51*(4), 373–380. doi:10.1111/j.1600-079X.2011.00899.x

107. Maldonado, M. D., Manfredi, M., Ribas-Serna, J., Garcia-Moreno, H., & Calvo, J. R. (2012). Melatonin administrated [administration] immediately before an intense exercise reverses oxidative stress, improves immunological defenses and lipid metabolism in football players. *Physiol Behav, 105*(5), 1099–1103. doi:10.1016/j.physbeh.2011.12.015

108. Chojnacki, C., Walecka-Kapica, E., Łokieć, K., Pawłowicz, M., Winczyk, K., Chojnacki, J., & Klupińska, G. (2013). Influence of melatonin on symptoms of irritable bowel syndrome in postmenopausal women. *Endokrynol Pol, 64*(2), 114–120.

CHAPTER 9: ARE GUT BACTERIA MAKING YOU FAT?

1. Mann, CC. 1493: Uncovering the New World Columbus Created. (2011). Vintage Books. ISBN: 978030727841

2. Ley, R. E. (2010). Obesity and the human microbiome. *Current Opinion in Gastroenterology, 26*(1), 5–11. doi:10.1097/MOG.0b013e328333d751

3. Tagliabue, A., & Elli, M. (2013). The role of gut microbiota in human obesity: recent findings and future perspectives. *Nutrition, metabolism, and cardiovascular diseases : NMCD, 23*(3), 160–168. doi:10.1016/j.numecd.2012.09.002

4. Vrieze, A., Holleman, F., Zoetendal, E. G., de Vos, W. M., Hoekstra, J. B. L., & Nieuwdorp, M. (2010). The environment within: how gut microbiota may influence metabolism and body composition. *Diabetologia, 53*(4), 606–613. doi:10.1007/s00125-010-1662-7

5. Turnbaugh, P. J., & Gordon, J. I. (2009). The core gut microbiome, energy balance and obesity. *The Journal of Physiology, 587*(Pt 17), 4153–4158. doi:10.1113/jphysiol.2009.174136

6. Brown, K., DeCoffe, D., Molcan, E., & Gibson, D. L. (2012). Diet-Induced Dysbiosis of the Intestinal Microbiota and the Effects on Immunity and Disease. *Nutrients, 4*(12), 1095–1119. doi:10.3390/nu4081095

7. Young, V. B. (2012). The intestinal microbiota in health and disease. *Current Opinion in Gastroenterology, 28*(1), 63–69. doi:10.1097/MOG.0b013e32834d61e9

8. Conterno, L., Fava, F., Viola, R., & Tuohy, K. M. (2011). Obesity and the gut microbiota: does up-regulating colonic fermentation protect against obesity and metabolic disease? *Genes & Nutrition, 6*(3), 241–260. doi:10.1007/s12263-011-0230-1

9.   Karlsson, C. L. J., Molin, G., Fåk, F., Johansson Hagslätt, M.-L., Jakesevic, M., Håkansson, Å., et al. (2011). Effects on weight gain and gut microbiota in rats given bacterial supplements and a high-energy-dense diet from fetal life through to 6 months of age. *British Journal of Nutrition, 106*(6), 887–895. doi:10.1017/S0007114511001036

10. Ehlers, S., Kaufmann, S. H. E., Participants of the 99(th) Dahlem Conference. (2010). Infection, inflammation, and chronic diseases: consequences of a modern lifestyle. *Trends in Immunology, 31*(5), 184–190. doi:10.1016/j.it.2010.02.003

11. Cani, P. D., & Delzenne, N. M. (2009). Interplay between obesity and associated metabolic disorders: new insights into the gut microbiota. *Current Opinion in Pharmacology, 9*(6), 737–743. doi:10.1016/j.coph.2009.06.016

12. Sonnenburg, J. L., Angenent, L. T., & Gordon, J. I. (2004). Getting a grip on things: how do communities of bacterial symbionts become established in our intestine? *Nature Immunology, 5*(6), 569–573. doi:10.1038/ni1079

13. Konkel, L. (2013, September). The environment within: exploring the role of the gut microbiome in health and disease. *Environmental Health Perspectives*, pp. A276–81. doi:10.1289/ehp.121-A276

14. Sommer, F., & Bäckhed, F. (2013). The gut microbiota--masters of host development and physiology. *Nature Reviews Microbiology, 11*(4), 227–238. doi:10.1038/nrmicro2974

15. Straub, R. H. (2011). Concepts of evolutionary medicine and energy regulation contribute to the etiology of systemic chronic inflammatory diseases. *Brain, Behavior, and Immunity, 25*(1), 1–5. doi:10.1016/j.bbi.2010.08.002

16. Geurts, L., Lazarevic, V., Derrien, M., Everard, A., Van Roye, M., Knauf, C., et al. (2011). Altered gut microbiota and endocannabinoid system tone in obese and diabetic leptin-resistant mice: impact on apelin regulation in adipose tissue. *Frontiers in Microbiology, 2*, 149–149. doi:10.3389/fmicb.2011.00149

17. Clemente-Postigo, M., Queipo-Ortuno, M. I., Murri, M., Boto-Ordonez, M., Perez-Martinez, P., Andres-Lacueva, C., et al. (2012). Endotoxin increase after fat overload is related to postprandial hypertriglyceridemia in morbidly obese patients. *The Journal of Lipid Research, 53*(5), 973–978. doi:10.1194/jlr.P020909

18. DiBaise, J. K., Frank, D. N., & Mathur, R. (2012). Impact of the Gut Microbiota on the Development of Obesity: Current Concepts. *The American Journal of Gastroenterology Supplements, 1*(1), 22–27. doi:10.1038/ajgsup.2012.5

19. Pendyala, S., Walker, J. M., & Holt, P. R. (2012). A High-Fat Diet Is Associated With Endotoxemia That Originates From the Gut. *YGAST, 142*(5), 1100–1101.e2. doi:10.1053/j.gastro.2012.01.034

20. Lugogo, N. L., Bappanad, D., & Kraft, M. (2011). Obesity, metabolic dysregulation and oxidative stress in asthma. *BBA - General Subjects*, *1810*(11), 1120–1126. doi:10.1016/j.bbagen.2011.09.004

21. Fernandez-Real, J. M., & Pickup, J. C. (2012). Innate immunity, insulin resistance and type 2 diabetes. *Diabetologia*, *55*(2), 273–278. doi:10.1007/s00125-011-2387-y

22. Gregor, M. F., & Hotamisligil, G. S. (2011). Inflammatory Mechanisms in Obesity. *Annual Review of Immunology*, *29*(1), 415–445. doi:10.1146/annurev-immunol-031210-101322

23. lez, M. G. A., del Mar Bibiloni, M., Pons, A., Llompart, I., & Tur, J. A. (2012). Inflammatory markers and metabolic syndrome among adolescents. *European Journal of Clinical Nutrition*, 1–5. doi:10.1038/ejcn.2012.112

24. Iyer, A., Fairlie, D. P., Prins, J. B., Hammock, B. D., & Brown, L. (2010). Inflammatory lipid mediators in adipocyte function and obesity. *Nature Reviews | Endocrinology*, *6*(2), 71–82. doi:10.1038/nrendo.2009.264

25. Stoppa-Vaucher, S., Dirlewanger, M. A., Meier, C. A., de Moerloose, P., Reber, G., Roux-Lombard, P., et al. (2012). Inflammatory and Prothrombotic States in Obese Children of European Descent. *Obesity*, *20*(8), 1662–1668. doi:10.1038/oby.2012.85

26. Nikolajczyk, B. S., Jagannathan-Bogdan, M., Shin, H., & Gyurko, R. (2011). State of the union between metabolism and the immune system in type 2 diabetes. *Genes and Immunity*, *12*(4), 239–250. doi:10.1038/gene.2011.14

27. Candela, M., Biagi, E., Maccaferri, S., Turroni, S., & Brigidi, P. (2012). Intestinal microbiota is a plastic factor responding to environmental changes. *Trends in Microbiology*, 1–7. doi:10.1016/j.tim.2012.05.003

28. Zhao, L., & Shen, J. (2010). Whole-body systems approaches for gut microbiota-targeted, preventive healthcare. *Journal of Biotechnology*, *149*(3), 183–190. doi:10.1016/j.jbiotec.2010.02.008

29. Cani, P. D., & Delzenne, N. M. (2009). The role of the gut microbiota in energy metabolism and metabolic disease. *Current Pharmaceutical Design*, *15*(13), 1546–1558.

30. Honda, K., & Littman, D. R. (2012). The microbiome in infectious disease and inflammation. *Annual Review of Immunology*, *30*, 759–795. doi:10.1146/annurev-immunol-020711-074937

31. Serino, M., Blasco-Baque, V., & Burcelin, R. (2012). Microbes on-air: gut and tissue microbiota as targets in type 2 diabetes. *J Clin Gastroenterol, 46 Suppl*, S27–8. doi:10.1097/MCG.0b013e318264e844

32. Diamant, M., Blaak, E. E., & de Vos, W. M. (2011). Do nutrient-gut-microbiota interactions play a role in human obesity, insulin resistance and type 2 diabetes? *Obesity reviews : an official journal of the International Association for the Study of Obesity*, *12*(4), 272–281. doi:10.1111/j.1467-789X.2010.00797.x

33. Scholtens, P. A. M. J., Oozeer, R., Martin, R., Amor, K. B., & Knol, J. (2012). The early settlers: intestinal microbiology in early life. *Annual review of food science and technology, 3*, 425–447. doi:10.1146/annurev-food-022811-101120

34. Fallani, M., Young, D., Scott, J., Norin, E., Amarri, S., Adam, R., et al. (2010). Intestinal Microbiota of 6-week-old Infants Across Europe: Geographic Influence Beyond Delivery Mode, Breast-feeding, and Antibiotics. *Journal of Pediatric Gastroenterology and Nutrition, 51*(1), 77–84. doi:10.1097/MPG.0b013e3181d1b11e

35. Ajslev, T. A., Andersen, C. S., Gamborg, M., Sørensen, T. I. A., & Jess, T. (2011). Childhood overweight after establishment of the gut microbiota: the role of delivery mode, pre-pregnancy weight and early administration of antibiotics. *International Journal of Obesity, 35*(4), 522–529. doi:10.1038/ijo.2011.27

36. Ray, K. (2012). Gut microbiota: Adding weight to the microbiota's role in obesity—exposure to antibiotics early in life can lead to increased adiposity. *Nature Reviews | Endocrinology, 8*(11), 623–623. doi:10.1038/nrendo.2012.173

37. Zoetendal, E. G., Raes, J., van den Bogert, B., Arumugam, M., Booijink, C. C. G. M., Troost, F. J., et al. (2012). The human small intestinal microbiota is driven by rapid uptake and conversion of simple carbohydrates. *The ISME Journal, 6*(7), 1415–1426. doi:10.1038/ismej.2011.212

38. Langlands, S. J., Hopkins, M. J., Coleman, N., & Cummings, J. H. (2004). Prebiotic carbohydrates modify the mucosa associated microflora of the human large bowel. *Gut, 53*(11), 1610–1616.

39. Spreadbury, I. (2012). Comparison with ancestral diets suggests dense acellular carbohydrates promote an inflammatory microbiota, and may be the primary dietary cause of leptin resistance and obesity. *Diabetes, Metabolic Syndrome and Obesity: Targets and Therapy, 5*, 175–189. doi:10.2147/DMSO.S33473

40. Pedersen, A. M., Bardow, A., Jensen, S. B., & Nauntofte, B. (2002). Saliva and gastrointestinal functions of taste, mastication, swallowing and digestion. *Oral Diseases, 8*(3), 117–129. doi:10.1034/j.1601-0825.2002.02851.x

41. Suzuki, H., Fukushima, M., Okamoto, S., Takahashi, O., Shimbo, T., Kurose, T., et al. (2005). Effects of thorough mastication on postprandial plasma glucose concentrations in nonobese Japanese subjects. *Metabolism, 54*(12), 1593–1599. doi:10.1016/j.metabol.2005.06.006

42. Fava, F., Gitau, R., Griffin, B. A., Gibson, G. R., Tuohy, K. M., & Lovegrove, J. A. (2012). The type and quantity of dietary fat and carbohydrate alter faecal microbiome and short-chain fatty acid excretion in a metabolic syndrome ‘at-risk’ population. *International Journal of Obesity*, 1–8. doi:10.1038/ijo.2012.33

43. Jumpertz, R., Le, D. S., Turnbaugh, P. J., Trinidad, C., Bogardus, C., Gordon, J. I., & Krakoff, J. (2011). Energy-balance studies reveal associations between gut microbes, caloric load, and nutrient absorption in humans. *American Journal of Clinical Nutrition, 94*(1), 58–65. doi:10.3945/ajcn.110.010132

44. Delzenne, N. M., Neyrinck, A. M., & Cani, P. D. (2011). Modulation of the gut microbiota by nutrients with prebiotic properties: consequences for host health in the context of obesity and metabolic syndrome. *Microbial Cell Factories, 10*(Suppl 1), S10. doi:10.1186/1475-2859-10-S1-S10

45. Lenz, A., & Diamond, F. B., Jr. (2008). Obesity: the hormonal milieu. *Current Opinion in Endocrinology, Diabetes and Obesity, 15*(1), 9–20. doi:10.1097/MED.0b013e3282f43a5b

46. Clarke, S. F., Murphy, E. F., Nilaweera, K., Ross, P. R., Shanahan, F., O'Toole, P. W., & Cotter, P. D. (2012). The gut microbiota and its relationship to diet and obesity: new insights. *Gut Microbes, 3*(3), 186–202. doi:10.4161/gmic.20168

47. Leclercq, S., Cani, P. D., Neyrinck, A. M., Stärkel, P., Jamar, F., Mikolajczak, M., et al. (2012). Role of intestinal permeability and inflammation in the biological and behavioral control of alcohol-dependent subjects. *Brain, Behavior, and Immunity*. doi:10.1016/j.bbi.2012.04.001

48. Isolauri, E. (2012). Development of healthy gut microbiota early in life. *Journal of Paediatrics and Child Health, 48*, 1–6. doi:10.1111/j.1440-1754.2012.02489.x

49. Thompson, A. L. (2012). Developmental origins of obesity: Early feeding environments, infant growth, and the intestinal microbiome. *American Journal of Human Biology, 24*(3), 350–360. doi:10.1002/ajhb.22254

50. Ley, R. E., Lozupone, C. A., Hamady, M., Knight, R., & Gordon, J. I. (2008). Worlds within worlds: evolution of the vertebrate gut microbiota. *Nature Reviews Microbiology, 6*(10), 776–788. doi:10.1038/nrmicro1978

51. Kanner, J., Gorelik, S., Roman, S., & Kohen, R. (2012). Protection by Polyphenols of Postprandial Human Plasma and Low-Density Lipoprotein Modification: The Stomach as a Bioreactor. *Journal of Agricultural and Food Chemistry*, 120503100206008. doi:10.1021/jf300193g

52. Huang, E. Y., Leone, V. A., Devkota, S., Wang, Y., Brady, M. J., & Chang, E. B. (2013). Composition of Dietary Fat Source Shapes Gut Microbiota Architecture and Alters Host Inflammatory Mediators in Mouse Adipose Tissue. *Journal of Parenteral and Enteral Nutrition, 37*(6), 746–754. doi:10.1177/0148607113486931

53. Jacobs, D. M., Gaudier, E., Duynhoven, J. V., & Vaughan, E. E. (2009). Non-digestible food ingredients, colonic microbiota and the impact on gut health and immunity: a role for metabolomics. *Current Drug Metabolism, 10*(1), 41–54.

54. Szic, K. K. S. V., Ndlovu, M. N. M., Haegeman, G. G., & Berghe, W. W. V. (2010). Nature or nurture: Let food be your epigenetic medicine in chronic inflammatory disorders. *Biochemical Pharmacology, 80*(12), 17–17. doi:10.1016/j.bcp.2010.07.029

55. Prior, I. A. I., Davidson, F. F., Salmond, C. E. C., & Czochanska, Z. Z. (1981). Cholesterol, coconuts, and diet on Polynesian atolls: a natural experiment: the Pukapuka and Tokelau island studies. *Am J Clin Nutr, 34*(8), 1552–1561.

56. Collison, K. S., Zaidi, M. Z., Saleh, S. M., Inglis, A., Mondreal, R., Makhoul, N. J., et al. (2011). Effect of trans-fat, fructose and monosodium glutamate feeding on feline weight gain, adiposity, insulin sensitivity, adipokine and lipid profile. *British Journal of Nutrition, 106*(2), 218–226. doi:10.1017/S000711451000588X

57. van Dorsten, F. A., Peters, S., Gross, G., Gomez-Roldan, V., Klinkenberg, M., de Vos, R. C., et al. (2012). Gut Microbial Metabolism of Polyphenols from Black Tea and Red Wine/Grape Juice Is Source-Specific and Colon-Region Dependent. *Journal of Agricultural and Food Chemistry, 60*(45), 11331–11342. doi:10.1021/jf303165w

58. Lacombe, A., Li, R. W., Klimis-Zacas, D., Kristo, A. S., Tadepalli, S., Krauss, E., et al. (2013). Lowbush Wild Blueberries have the Potential to Modify Gut Microbiota and Xenobiotic Metabolism in the Rat Colon. *PLoS ONE, 8*(6), e67497. doi:10.1371/journal.pone.0067497.t003

59. Bischoff, S. C. (2011). "Gut health": a new objective in medicine? *BMC Medicine, 9*, 24. doi:10.1186/1741-7015-9-24

60. Cani, P. D., & Delzenne, N. M. (2011). The gut microbiome as therapeutic target. *Pharmacology and Therapeutics, 130*(2), 202–212. doi:10.1016/j.pharmthera.2011.01.012

61. Walker, A. W., & Lawley, T. D. (2013). Therapeutic modulation of intestinal dysbiosis. *Pharmacological research : the official journal of the Italian Pharmacological Society, 69*(1), 75–86. doi:10.1016/j.phrs.2012.09.008

62. Round, J. L., & Mazmanian, S. K. (2009). The gut microbiota shapes intestinal immune responses during health and disease. *Nature Reviews Immunology, 9*(5), 313–323.

63. Duboc, H., Rajca, S., Rainteau, D., Benarous, D., Maubert, M. A., Quervain, E., et al. (2012). Connecting dysbiosis, bile-acid dysmetabolism and gut inflammation in inflammatory bowel diseases. *Gut.* doi:10.1136/gutjnl-2012-302578

64. Shelton, R. C., & Miller, A. H. (2010). Eating ourselves to death (and despair): the contribution of adiposity and inflammation to depression. *Progress in Neurobiology, 91*(4), 275–299. doi:10.1016/j.pneurobio.2010.04.004

65. Bowe, W. P., & Logan, A. C. (2011). Acne vulgaris, probiotics and the gut-brain-skin axis - back to the future? *Gut Pathogens, 3*(1), 1. doi:10.1186/1757-4749-3-1

66. Tremellen, K., & Pearce, K. (2012). Dysbiosis of Gut Microbiota (DOGMA)–A novel theory for the development of Polycystic Ovarian Syndrome. *Medical Hypotheses, 79*(1), 104–112. doi:10.1016/j.mehy.2012.04.016

67. Xiao, S., Fei, N., Pang, X., Shen, J., & Wang, L. (2013). A gut microbiota-targeted dietary intervention for amelioration of chronic inflammation underlying metabolic syndrome. *FEMS microbiology* doi:10.1111/1574-6941.12228

68. Bäckhed, F., Ding, H., Wang, T., Hooper, L. V., Koh, G. Y., Nagy, A., et al. (2004). The gut microbiota as an environmental factor that regulates fat storage. *Proceedings of the National Academy of Sciences of the United States of America, 101*(44), 15718–15715723. doi:10.1073/pnas.0407076101

69. Sears, C. L. (2005). A dynamic partnership: celebrating our gut flora. *Anaerobe, 11*(5), 247–251.

70. Qin, J., Li, R., Raes, J., Arumugam, M., Burgdorf, K. S., Manichanh, C., et al. (2010). A human gut microbial gene catalogue established by metagenomic sequencing. *Nature, 464*(7285), 59–65.

71. Pandeya, D. R., D'Souza, R., Rahman, M. M., Akhter, S., Kim, H.-J., & Hong, S.-T. (2012). Host-microbial interaction in the mammalian intestine and their metabolic role inside. *Biomedical Research, 23*(1), 9–21.

72. Evans, J. M., Morris, L. S., & Marchesi, J. R. (2013). The gut microbiome: the role of a virtual organ in the endocrinology of the host. *Journal of Endocrinology, 218*(3), R37–R47. doi:10.1530/JOE-13-0131

73. Lin, H. V., Frassetto, A., Kowalik, E. J., Jr, Nawrocki, A. R., Lu, M. M., Kosinski, J. R., et al. (2012). Butyrate and Propionate Protect against Diet-Induced Obesity and Regulate Gut Hormones via Free Fatty Acid Receptor 3-Independent Mechanisms. *PLoS ONE, 7*(4), e35240. doi:10.1371/journal.pone.0035240.g006

74. Meijer, K., de Vos, P., & Priebe, M. G. (2010). Butyrate and other short-chain fatty acids as modulators of immunity: what relevance for health? *Current Opinion in Clinical Nutrition and Metabolic Care, 13*(6), 715–721. doi:10.1097/MCO.0b013e32833eebe5

75. Bäckhed, F., Ding, H., Wang, T., Hooper, L. V., Koh, G. Y., Nagy, A., et al. (2004). The gut microbiota as an environmental factor that regulates fat storage. *Proceedings of the National Academy of Sciences of the United States of America, 101*(44), 15718–15715723. doi:10.1073/pnas.0407076101

76. Harris, K., Kassis, A., Major, G., & Chou, C. J. (2012). Is the gut microbiota a new factor contributing to obesity and its metabolic disorders? *Journal of Obesity, 2012*, 879151. doi:10.1155/2012/879151

77. Musso, G., Gambino, R., & Cassader, M. (2010). Obesity, Diabetes, and Gut Microbiota: The hygiene hypothesis expanded? *Diabetes Care, 33*(10), 2277–2284. doi:10.2337/dc10-0556

78. Murphy, E. F., Cotter, P. D., Healy, S., Marques, T. M., O'sullivan, O., Fouhy, F., et al. (2010). Composition and energy harvesting capacity of the gut microbiota: relationship to diet, obesity and time in mouse models. *Gut, 59*(12), 1635–1642. doi:10.1136/gut.2010.215665

79. Kallus, S. J., & Brandt, L. J. (2012). The intestinal microbiota and obesity. *J Clin Gastroenterol, 46*(1), 16–24. doi:10.1097/MCG.0b013e31823711fd

80. Basseri, R. J., Basseri, B., Pimentel, M., Chong, K., Youdim, A., Low, K., et al. (2012). Intestinal methane production in obese individuals is associated with a higher body mass index. *Gastroenterology & hepatology, 8*(1), 22.

81. Baboota, R. K., Bishnoi, M., Ambalam, P., Kondepudi, K. K., Sarma, S. M., Boparai, R. K., & Podili, K. (2013). Functional food ingredients for the management of obesity and associated co-morbidities – A review. *Journal of Functional Foods, 5*(3), 997–1012. doi:10.1016/j.jff.2013.04.014

82. Turnbaugh, P. J., Ley, R. E., Mahowald, M. A., Magrini, V., Mardis, E. R., & Gordon, J. I. (2006). An obesity-associated gut microbiome with increased capacity for energy harvest. *Nature, 444*(7122), 1027–131. doi:10.1038/nature05414

83. Cani, P. D., Amar, J., Iglesias, M. A., Poggi, M., Knauf, C., Bastelica, D., et al. (2007). Metabolic Endotoxemia Initiates Obesity and Insulin Resistance. *Diabetes, 56*(7), 1761–1772. doi:10.2337/db06-1491

84. Amar, J., Chabo, C., Waget, A., Klopp, P., Vachoux, C., Bermúdez-Humarán, L. G., et al. (2012). Intestinal mucosal adherence and translocation of commensal bacteria at the early onset of type 2 diabetes: molecular mechanisms and probiotic treatment. *EMBO Molecular Medicine, 3*(9), 559–572. doi:10.1002/emmm.201100159

85. Amar, J., Lange, C., Payros, G., Garret, C., Chabo, C., Lantieri, O., et al. (2013). Blood Microbiota Dysbiosis Is Associated with the Onset of Cardiovascular Events in a Large General Population: The D.E.S.I.R. Study. *PLoS ONE, 8*(1), e54461. doi:10.1371/journal.pone.0054461.t004

86. Caesar, R., Fåk, F., & Backhed, F. (2010). Effects of gut microbiota on obesity and atherosclerosis via modulation of inflammation and lipid metabolism. *Journal of Internal Medicine, 268*(4), 320–328. doi:10.1111/j.1365-2796.2010.02270.x

87. Turnbaugh, P. J., Ridaura, V. K., Faith, J. J., Rey, F. E., Knight, R., & Gordon, J. I. (2009). The effect of diet on the human gut microbiome: a metagenomic analysis in humanized gnotobiotic mice. *Science Translational Medicine, 1*(6), 6ra14. doi:10.1126/scitranslmed.3000322

88. McFall-Ngai, M., Hadfield, M. G., Bosch, T. C., Carey, H. V., Domazet-Lošo, T., Douglas, A. E., et al. (2013). Animals in a bacterial world, a new imperative for the life sciences. *Proceedings of the National Academy of Sciences of the United States of America, 110*(9), 3229–3236. doi:10.1073/pnas.1218525110/-/DCSupplemental

89. Burcelin, R. (2012). Regulation of Metabolism: A Cross Talk Between Gut Microbiota and Its Human Host. *Physiology, 27*(5), 300–307. doi:10.1152/physiol.00023.2012

90. Cahenzli, J., Balmer, M. L., & McCoy, K. D. (2013). Microbial-immune cross-talk and regulation of the immune system. *Immunology, 138*(1), 12–22. doi:10.1111/j.1365-2567.2012.03624.x

91. Grenham, S., Clarke, G., Cryan, J. F., & Dinan, T. G. (2011). Brain-gut-microbe communication in health and disease. *Frontiers in Physiology, 2*, 94–94. doi:10.3389/fphys.2011.00094

92. Aron-Wisnewsky, J., Doré, J., & Clément, K. (2012). The importance of the gut microbiota after bariatric surgery. *Nature Reviews Gastroenterology and Hepatology, 9*(10), 590–598. doi:10.1038/nrgastro.2012.161

93. Li, J. V., Ashrafian, H., Bueter, M., Kinross, J., Sands, C., le Roux, C. W., et al. (2011). Metabolic surgery profoundly influences gut microbial-host metabolic cross-talk. *Gut, 60*(9), 1214–1223. doi:10.1136/gut.2010.234708

94. Cani, P. D., & Delzenne, N. M. (2011). Benefits of bariatric surgery: an issue of microbial-host metabolism interactions? *Gut, 60*(9), 1166–1167. doi:10.1136/gut.2011.242503

95. Liu, Z. H., Huang, M. J., Zhang, X. W., Wang, L., Huang, N. Q., Peng, H., et al. (2012). The effects of perioperative probiotic treatment on serum zonulin concentration and subsequent postoperative infectious complications after colorectal cancer surgery: a double-center and double-blind randomized clinical trial. *American Journal of Clinical Nutrition, 97*(1), 117–126. doi:10.3945/ajcn.112.040949

96. Lecerf, J.-M., Dépeint, F., Clerc, E., Dugenet, Y., Niamba, C. N., Rhazi, L., et al. (2012). Xylo-oligosaccharide (XOS) in combination with inulin modulates both the intestinal environment and immune status in healthy subjects, while XOS alone only shows prebiotic properties. *British Journal of Nutrition, 108*(10), 1847–1858. doi:10.1017/S0007114511007252

97. Dewulf, E. M., Cani, P. D., Claus, S. P., Fuentes, S., Puylaert, P. G. B., Neyrinck, A. M., et al. (2013). Insight into the prebiotic concept: lessons from an exploratory, double blind intervention study with inulin-type fructans in obese women. *Gut, 62*(8), 1112–1121. doi:10.1136/gutjnl-2012-303304

98. Pourghassem Gargari, B., Dehghan, P., Aliasgharzadeh, A., & Asghari Jafar-abadi, M. (2013). Effects of High Performance Inulin Supplementation on Glycemic Control and Antioxidant Status in Women with Type 2 Diabetes. *Diabetes & Metabolism Journal, 37*(2), 140. doi:10.4093/dmj.2013.37.2.140

99. Geraedts, M. C. P., Troost, F. J., Munsters, M. J. M., Stegen, J. H. C. H., de Ridder, R. J., Conchillo, J. M., et al. (2011). Intraduodenal Administration of Intact Pea Protein Effectively Reduces Food Intake in Both Lean and Obese Male Subjects. *PLoS ONE, 6*(9), e24878. doi:10.1371/journal.pone.0024878.t001

100. Geraedts, M. C. P., Troost, F. J., Tinnemans, R., Söderholm, J. D., Brummer, R.-J., & Saris, W. H. M. (2010). Release of satiety hormones in response to specific dietary proteins is different between human and murine small intestinal mucosa. *Annals of nutrition & metabolism, 56*(4), 308–313. doi:10.1159/000312664

101. Turnbaugh, P. J., Hamady, M., Yatsunenko, T., Cantarel, B. L., Duncan, A., Ley, R. E., et al. (2009). A core gut microbiome in obese and lean twins. *Nature, 457*(7228), 480–484. doi:10.1038/nature07540

102. Samuel, B. S., Shaito, A., Motoike, T., Rey, F. E., Bäckhed, F., Manchester, J. K., et al. (2008). Effects of the gut microbiota on host adiposity are modulated by the short-chain fatty-acid binding G protein-coupled receptor, Gpr41. *PNAS, 105*(43), 16767–16772.

103. Ley, R. E., Turnbaugh, P. J., Klein, S., & Gordon, J. I. (2006). Microbial ecology: human gut microbes associated with obesity. *Nature, 444*(7122), 1022–1023. doi:10.1038/nature4441021a

104. Kaplan, J. L., & Walker, W. A. (2012). Early gut colonization and subsequent obesity risk. *Current Opinion in Clinical Nutrition and Metabolic Care, 15*(3), 278–284. doi:10.1097/MCO.0b013e32835133cb

105. Azad, M. B., & Kozyrskyj, A. L. (2012). Perinatal Programming of Asthma: The Role of Gut Microbiota. *Clinical and Developmental Immunology, 2012*, 1–9. doi:10.1155/2012/932072

106. Sartor, R. B. (2011). Key questions to guide a better understanding of host-commensal microbiota interactions in intestinal inflammation. *Mucosal Immunology, 4*(2), 127–132. doi:10.1038/mi.2010.87

107. Dominguez-Bello, M. G., Costello, E. K., Contreras, M., Magris, M., Hidalgo, G., Fierer, N., & Knight, R. (2010). Delivery mode shapes the acquisition and structure of the initial microbiota across multiple body habitats in newborns. *Proceedings of the National Academy of Sciences of the United States of America, 107*(26), 11971–11975. doi:10.1073/pnas.1002601107/-/DC Supplemental

108. van Nimwegen MSc, F. A., PhD, J. P., PhD, E. E. S., PhD, D. S. P. M., PhD, G. H. K. M., PhD, M. K. M., et al. (2011). Mode and place of delivery, gastrointestinal microbiota, and their influence on asthma and atopy. *Journal of Allergy and Clinical Immunology, 128*(5), 948–955.e3. doi:10.1016/j.jaci.2011.07.027

109. Kalliomäki, M., Collado, M. C., Salminen, S., & Isolauri, E. (2008). Early differences in fecal microbiota composition in children may predict overweight. *Am J Clin Nutr, 87*(3), 534–538.

110. Collado, M. C., Isolauri, E., Laitinen, K., & Salminen, S. (2008). Distinct composition of gut microbiota during pregnancy in overweight and normal-weight women. *Am J Clin Nutr, 88*(4), 894–899.

111. Santacruz, A., Collado, M. C., García-Valdés, L., Segura, M. T., Martín-Lagos, J. A., Anjos, T., et al. (2010). Gut microbiota composition is associated with body weight, weight gain and biochemical parameters in pregnant women. *The British journal of nutrition, 104*(1), 83.

112. Huh, S. Y., Rifas-Shiman, S. L., Zera, C. A., Edwards, J. W. R., Oken, E., Weiss, S. T., & Gillman, M. W. (2012). Delivery by caesarean section and risk of obesity in preschool age children: a prospective cohort study. *Archives of Disease in Childhood, 97*(7), 610–616. doi:10.1136/archdischild-2011-301141

113. Blustein, J., Attina, T., Liu, M., Ryan, A. M., Cox, L. M., Blaser, M. J., & Trasande, L. (2013). Association of caesarean delivery with child adiposity from age 6 weeks to 15 years. *International Journal of Obesity, 37*(7), 900–906. doi:10.1038/ijo.2013.49

114. Mesquita, D. N., Barbieri, M. A., Goldani, H., & Cardoso, V. C. (2013). Cesarean Section Is Associated with Increased Peripheral and Central Adiposity in Young Adulthood: Cohort Study. *PLoS ONE, 8*(6), e66827.

115. Horta, B. L., Gigante, D. P., Lima, R. C., Barros, F. C., & Victora, C. G. (2013). Birth by Caesarean Section and Prevalence of Risk Factors for Non-Communicable Diseases in Young Adults: A Birth Cohort Study. *PLoS ONE, 8*(9), e74301. doi:10.1371/journal.pone.0074301.t007

116. Goldani, M. Z., Barbieri, M. A., da Silva, A. N. A. M., Gutierrez, M. R. P., Bettiol, H., & Goldani, H. A. S. (2013). Cesarean section and increased body mass index in school children: two cohort studies from distinct socioeconomic background areas in Brazil. *Nutrition Journal, 12*(1), 1–1. doi:10.1186/1475-2891-12-104

117. Karlsson, C. L. J., Önnerfält, J., Xu, J., Molin, G., Ahrné, S., & Thorngren-Jerneck, K. (2012). The Microbiota of the Gut in Preschool Children With Normal and Excessive Body Weight. *Obesity, 20*(11), 2257–2261. doi:10.1038/oby.2012.110

118. Martin, J. A., Hamilton, B. E., & Ventura, S. J. (2013). Births: Final data for 2011. *National Vital Statistics Reports, 62*(1), 1–70.

119. Gueimonde, M., Laitinen, K., Salminen, S., & Isolauri, E. (2007). Breast Milk: A Source of Bifidobacteria for Infant Gut Development and Maturation? *Neonatology, 92*(1), 64–66.

120. Savino, F., Liguori, S. A., Fissore, M. F., & Oggero, R. (2009). Breast Milk Hormones and Their Protective Effect on Obesity. *International Journal of Pediatric Endocrinology, 2009*, 1–8. doi:10.1155/2009/327505

121. Cani, P. D., Neyrinck, A. M., Fava, F., Knauf, C., Burcelin, R. G., Tuohy, K. M., et al. (2007). Selective increases of bifidobacteria in gut microflora improve high-fat-diet-induced diabetes in mice through a mechanism associated with endotoxaemia. *Diabetologia, 50*(11), 2374–2383. doi:10.1007/s00125-007-0791-0

122. Blaut, M., & Bischoff, S. C. (2010). Probiotics and obesity. *Annals of nutrition & metabolism, 57 Suppl*, 20–23. doi:10.1159/000309079

123. Million, M., Maraninchi, M., Henry, M., Armougom, F., Richet, H., Carrieri, P., et al. (2011). Obesity-associated gut microbiota is enriched in Lactobacillus reuteri and depleted in Bifidobacterium animalis and Methanobrevibacter smithii, 1–9. doi:10.1038/ijo.2011.153

124. Barranco, C. (2012). Nutrition: Breast is best for avoiding obesity. Nature Reviews | *Endocrinology*, 1–1. doi:10.1038/nrendo.2012.80

125. Crume, T. L., Bahr, T. M., Mayer-Davis, E. J., Hamman, R. F., Scherzinger, A. L., Stamm, E., & Dabelea, D. (2012). Selective protection against extremes in childhood body size, abdominal fat deposition, and fat patterning in breastfed children. *Archives of Pediatrics & Adolescent Medicine, 166*(5), 437–443. doi:10.1001/archpediatrics.2011.1488

126. De Palma, G., Capilla, A., Nova, E., Castillejo, G., Varea, V., Pozo, T., et al. (2012). Influence of Milk-Feeding Type and Genetic Risk of Developing Coeliac Disease on Intestinal Microbiota of Infants: The PROFICEL Study. *PLoS ONE, 7*(2), e30791. doi:10.1371/journal.pone.0030791.t010

127. Bergmann, K. E., Bergmann, R. L., Kries, von, R., Böhm, O., Richter, R., Dudenhausen, J. W., & Wahn, U. (2003). Early determinants of childhood overweight and adiposity in a birth cohort study: role of breast-feeding. *International Journal of Obesity, 27*(2), 162–172. doi:10.1038/sj.ijo.802200

128. Glickman, D., & Shalala, D. (2012) *Lots to Lose: How america's Health and Obesity crisis Threatens our economic Future* (pp. 1–110). Bipartisan Policy Center.

129. Guaraldi, F., & Salvatori, G. (2012). Effect of breast and formula feeding on gut microbiota shaping in newborns. *Frontiers in cellular and infection microbiology, 2*, 94. doi:10.3389/fcimb.2012.00094

130. Blaser, M. J., & Falkow, S. (2009). What are the consequences of the disappearing human microbiota? *Nature Reviews Microbiology, 7*(12), 887–894. doi:10.1038/nrmicro2245

131. Blaser, M. (2011). Antibiotic overuse: Stop the killing of beneficial bacteria. *Nature, 476*(7361), 393–394. doi:10.1038/476393a

132. Trasande, L., Blustein, J., Liu, M., Corwin, E., Cox, L. M., & Blaser, M. J. (2013). Infant antibiotic exposures and early-life body mass. *International Journal of Obesity, 37*(1), 16–23. doi:10.1038/ijo.2012.132

133. Thuny, F., Richet, H., Casalta, J.-P., Angelakis, E., Habib, G., & Raoult, D. (2010). Vancomycin Treatment of Infective Endocarditis Is Linked with Recently Acquired Obesity. *PLoS ONE, 5*(2), e9074. doi:10.1371/journal.pone.0009074.t003

134. Gustafson, R. H., & Bowen, R. E. (1997). Antibiotic use in animal agriculture. *Journal of applied microbiology, 83*(5), 531–541.

135. Million, M., & Raoult, D. (2013). The role of the manipulation of the gut microbiota in obesity. *Current infectious disease reports, 15*(1), 25–30. doi:10.1007/s11908-012-0301-5

136. Haight, T. H., & Pierce, W. E. (1955). Effect of Prolonged Antibiotic Administration on the Weight of Healthy Young Males One Figure. *The Journal of Nutrition*, *56*(1), 151–161.

137. Antimicrobials Sold or Distributed for Use in Food-Producing Animals (2011). *Summary Report* (pp. 1–4). Food and Drug Administration, Department of Health and Human Services.

138. Cho, I., Yamanishi, S., Cox, L., Methé, B. A., Zavadil, J., Li, K., et al. (2012). Antibiotics in early life alter the murine colonic microbiome and adiposity. *Nature*, 1–9. doi:10.1038/nature11400

139. Fei, N., & Zhao, L. (2012). An opportunistic pathogen isolated from the gut of an obese human causes obesity in germfree mice. *The ISME Journal*, *7*(4), 880–884. doi:10.1038/ismej.2012.153

140. Hvistendahl, M. (2012). My microbiome and me. *Science Magazine*, *336*(6086), 1248–1250. doi:10.1126/science.336.6086.1248

141. Qin, J., Li, Y., Cai, Z., Li, S., Zhu, J., Zhang, F., et al. (2012). A metagenome-wide association study of gut microbiota in type 2 diabetes. *Nature*, *490*(7418), 55–60. doi:10.1038/nature11450

142. Amar, J., Serino, M., Lange, C., Chabo, C., Iacovoni, J., Mondot, S., et al. (2011). Involvement of tissue bacteria in the onset of diabetes in humans: evidence for a concept. *Diabetologia*, *54*(12), 3055–3061. doi:10.1007/s00125-011-2329-8

143. Mohammed, N., Tang, L., Jahangiri, A., de Villiers, W., & Eckhardt, E. (2012). Elevated IgG levels against specific bacterial antigens in obese patients with diabetes and in mice with diet-induced obesity and glucose intolerance. *Metabolism: clinical and experimental*, *61*(9), 1211–1214. doi:10.1016/j.metabol.2012.02.007

144. Beutler, B., & Rietschel, E. T. (2003). Innate immune sensing and its roots: the story of endotoxin. *Nature Reviews Immunology*, *3*(2), 169–176. doi:10.1038/nri1004

145. Amar, J., Burcelin, R., Ruidavets, J. B., Cani, P. D., Fauvel, J., Alessi, M. C., et al. (2008). Energy intake is associated with endotoxemia in apparently healthy men. *American Journal of Clinical Nutrition*, *87*(5), 1219–1223.

146. Cani, P. D., Bibiloni, R., Knauf, C., Waget, A., Neyrinck, A. M., Delzenne, N. M., & Burcelin, R. (2008). Changes in gut microbiota control metabolic endotoxemia-induced inflammation in high-fat diet-induced obesity and diabetes in mice. *Diabetes*, *57*(6), 1470–1481. doi:10.2337/db07-1403

147. Lassenius, M. I., Pietilainen, K. H., Kaartinen, K., Pussinen, P. J., Syrjanen, J., Forsblom, C., et al. (2011). Bacterial Endotoxin Activity in Human Serum Is Associated With Dyslipidemia, Insulin Resistance, Obesity, and Chronic Inflammation. *Diabetes Care*, *34*(8), 1809–1815. doi:10.2337/dc10-2197

148. Basu, S., Haghiac, M., Surace, P., Challier, J.-C., Guerre-Millo, M., Singh, K., et al. (2011). Pregravid obesity associates with increased maternal endotoxemia and metabolic inflammation. *Obesity, 19*(3), 476–482. doi:10.1038/oby.2010.215

149. Sun, L., Yu, Z., Ye, X., Zou, S., Li, H., Yu, D., et al. (2010). A marker of endotoxemia is associated with obesity and related metabolic disorders in apparently healthy Chinese. *Diabetes Care, 33*(9), 1925–1932. doi:10.2337/dc10.0340

150. Gonzalez-Quintela, A., Alonso, M., Campos, J., Vizcaino, L., Loidi, L., & Gude, F. (2013). Determinants of Serum Concentrations of Lipopolysaccharide-Binding Protein (LBP) in the Adult Population: The Role of Obesity. *PLoS ONE, 8*(1), e54600. doi:10.1371/journal. pone.0054600.t005

151. Moreno-Navarrete, J. M., Escoté, X., Ortega, F., Serino, M., Campbell, M., Michalski, M.-C., et al. (2013). A role for adipocyte-derived lipopolysaccharide-binding protein in inflammation- and obesity-associated adipose tissue dysfunction. *Diabetologia, 56*(11), 2524–2537. doi:10.1007/ s00125-013-3015-9

152. Hawkesworth, S., Moore, S. E., Fulford, A. J. C., Barclay, G. R., Darboe, A. A., Mark, H., et al. (2013). Evidence for metabolic endotoxemia in obese and diabetic Gambian women. *Nutrition and Diabetes, 3*(8), e83–6. doi:10.1038/nutd.2013.24

153. Requena, T., Cotter, P., Shahar, D. R., & Kleiveland, C. R. (2013). Interactions between gut microbiota, food and the obese host. *Trends in Food Science* doi:10.1016/j.tifs.2013.08.007

154. Martins dos Santos, V., Müller, M., & de Vos, W. M. (2010). Systems biology of the gut: the interplay of food, microbiota and host at the mucosal interface. *Current Opinion in Biotechnology, 21*(4), 539–550. doi:10.1016/j. copbio.2010.08.003

155. Jialal, I., Kaur, H., & Devaraj, S. (2013). Toll-like Receptor Status in Obesity and Metabolic Syndrome: A Translational Perspective. *The Journal of Clinical Endocrinology and Metabolism.* doi:10.1210/jc.2013-3092

156. Bengmark, S. (2013). Processed Foods, Dysbiosis, Systemic Inflammation, and Poor Health. *Current Nutrition & Food Science, 9*(2), 113–143.

157. Ding, S., Chi, M. M., Scull, B. P., Rigby, R., Schwerbrock, N. M. J., Magness, S., et al. (2010). High-Fat Diet: Bacteria Interactions Promote Intestinal Inflammation Which Precedes and Correlates with Obesity and Insulin Resistance in Mouse. *PLoS ONE, 5*(8), e12191. doi:10.1371/ journal.pone.0012191.t005

158. Ding, S., & Lund, P. K. (2011). Role of intestinal inflammation as an early event in obesity and insulin resistance. *Current Opinion in Clinical Nutrition and Metabolic Care, 14*(4), 328–333. doi:10.1097/ MCO.0b013e3283478727

159. Dalmas, E., Rouault, C., Abdennour, M., Rovere, C., Rizkalla, S., Bar-Hen, A., et al. (2011). Variations in circulating inflammatory factors are related to changes in calorie and carbohydrate intakes early in the course of surgery-induced weight reduction. *American Journal of Clinical Nutrition*, *94*(2), 450–458. doi:10.3945/ajcn.111.013771

160. Spagnuolo, M. I., Cicalese, M. P., Caiazzo, M. A., Franzese, A., Squeglia, V., Assante, L. R., et al. (2010). Relationship between severe obesity and gut inflammation in children: what's next? *Italian Journal of Pediatrics*, *36*(1), 66. doi:10.1186/1824-7288-36-66

161. Kant, P., Fazakerley, R., & Hull, M. A. (2012). Faecal calprotectin levels before and after weight loss in obese and overweight subjects. *International Journal of Obesity*, 1–3. doi:10.1038/ijo.2012.38

162. Mehta, N. N., McGillicuddy, F. C., Anderson, P. D., Hinkle, C. C., Shah, R., Pruscino, L., et al. (2009). Experimental endotoxemia induces adipose inflammation and insulin resistance in humans. *Diabetes*, *59*(1), 172–181. doi:10.2337/db09-0367

163. Pussinen, P. J., Havulinna, A. S., Lehto, M., Sundvall, J., & Salomaa, V. (2011). Endotoxemia is associated with an increased risk of incident diabetes. *Diabetes Care*, *34*(2), 392–397. doi:10.2337/dc10-1676

164. Kaliannan, K., Hamarneh, S. R., Economopoulos, K. P., Nasrin Alam, S., Moaven, O., Patel, P., et al. (2013). Intestinal alkaline phosphatase prevents metabolic syndrome in mice. *Proceedings of the National Academy of Sciences*, *110*(17), 7003–7008. doi:10.1073/pnas.1220180110

165. Malo, M. S., Alam, S. N., Mostafa, G., Zeller, S. J., Johnson, P. V., Mohammad, N., et al. (2010). Intestinal alkaline phosphatase preserves the normal homeostasis of gut microbiota. *Gut*, *59*(11), 1476–1484. doi:10.1136/gut.2010.211706

166. Sánchez de Medina, F., Martínez-Augustin, O., González, R., Ballester, I., Nieto, A., Gálvez, J., & Zarzuelo, A. (2004). Induction of alkaline phosphatase in the inflamed intestine: a novel pharmacological target for inflammatory bowel disease. *Biochemical Pharmacology*, *68*(12), 2317–2326. doi:10.1016/j.bcp.2004.07.045

167. Munford, R. S. (2005). Invited review: Detoxifying endotoxin: time, place and person. *Journal of Endotoxin Research*, *11*(2), 69–84. doi:10.1177/0968 0519050110020201

168. Chen, K. T., Malo, M. S., Moss, A. K., Zeller, S., Johnson, P., Ebrahimi, F., et al. (2010). Identification of specific targets for the gut mucosal defense factor intestinal alkaline phosphatase. *AJP: Gastrointestinal and Liver Physiology*, *299*(2), G467–75. doi:10.1152/ajpgi.00364.2009

169. Joanne Whitehead. (2009). Intestinal alkaline phosphatase: The molecular link between rosacea and gastrointestinal disease? *Medical Hypotheses*, *73*(6), 1019–1022. doi:10.1016/j.mehy.2009.02.049

170. La Serre, de, C. B., Ellis, C. L., Lee, J., Hartman, A. L., Rutledge, J. C., & Raybould, H. E. (2010). Propensity to high-fat diet-induced obesity in rats is associated with changes in the gut microbiota and gut inflammation. *AJP: Gastrointestinal and Liver Physiology, 299*(2), G440–G448. doi:10.1152/ajpgi.00098.2010

171. Tremaroli, V., & Bäckhed, F. (2012). Functional interactions between the gut microbiota and host metabolism. *Nature, 489*(7415), 242–249. doi:10.1038/nature11552

172. Fasano, A. (2011). Zonulin and its regulation of intestinal barrier function: the biological door to inflammation, autoimmunity, and cancer. *Physiological Reviews, 91*(1), 151–175. doi:10.1152/physrev.00003.2008

173. Fasano, A. (2012). Leaky gut and autoimmune diseases. *Clinical reviews in allergy and immunology, 42*(1), 71–78. doi:10.1007/s12016-011-8291-x

174. Bested, A. C., Logan, A. C., & Selhub, E. M. (2013). Intestinal microbiota, probiotics and mental health: from Metchnikoff to modern advances:Part II – contemporary contextual research. *Gut Pathogens, 5*(1), 1–1. doi:10.1186/1757-4749-5-3

175. Brandtzaeg, P. (2011). The gut as communicator between environment and host: Immunological consequences. *European Journal of Pharmacology, 668*(S1), S16–S32. doi:10.1016/j.ejphar.2011.07.006

176. Devaraj, S., Hemarajata, P., & Versalovic, J. (2013). The human gut microbiome and body metabolism: implications for obesity and diabetes. *Clinical Chemistry, 59*(4), 617–628. doi:10.1373/clinchem.2012.187617

177. Trøseid, M., Nestvold, T. K., Rudi, K., Thoresen, H., Nielsen, E. W., & Lappegård, K. T. (2013). Plasma Lipopolysaccharide Is Closely Associated With Glycemic Control and Abdominal Obesity. *Diabetes Care, 36*(11), 3627–3632.

178. Żak-Gołąb, A., Kocełak, P., Aptekorz, M., Zientara, M., Juszczyk, Ł., Martirosian, G., et al. (2012). Gut microbiota, microinflammation, metabolic profile and zonulin concentration in obese and normal weight subjects. *Cardiovascular Diabetology, 11*(1), 116. doi:10.1038/oby.2009.319

179. Lam, Y. Y., Mitchell, A. J., Holmes, A. J., Denyer, G. S., Gummesson, A., Caterson, I. D., et al. (2011). Role of the Gut in Visceral Fat Inflammation and Metabolic Disorders. *Obesity, 19*(11), 2113–2120. doi:10.1038/oby.2011.68

180. Gummesson, A., Carlsson, L. M. S., Storlien, L. H., Bäckhed, F., Lundin, P., Löfgren, L., et al. (2011). Intestinal Permeability Is Associated With Visceral Adiposity in Healthy Women. *Obesity, 19*(11), 2280–2282. doi:10.1038/oby.2011.251

181. Żak-Gołąb, A., Kocełak, P., Aptekorz, M., Zientara, M., Juszczyk, Ł., Martirosian, G., et al. (2012). Gut microbiota, microinflammation, metabolic profile and zonulin concentration in obese and normal weight subjects. *Cardiovascular Diabetology, 11*(1), 116. doi:10.1038/oby.2009.319

182. Teixeira, T. F. S., Souza, N. C. S., Chiarello, P. G., Franceschini, S. C. C., Bressan, J., Ferreira, C. L. L. F., & do Carmo G Peluzio, M. (2012). Intestinal permeability parameters in obese patients are correlated with metabolic syndrome risk factors. *Clinical Nutrition, 31*(5), 735–740. doi:10.1016/j.clnu.2012.02.009

183. Moreno-Navarrete, J. M., Sabater, M., Ortega, F., Ricart, W., & Fernández-Real, J.-M. (2012). Circulating Zonulin, a Marker of Intestinal Permeability, Is Increased in Association with Obesity-Associated Insulin Resistance. *PLoS ONE, 7*(5), e37160. doi:10.1371/journal.pone.0037160. t003

184. Kunisawa, J., & Kiyono, H. (2013). Immune regulation and monitoring at the epithelial surface of the intestine. *Drug Discovery Today, 18*(1-2), 87–92. doi:10.1016/j.drudis.2012.08.001

185. Visser, J., Rozing, J., Sapone, A., Lammers, K., & Fasano, A. (2009). Tight junctions, intestinal permeability, and autoimmunity. *Annals of the New York Academy of Sciences, 1165*(1), 195–205.

186. Tlaskalova-Hogenova, H., Tuckova, L., Mestecky, J., Kolinska, J., Rossmann, P., Stepankova, R., et al. (2005). Interaction of mucosal microbiota with the innate immune system. *Scandinavian journal of immunology, 62 Suppl 1*, 106–113. doi:10.1111/j.1365-3083.2005.01618.x

187. Fasano, A. (2001). Intestinal zonulin: open sesame! *Gut, 49*(2), 159–162. doi:10.1136/gut.49.2.159

188. Pickup, J. C., Mattock, M. B., Chusney, G. D., & Burt, D. (1997). NIDDM as a disease of the innate immune system: association of acute-phase reactants and interleukin-6 with metabolic syndrome X. *Diabetologia, 40*(11), 1286–1292. doi:10.1007/s001250050822

189. Pickup, J. C., & Crook, M. A. (1998). Is Type II diabetes mellitus a disease of the innate immune system? *Diabetologia, 41*(10), 1241–1248. doi:10.1007/s001250051058

190. Pradhan, A. D., Manson, J. E., Rifai, N., Buring, J. E., & Ridker, P. M. (2001). C-reactive protein, interleukin 6, and risk of developing type 2 diabetes mellitus. *JAMA: The Journal of the American Medical Association, 286*(3), 327–334. doi:10.1001/jama.286.3.327

191. Kelly, C. J., Colgan, S. P., & Frank, D. N. (2012). Of microbes and meals: the health consequences of dietary endotoxemia. *Nutrition in Clinical Practice, 27*(2), 215–225. doi:10.1177/0884533611434934

192. Harte, A. L., Varma, M. C., Tripathi, G., McGee, K. C., Al-Daghri, N. M., Al-Attas, O. S., et al. (2012). High Fat Intake Leads to Acute Postprandial Exposure to Circulating Endotoxin in Type 2 Diabetic Subjects. *Diabetes Care, 35*(2), 375–382. doi:10.2337/dc11-1593

193. Waligora-Dupriet, A.-J., Campeotto, F., Nicolis, I., Bonet, A., Soulaines, P., Dupont, C., & Butel, M.-J. (2007). Endotoxin increase after fat overload is related to postprandial hypertriglyceridemia in morbidly obese patients. *International Journal of Food Microbiology, 113*(1), 108–113. doi:10.1016/j. ijfoodmicro.2006.07.009

194. Lumeng, C. N., & Saltiel, A. R. (2011). Inflammatory links between obesity and metabolic disease. *The Journal of Clinical Investigation, 121*(6), 2111–2117. doi:10.1172/JCI57132

195. Lumeng, C. N. (2013). Innate immune activation in obesity. *Molecular Aspects of Medicine, 34*(1), 12–29. doi:10.1016/j.mam.2012.10.002

196. Skinner, A. C., Steiner, M. J., Henderson, F. W., & Perrin, E. M. (2010). Multiple markers of inflammation and weight status: cross-sectional analyses throughout childhood. *Pediatrics, 125*(4), e801–9. doi:10.1542/ peds.2009-2182

197. Egger, G., & Dixon, J. (2008). Should obesity be the main game? Or do we need an environmental makeover to combat the inflammatory and chronic disease epidemics? *Obesity reviews : an Official Journal of the International Association for the Study of Obesity, 10*(2), 237–249. doi:10.1111/j.1467-789X.2008.00542.x

CHAPTER 10: GUT TREATMENT

1. Grace, E., Shaw, C., Whelan, K., & Andreyev, H. J. N. (2013). Review article: small intestinal bacterial overgrowth - prevalence, clinical features, current and developing diagnostic tests, and treatment. *Alimentary Pharmacology & Therapeutics, 38*(7), 674–688. doi:10.1111/apt.12456

2. Shanab, A. A., Scully, P., Crosbie, O., Buckley, M., O'mahony, L., Shanahan, F., et al. (2011). Small intestinal bacterial overgrowth in nonalcoholic steatohepatitis: association with toll-like receptor 4 expression and plasma levels of interleukin 8. *Digestive Diseases and Sciences, 56*(5), 1524–1534. doi:10.1007/s10620-010-1447-3

3. Sabate, J.-M., Jouet, P., Harnois, F., Mechler, C., Msika, S., Grossin, M., & Coffin, B. (2008). High Prevalence of Small Intestinal Bacterial Overgrowth in Patients with Morbid Obesity: A Contributor to Severe Hepatic Steatosis. *Obesity Surgery, 18*(4), 371–377. doi:10.1007/s11695-007-9398-2

4. Jouet, P., Coffin, B., & Sabate, J.-M. (2011). Small intestinal bacterial overgrowth in patients with morbid obesity. *Digestive Diseases and Sciences, 56*(2), 615–author reply 615–6. doi:10.1007/s10620-010-1356-5

5. Madrid, A. M., Poniachik, J., Quera, R., & Defilippi, C. (2010). Small Intestinal Clustered Contractions and Bacterial Overgrowth: A Frequent Finding in Obese Patients. *Digestive Diseases and Sciences, 56*(1), 155–160. doi:10.1007/s10620-010-1239-9

6. Frank, D. N., Zhu, W., Sartor, R. B., & Li, E. (2011). Investigating the biological and clinical significance of human dysbioses. *Trends in Microbiology, 19*(9), 427–434. doi:10.1016/j.tim.2011.06.005

7. Pendyala, S., Walker, J. M., & Holt, P. R. (2012). A High-Fat Diet Is Associated With Endotoxemia That Originates From the Gut. *YGAST, 142*(5), 1100–1101.e2. doi:10.1053/j.gastro.2012.01.034

8. Serino, M., Fernández-Real, J.-M., Fuentes, E. G., Queipo-Ortuño, M., Moreno-Navarrete, J. M., Sánchez, Á., et al. (2013). The gut microbiota profile is associated with insulin action in humans. *Acta Diabetologica, 50*(5), 753–761. doi:10.1007/s00592-012-0410-5

9. Moreira, A. P. B., Texeira, T. F. S., Ferreira, A. B., Peluzio, M. D. C. G., & Alfenas, R. de C. G. (2012). Influence of a high-fat diet on gut microbiota, intestinal permeability and metabolic endotoxaemia. *British Journal of Nutrition, 108*(5), 801–809. doi:10.1017/S0007114512001213

10. Boroni Moreira, A. P., Fiche Salles Teixeira, T., do C Gouveia Peluzio, M., & de Cássia Gonçalves Alfenas, R. (2012). Gut microbiota and the development of obesity. *Nutrición hospitalaria, 27*(5), 1408–1414. doi:10.3305/nh.2012.27.5.5887

11. Cani, P. D., Everard, A., & Duparc, T. (2013). ScienceDirectGut microbiota, enteroendocrine functions and metabolism. *Current Opinion in Pharmacology, 13*, 1–6. doi:10.1016/j.coph.2013.09.008

12. Fei, N., & Zhao, L. (2012). An opportunistic pathogen isolated from the gut of an obese human causes obesity in germfree mice. *The ISME Journal, 7*(4), 880–884. doi:10.1038/ismej.2012.153

13. Manco, M., Putignani, L., & Bottazzo, G. F. (2010). Gut Microbiota, Lipopolysaccharides, and Innate Immunity in the Pathogenesis of Obesity and Cardiovascular Risk. *Endocrine Reviews, 31*(6), 817–844. doi:10.1210/er.2009-0030

14. Ilan, Y. (2012). Leaky gut and the liver: a role for bacterial translocation in nonalcoholic steatohepatitis. *World Journal of Gastroenterology, 18*(21), 2609–2618. doi:10.3748/wjg.v18.i21.2609

15. Munukka, E., Wiklund, P., Pekkala, S., Völgyi, E., Xu, L., Cheng, S., et al. (2009). Women With and Without Metabolic Disorder Differ in Their Gut Microbiota Composition. *Obesity, 20*(5), 1082–1087. doi:10.1038/oby.2012.8

16. Ley, R. E., Turnbaugh, P. J., Klein, S., & Gordon, J. I. (2006). Microbial ecology: human gut microbes associated with obesity. *Nature, 444*(7122), 1022–1023. doi:10.1038/nature4441021a

17. Bervoets, L., Van Hoorenbeeck, K., Kortleven, I., Van Noten, C., Hens, N., Vael, C., et al. (2013). Differences in gut microbiota composition between obese and lean children: a cross-sectional study. *Gut Pathogens, 5*(1), 10. doi:10.1186/1757-4749-5-10

18. Verdam, F. J., Fuentes, S., de Jonge, C., Zoetendal, E. G., Erbil, R., Greve, J. W., et al. (2013). Human intestinal microbiota composition is associated with local and systemic inflammation in obesity. *Obesity, 21*(12), E607–15. doi:10.1002/oby.20466

19. Kootte, R. S., Vrieze, A., Holleman, F., Dallinga-Thie, G. M., Zoetendal, E. G., de Vos, W. M., et al. (2012). The therapeutic potential of manipulating gut microbiota in obesity and type 2 diabetes mellitus. *Diabetes, Obesity and Metabolism, 14*(2), 112–120. doi:10.1111/j.1463-1326.2011.01483.x

20. Vrieze, A., Van Nood, E., Holleman, F., Salojärvi, J., Kootte, R. S., Bartelsman, J. F. W. M., et al. (2012). Transfer of Intestinal Microbiota From Lean Donors Increases Insulin Sensitivity in Individuals With Metabolic Syndrome. *Gastroenterology, 143*(4), 913–916.e7. doi:10.1053/j.gastro.2012.06.031

21. Hamer, H. M., Jonkers, D. M. A. E., Bast, A., Vanhoutvin, S. A. L. W., Fischer, M. A. J. G., Kodde, A., et al. (2009). Butyrate modulates oxidative stress in the colonic mucosa of healthy humans. *Clinical Nutrition, 28*(1), 88–93. doi:10.1016/j.clnu.2008.11.002

22. Lewis, K., Lutgendorff, F., Phan, V., Söderholm, J. D., Sherman, P. M., & McKay, D. M. (2010). Enhanced translocation of bacteria across metabolically stressed epithelia is reduced by butyrate. *Inflamm Bowel Dis, 16*(7), 1138–1148. doi:10.1002/ibd.2117

23. Brahe, L. K., Astrup, A., & Larsen, L. H. (2013). Is butyrate the link between diet, intestinal microbiota and obesity-related metabolic diseases? *Obesity Reviews, 14*(12), 950–959. doi:10.1111/obr.12068

24. Serino, M., Fernández-Real, J.-M., Fuentes, E. G., Queipo-Ortuño, M., Moreno-Navarrete, J. M., Sánchez, Á., et al. (2013). The gut microbiota profile is associated with insulin action in humans. *Acta Diabetologica, 50*(5), 753–761. doi:10.1007/s00592-012-0410-5

25. Million, M., Maraninchi, M., Henry, M., Armougom, F., Richet, H., Carrieri, P., et al. (2011). Obesity-associated gut microbiota is enriched in Lactobacillus reuteri and depleted in Bifidobacterium animalis and Methanobrevibacter smithii, 1–9. doi:10.1038/ijo.2011.153

26. Chen, J. J., Wang, R., Li, X.-F., & Wang, R.-L. (2011). Bifidobacterium longum supplementation improved high-fat-fed-induced metabolic syndrome and promoted intestinal Reg I gene expression. *Experimental Biology and Medicine, 236*(7), 823–831. doi:10.1258/ebm.2011.010399

27. Walker, A. W., & Lawley, T. D. (2013). Therapeutic modulation of intestinal dysbiosis. *Pharmacological research : the official journal of the Italian Pharmacological Society, 69*(1), 75–86. doi:10.1016/j.phrs.2012.09.008

28. Cani, P. D., Possemiers, S., Van De Wiele, T., Guiot, Y., Everard, A., Rottier, O., et al. (2009). Changes in gut microbiota control inflammation in obese mice through a mechanism involving GLP-2-driven improvement of gut permeability. *Gut, 58*(8), 1091–1103. doi:10.1136/gut.2008.165886

29. Furet, J.-P., Kong, L.-C., Tap, J., Poitou, C., Basdevant, A., Bouillot, J.-
     L., et al. (2010). Differential adaptation of human gut microbiota to
     bariatric surgery-induced weight loss: links with metabolic and low-grade
     inflammation markers. *Diabetes, 59*(12), 3049–3057. doi:10.2337/db10-
     0253

30. Liou, A. P., Paziuk, M., Luevano, J. M., Machineni, S., Turnbaugh, P. J., &
     Kaplan, L. M. (2013). Conserved Shifts in the Gut Microbiota Due to
     Gastric Bypass Reduce Host Weight and Adiposity. *Science Translational
     Medicine, 5*(178), 178ra41–178ra41. doi:10.1126/scitranslmed.3005687

31. Everard, A., Belzer, C., Geurts, L., Ouwerkerk, J. P., Druart, C., Bindels,
     L. B., et al. (2013). Cross-talk between Akkermansia muciniphila and
     intestinal epithelium controls diet-induced obesity. *Proceedings of the
     National Academy of Sciences of the United States of America, 110*(22), 9066–
     9071. doi:10.1073/pnas.1219451110/-/DCSupplemental

32. Tagliabue, A., & Elli, M. (2013). The role of gut microbiota in human
     obesity: recent findings and future perspectives. *Nutrition, metabolism,
     and cardiovascular diseases : NMCD, 23*(3), 160–168. doi:10.1016/j.
     numecd.2012.09.002

33. Mathur, R., Amichai, M., Chua, K. S., Mirocha, J., Barlow, G. M., &
     Pimentel, M. (2013). Methane and hydrogen positivity on breath test
     is associated with greater body mass index and body fat. *The Journal of
     Clinical Endocrinology and Metabolism, 98*(4), E698–702. doi:10.1210/
     jc.2012-3144

34. Clarke, S. F., Murphy, E. F., Nilaweera, K., Ross, P. R., Shanahan, F., O'Toole,
     P. W., & Cotter, P. D. (2012). The gut microbiota and its relationship to
     diet and obesity: new insights. *Gut Microbes, 3*(3), 186–202. doi:10.4161/
     gmic.20168

35. Greiner, T., & Bäckhed, F. (2011). Effects of the gut microbiota on obesity
     and glucose homeostasis. *Trends in Endocrinology & Metabolism, 22*(4),
     117–123. doi:10.1016/j.tem.2011.01.002

36. Zhang, H., DiBaise, J. K., Zuccolo, A., Kudrna, D., Braidotti, M., Yu, Y.,
     et al. (2009). Human gut microbiota in obesity and after gastric bypass.
     Proceedings of the National Academy of Sciences, 106(7), 2365–2370.
     doi:10.1073/pnas.0812600106

37. Costabile, A., Kolida, S., Klinder, A., Gietl, E., Bäuerlein, M., Frohberg,
     C., et al. (2007). A double-blind, placebo-controlled, cross-over study
     to establish the bifidogenic effect of a very-long-chain inulin extracted
     from globe artichoke (Cynara scolymus) in healthy human subjects.
     European Journal of Clinical Nutrition, 104(10), 1189–1195. doi:10.1017/
     S0007114510001571

38. Ravussin, Y., Koren, O., Spor, A., LeDuc, C., Gutman, R., Stombaugh, J., et
     al. (2009). Responses of Gut Microbiota to Diet Composition and Weight
     Loss in Lean and Obese Mice. *Obesity, 20*(4), 738–747. doi:10.1038/
     oby.2011.111

39. Qin, J., Li, Y., Cai, Z., Li, S., Zhu, J., Zhang, F., et al. (2012). A metagenome-wide association study of gut microbiota in type 2 diabetes. *Nature, 490*(7418), 55–60. doi:10.1038/nature11450

40. Claesson, M. J., Jeffery, I. B., Conde, S., Power, S. E., O'Connor, E. M., Cusack, S., et al. (2012). Gut microbiota composition correlates with diet and health in the elderly. *Nature,* 1–8. doi:10.1038/nature11319

41. Million, M., & Raoult, D. (2013). The role of the manipulation of the gut microbiota in obesity. *Current infectious disease reports, 15*(1), 25–30. doi:10.1007/s11908-012-0301-5

42. Ismail, N. A., Ragab, S. H., ElBaky, A. A., Shoeib, A. R. S., Alhosary, Y., & Fekry, D. (2011). Frequency of Firmicutes and Bacteroidetes in gut microbiota in obese and normal weight Egyptian children and adults. *Archives of Medical Science, 3,* 501–507. doi:10.5114/aoms.2011.23418

43. Ismail, N. A., Ragab, S. H., ElBaky, A. A., Shoeib, A. R. S., Alhosary, Y., & Fekry, D. (2011). Frequency of Firmicutes and Bacteroidetes in gut microbiota in obese and normal weight Egyptian children and adults. *Archives of Medical Science, 3,* 501–507. doi:10.5114/aoms.2011.23418

44. Teixeira, T. F. S., Souza, N. C. S., Chiarello, P. G., Franceschini, S. C. C., Bressan, J., Ferreira, C. L. L. F., & do Carmo G Peluzio, M. (2012). Intestinal permeability parameters in obese patients are correlated with metabolic syndrome risk factors. *Clinical Nutrition, 31*(5), 735–740. doi:10.1016/j.clnu.2012.02.009

45. Moreno-Navarrete, J. M., Sabater, M., Ortega, F., Ricart, W., & Fernández-Real, J.-M. (2012). Circulating Zonulin, a Marker of Intestinal Permeability, Is Increased in Association with Obesity-Associated Insulin Resistance. *PLoS ONE, 7*(5), e37160. doi:10.1371/journal.pone.0037160. t003

46. Abraham, C., & Cho, J. H. (2009). Inflammatory Bowel Disease. *New England Journal of Medicine, 361*(21), 2066–2078. doi:10.1056/NEJMra0804647

47. Wershil, B. K., & Furuta, G. T. (2008). 4. Gastrointestinal mucosal immunity. *J Allergy Cln Immunol, 121*(2 Suppl), S380–3– quiz S415. doi:10.1016/j.jaci.2007.10.023

48. Zimmermann, K., Haas, A., & Oxenius, A. (2012). Systemic antibody responses to gut microbes in health and disease. *Gut Microbes, 3*(1), 42–47. doi:10.4161/gmic.19344

49. Vighi, G., Marcucci, F., Sensi, L., Di Cara, G., & Frati, F. (2008). Allergy and the gastrointestinal system. *Clinical and Experimental Immunology, 153 Suppl 1,* 3–6. doi:10.1111/j.1365-2249.2008.03713.x

50. Sonier, B., Patrick, C., Ajjikuttira, P., & Scott, F. W. (2009). Intestinal immune regulation as a potential diet-modifiable feature of gut inflammation and autoimmunity. *International Reviews of Immunology, 28*(6), 414–445. doi:10.3109/08830180903208329

51. Brandtzaeg, P. (2010). Food allergy: separating the science from the mythology. *Nature Reviews Gastroenterology and Hepatology, 7*(7), 380–400. doi:10.1038/nrgastro.2010.80

52. Shimizu, M. (2010). Interaction between Food Substances and the Intestinal Epithelium. *Biosci, Biotechnol, Biochem, 74*(2), 232–241. doi:10.1271/bbb.90730

53. Bengmark, S. (2013). Processed Foods, Dysbiosis, Systemic Inflammation, and Poor Health. *Current Nutrition & Food Science, 9*(2), 113–143.

54. Clemente, M. G., De Virgiliis, S., Kang, J. S., Macatagney, R., Musu, M. P., Di Pierro, M. R., et al. (2003). Early effects of gliadin on enterocyte intracellular signalling involved in intestinal barrier function. *Gut, 52*(2), 218–223.

55. Groschwitz, K. R., & Hogan, S. P. (2009). Intestinal barrier function: molecular regulation and disease pathogenesis. J. Allergy Clin Immunol, *124*(1), 3–20– quiz 21–2. doi:10.1016/j.jaci.2009.05.038

56. Fasano, A., & Shea-Donohue, T. (2005). Mechanisms of disease: the role of intestinal barrier function in the pathogenesis of gastrointestinal autoimmune diseases. Nature Clinical Practice Gastroenterolology & Hepatology, *2*(9), 416–422. doi:10.1038/ncpgasthep0259

57. Fasano, A. (2011). Zonulin and its regulation of intestinal barrier function: the biological door to inflammation, autoimmunity, and cancer. *Physiological Reviews, 91*(1), 151–175. doi:10.1152/physrev.00003.2008

58. Tlaskalová-Hogenová, H., Štěpánková, R., Kozáková, H., Hudcovic, T., Vannucci, L., Tučková, L., et al. (2011). The role of gut microbiota (commensal bacteria) and the mucosal barrier in the pathogenesis of inflammatory and autoimmune diseases and cancer: contribution of germ-free and gnotobiotic animal models of human diseases. *Cellular and Molecular Immunology, 8*(2), 110–120. doi:10.1038/cmi.2010.67

59. Karczewski, J., Troost, F. J., Konings, I., Dekker, J., Kleerebezem, M., Brummer, R. J. M., & Wells, J. M. (2010). Regulation of human epithelial tight junction proteins by Lactobacillus plantarum in vivo and protective effects on the epithelial barrier. *AJP: Gastrointestinal and Liver Physiology, 298*(6), G851–G859. doi:10.1152/ajpgi.00327.2009

60. Sharma, R., Young, C., & Neu, J. (2010). Molecular modulation of intestinal epithelial barrier: contribution of microbiota. *Journal of Biomedicine and Biotechnology, 2010.* doi:10.1155/2010/305879

61. Delzenne, N. M., Neyrinck, A. M., & Cani, P. D. (2011). Modulation of the gut microbiota by nutrients with prebiotic properties: consequences for host health in the context of obesity and metabolic syndrome. *Microbial Cell Factories, 10*(Suppl 1), S10. doi:10.1186/1475-2859-10-S1-S10

62. Bäckhed, F. (2011). Programming of host metabolism by the gut microbiota. *Annals of nutrition & metabolism, 58 Suppl 2,* 44–52. doi:10.1159/000328042

63. Hoerauf, A. (2010). Microflora, helminths, and the immune system-who controls whom. *N Engl J Med, 363*(15), 1476–1478.

64. Ege, M. J., Mayer, M., Normand, A.-C., Genuneit, J., Cookson, W. O., Braun-Fahrländer, C., et al. (2011). Exposure to environmental microorganisms and childhood asthma. *N Engl J Med, 364*(8), 701–709.

65. Ege, M. J. (2011). Intestinal microbial diversity in infancy and allergy risk at school age. *Journal of Allergy and Clinical Immunology, 128*(3), 653–654. doi:10.1016/j.jaci.2011.06.044

66. Penders, J., Thijs, C., Vink, C., Stelma, F. F., Snijders, B., Kummeling, I., et al. (2006). Factors influencing the composition of the intestinal microbiota in early infancy. *Pediatrics, 118*(2), 511–521. doi:10.1542/peds.2005-2824

67. Tanaka, S., Kobayashi, T., Songjinda, P., Tateyama, A., Tsubouchi, M., Kiyohara, C., et al. (2009). Influence of antibiotic exposure in the early postnatal period on the development of intestinal microbiota. *FEMS Immunology & Medical Microbiology, 56*(1), 80–87. doi:10.1111/j.1574-695X.2009.00553.x

68. de, K. L., Duffaut, C., Zakaroff-Girard, A., & Bouloumié, A. (2011). Immune cells in adipose tissue: Key players in metabolic disorders. *Diabetes & Metabolism, 37*(4), 283–290. doi:10.1016/j.diabet.2011.03.002

69. Spies, C. M., Straub, R. H., & Buttgereit, F. (2012). Energy metabolism and rheumatic diseases: from cell to organism. *Arthritis Research & Therapy, 14*(3), 216. doi:10.1186/ar3885

70. Khovidhunkit, W., Kim, M.-S., Memon, R. A., Shigenaga, J. K., Moser, A. H., Feingold, K. R., & Grunfeld, C. (2004). Effects of infection and inflammation on lipid and lipoprotein metabolism: mechanisms and consequences to the host. *The Journal of Lipid Research, 45*(7), 1169–1196.

71. Cottrell, L., Neal, W. A., Ice, C., Perez, M. K., & Piedimonte, G. (2011). Metabolic Abnormalities in Children with Asthma. *American Journal of Respiratory and Critical Care Medicine, 183*(4), 441–448. doi:10.1164/rccm.201004-0603OC

72. Goldszmid, R. S., & Trinchieri, G. (2012). The price of immunity. *Nature Immunology, 13*(10), 932–938.

73. Marques, T. M., Wall, R., Ross, R. P., Fitzgerald, G. F., Ryan, C. A., & Stanton, C. (2010). Programming infant gut microbiota: influence of dietary and environmental factors. *Current Opinion in Biotechnology, 21*(2), 149–156. doi:10.1016/j.copbio.2010.03.020

74. Le Chatelier, E., Nielsen, T., Qin, J., Prifti, E., Hildebrand, F., Falony, G., et al. (2013). Richness of human gut microbiome correlates with metabolic markers. *Nature, 500*(7464), 541–546. doi:doi:10.1038/nature12506

75. Ostaff, M. J., Stange, E. F., & Wehkamp, J. (2013). Antimicrobial peptides and gut microbiota in homeostasis and pathology. *EMBO Molecular Medicine.* doi:10.1002/emmm.201201773

76. Hooper, L. V., Littman, D. R., & Macpherson, A. J. (2012). Interactions Between the Microbiota and the Immune System. *Science*, *336*(6086), 1268–1273. doi:10.1126/science.1223490

77. Duerkop, B. A., Vaishnava, S., & Hooper, L. V. (2009). Immune Responses to the Microbiota at the Intestinal Mucosal Surface. *Immunity*, *31*(3), 368–376. doi:10.1016/j.immuni.2009.08.009

78. Vickery, B. P., Scurlock, A. M., Jones, S. M., & Burks, A. (2011). Mechanisms of immune tolerance relevant to food allergy. *Journal of Allergy and Clinical Immunology*, *127*(3), 576–584. doi:10.1016/j.jaci.2010.12.1116

79. Ilan, Y. (2009). Oral tolerance: can we make it work? *HIM*, *70*(10), 768–776.

80. Bluestone, J. A. (2011). Mechanisms of tolerance. *Immunological Reviews*, *241*(1), 5–19.

81. Nutsch, K. M., & Hsieh, C.-S. (2012). T cell tolerance and immunity to commensal bacteria. *Current Opinion in Immunology*, *24*(4), 385–391. doi:10.1016/j.coi.2012.04.009

82. Procaccini, C., Galgani, M., De Rosa, V., & Matarese, G. (2012). Intracellular metabolic pathways control immune tolerance. *TRENDS in Immunology*, *33*(1), 1–7. doi:10.1016/j.it.2011.09.002

83. Coombes, J. L., & Powrie, F. (2008). Dendritic cells in intestinal immune regulation. *Nature Reviews Immunology*, *8*(6), 435–446. doi:10.1038/nri2335

84. Barbi, J., Pardoll, D., & Pan, F. (2013). Metabolic control of the Treg/Th17 axis. *Immunological Reviews*, *252*(1), 52–77. doi:10.1111/imr.12029

85. Yu, L. C.-H. (2012). Intestinal Epithelial barrier dysfunction in food hypersensitivity. *Journal of Allergy*, *2012*(2), 1–11. doi:10.1056/NEJMoa022613

86. Theoharides, T. C., Alysandratos, K. D., Angelidou, A., Delivanis, D. A., Sismanopoulos, N., Zhang, B., et al. (2012). Mast cells and inflammation. *BBA – Molecular Basis of Disease*, *1822*(1), 21–33. doi:10.1016/j.bbadis.2010.12.014

87. Xu, J. M., & Shi, G. P. (2012). Emerging role of mast cells and macrophages in cardiovascular and metabolic diseases. *Endocrine Reviews*, *33*(1), 71–108. doi:10.1210/er.2011-0013

88. Walker, M. E., Hatfield, J. K., & Brown, M. A. (2012). New insights into the role of mast cells in autoimmunity: Evidence for a common mechanism of action? *BBA – Molecular Basis of Disease*, 1822(1), 57–65. doi:10.1016/j.bbadis.2011.02.009

89. De Winter, B. Y., van den Wijngaard, R. M., & de Jonge, W. J. (2012). Intestinal mast cells in gut inflammation and motility disturbances. *BBA - Molecular Basis of Disease*, *1822*(1), 66–73. doi:10.1016/j.bbadis.2011.03.016

90. Theoharides, T. C., Sismanopoulos, N., Delivanis, D. A., Zhang, B., Hatziagelaki, E. E., & Kalogeromitros, D. (2011). Mast cells squeeze the heart and stretch the gird: their role in atherosclerosis and obesity. *Trends in Pharmacological Sciences, 32*(9), 534–542. doi:10.1016/j.tips.2011.05.005

91. Maintz, L., & Novak, N. (2007). Histamine and histamine intolerance. *Am J Clin Nutr, 85*(5), 1185–1196.

92. Schwelberger, H. G. (2010). Histamine intolerance: a metabolic disease? *Inflammation Research, 59*(2), 219–221. doi:10.1007/s00011-009-0134-3

93. Ji, Y., Sakata, Y., & Tso, P. (2011). Nutrient-induced inflammation in the intestine. *Current Opinion in Clinical Nutrition and Metabolic Care, 14*(4), 315–321. doi:10.1097/MCO.0b013e3283476e74

94. Hilsden, R. J., Meddings, J. B., Hardin, J., Gall, D. G., & Sutherland, L. R. (1999). Intestinal permeability and postheparin plasma diamine oxidase activity in the prediction of Crohn's disease relapse. *Inflamm Bowel Dis, 5*(2), 85–91.

95. Wigand, P., Blettner, M., Saloga, J., & Decker, H. (2012). Prevalence of wine intolerance: results of a survey from Mainz, Germany. *Deutsches Ärzteblatt International, 109*(25), 437. doi:10.3238/arztebl.2012.0437

96. Matteoli, G., Mazzini, E., Iliev, I. D., Mileti, E., Fallarino, F., Puccetti, P., et al. (2010). Gut CD103+ dendritic cells express indoleamine 2,3-dioxygenase which influences T regulatory/T effector cell balance and oral tolerance induction. *Gut, 59*(5), 595–604. doi:10.1136/gut.2009.185108

97. Capuron, L., Schroecksnadel, S., Féart, C., Aubert, A., Higueret, D., Barberger-Gateau, P., et al. (2011). Chronic low-grade inflammation in elderly persons is associated with altered tryptophan and tyrosine metabolism: role in neuropsychiatric symptoms. *BPS, 70*(2), 175–182. doi:10.1016/j.biopsych.2010.12.006

98. Sublette, M. E., & Postolache, T. T. (2012). Neuroinflammation and depression: the role of indoleamine 2,3-dioxygenase (IDO) as a molecular pathway. *Psychosomatic medicine, 74*(7), 668–672. doi:10.1097/PSY.0b013e318268de9f

99. Leonard, B. E., Schwarz, M., & Myint, A. M. (2012). The metabolic syndrome in schizophrenia: is inflammation a contributing cause? *Journal of Psychopharmacology, 26*(5 suppl), 33–41. doi:10.1177/0269881111431622

100. Shelton, R. C., & Miller, A. H. (2010). Eating ourselves to death (and despair): the contribution of adiposity and inflammation to depression. *Progress in Neurobiology, 91*(4), 275–299. doi:10.1016/j.pneurobio.2010.04.004

101. Saransaari, P., & Oja, S. S. (2009). Modulation of taurine release in ischemia by glutamate receptors in mouse brain stem slices. *Amino Acids, 38*(3), 739–746. doi:10.1007/s00726-009-0278-z

102. Anand, P., Thomas, S. G., Kunnumakkara, A. B., Sundaram, C., Harikumar, K. B., Sung, B., et al. (2008). Biological activities of curcumin and its analogues (Congeners) made by man and Mother Nature. *Biochemical Pharmacology*, *76*(11), 1590–1611. doi:10.1016/j.bcp.2008.08.008

103. Bengmark, S. (2012). Gut microbiota, immune development and function. *Pharmacological Research*, *69*(1), 87–113. doi:10.1016/j.phrs.2012.09.002

104. Bollrath, J., & Powrie, F. (2013). Feed Your Tregs More Fiber. *Science*, *341*(6145), 463–464. doi:10.1126/science.1242674

105. Issazadeh-Navikas, S., & Teimer, R. (2012). Influence of Dietary Components on Regulatory T Cells. *Molecular Medicine*, *18*(1), 1. doi:10.2119/molmed.2011.00311

106. Vaishnava, S., & Hooper, L. V. (2011). Eat your carrots! T cells are RARing to go. *Immunity*, *34*(3), 290–292. doi:10.1016/j.immuni.2011.03.007

107. Ooi, J. H., Chen, J., & Cantorna, M. T. (2011). Vitamin D regulation of immune function in the gut: Why do T cells have vitamin D receptors? Journal of Molecular Aspects of Medicine, 1–6. doi:10.1016/j.mam.2011.10.014

108. Brehm, J. M., Celedón, J. C., Soto-Quiros, M. E., Avila, L., Hunninghake, G. M., Forno, E., et al. (2009). Serum vitamin D levels and markers of severity of childhood asthma in Costa Rica. *American Journal of Respiratory and Critical Care Medicine*, *179*(9), 765.

109. McGill, A.-T., Stewart, J. M., Lithander, F. E., Strik, C. M., & Poppitt, S. D. (2008). Relationships of low serum vitamin D3 with anthropometry and markers of the metabolic syndrome and diabetes in overweight and obesity. *Nutrition Journal*, *7*(1), 4. doi:10.1186/1475-2891-7-4

110. Harris, S. S., & Dawson-Hughes, B. (2007). Reduced Sun Exposure Does Not Explain the Inverse Association of 25-Hydroxyvitamin D with Percent Body Fat in Older Adults. *Journal of Clinical Endocrinology & Metabolism*, *92*(8), 3155–3157. doi:10.1210/jc.2007-0722

111. Saneei, P., Salehi-Abargouei, A., & Esmaillzadeh, A. (2013). Serum 25-hydroxy vitamin D levels in relation to body mass index: a systematic review and meta-analysis. *Obesity Reviews*, *14*(5), 393–404. doi:10.1111/obr.12016

112. Jacobs, E. T., Alberts, D. S., Foote, J. A., Green, S. B., Hollis, B. W., Yu, Z., & Martínez, M. E. (2008). Vitamin D insufficiency in southern Arizona. *Am J Clin Nutr*, *87*(3), 608–613.

113. Palacios, C., Gil, K., Pérez, C. M., & Joshipura, K. (2012). Determinants of Vitamin D Status among Overweight and Obese Puerto Rican Adults. *Annals of nutrition & metabolism*, *60*(1), 35–43. doi:10.1159/000335282

114. Goodman, W. A., & Pizarro, T. T. (2013). Regulatory cell populations in the intestinal mucosa. *Current Opinion in Gastroenterology*, *29*(6), 614–620. doi:10.1097/MOG.0b013e328365d30f

115. Field, C. J., Clandinin, M. T., & Aerde, J. E. (2001). Polyunsaturated fatty acids and T-cell function: Implications for the neonate. *Lipids*, *36*(9), 1025–1032. doi:10.1007/s11745-001-0813-6

116. Betiati, D. D. S. B., Oliveira, P. F. de, Camargo, C. de Q., Nunes, E. A., & Trindade, E. B. S. de M. (2013). Effects of omega-3 fatty acids on regulatory T cells in hematologic neoplasms. *Revista Brasileira de Hematologia e Hemoterapia*, *35*(2). doi:10.5581/1516-8484.20130033

117. Kong, W., Yen, J.-H., & Ganea, D. (2011). Docosahexaenoic acid prevents dendritic cell maturation, inhibits antigen-specific Th1/Th17 differentiation and suppresses experimental autoimmune encephalomyelitis. *Brain, Behavior, and Immunity*, *25*(5), 872–882. doi:10.1016/j.bbi.2010.09.012

118. Arora, T., & Singh, S. (2013). Probiotics: Interaction with gut microbiome and antiobesity potential. *Nutrition*. doi:10.1016/j.nut.2012.07.017

119. Baboota, R. K., Bishnoi, M., Ambalam, P., Kondepudi, K. K., Sarma, S. M., Boparai, R. K., & Podili, K. (2013). Functional food ingredients for the management of obesity and associated co-morbidities–A review. *Journal of Functional Foods*. doi:10.1016/j.jff.2013.04.014

120. Saad, N., Delattre, C., Urdaci, M., Schmitter, J. M., & Bressollier, P. (2012). An overview of the last advances in probiotic and prebiotic field. *LWT - Food Science and Technology*, *50*(1), 1–16. doi:10.1016/j.lwt.2012.05.014

121. Saulnier, D. M., Ringel, Y., Heyman, M. B., Foster, J. A., Bercik, P., Shulman, R. J., et al. (2013). The intestinal microbiome, probiotics and prebiotics in neurogastroenterology. *Gut Microbes*, *4*(1), 17–27. doi:10.4161/gmic.22973

122. Tillisch, K., information, C. A. C., author, E.-M. T. C., Labus, J., Kilpatrick, L., Jiang, Z., et al. (2013). Consumption of Fermented Milk Product With Probiotic Modulates Brain Activity. *Gastroenterology*, *144*(7), 1394–1401.

123. Lammers, K. M., Brigidi, P., Vitali, B., Gionchetti, P., Rizzello, F., Caramelli, E., et al. (2003). Immunomodulatory effects of probiotic bacteria DNA: IL-1 and IL-10 response in human peripheral blood mononuclear cells. *FEMS Immunology & Medical Microbiology*, *38*(2), 165–172. doi:10.1016/S0928-8244(03)00144-5

124. Ghadimi, D., Folsterholst, R., Devrese, M., Winkler, P., Heller, K., & Schrezenmeir, J. (2008). Effects of probiotic bacteria and their genomic DNA on TH1/TH2-cytokine production by peripheral blood mononuclear cells (PBMCs) of healthy and allergic subjects. *Immunobiology*, *213*(8), 677–692. doi:10.1016/j.imbio.2008.02.001

125. Bell, B. P. (1994). A Multistate Outbreak of Escherichia coli O157:H7— Associated Bloody Diarrhea and Hemolytic Uremic Syndrome From Hamburgers. *JAMA: The Journal of the American Medical Association*, *272*(17), 1349–1353. doi:10.1001/jama.1994.03520170059036

126. Kruis, W., Fric, P., Pokrotnieks, J., Lukás, M., Fixa, B., Kascák, M., et al. (2004). Maintaining remission of ulcerative colitis with the probiotic Escherichia coli Nissle 1917 is as effective as with standard mesalazine. *Gut*, *53*(11), 1617–1623. doi:10.1136/gut.2003.037747

127. Takahashi, N., Kitazawa, H., Iwabuchi, N., Xiao, J.-Z., MIYAJI, K., Iwatsuki, K., & Saito, T. (2006). Oral Administration of an Immunostimulatory DNA Sequence from Bifidobacterium longum Improves Th1/Th2 Balance in a Murine Model. *Biosci, Biotechnol, Biochem*, *70*(8), 2013–2017. doi:10.1271/bbb.60260

128. Medina, M., Izquierdo, E., Ennahar, S., & Sanz, Y. (2007). Differential immunomodulatory properties of Bifidobacterium logum strains: relevance to probiotic selection and clinical applications. *Clinical and Experimental Immunology*, *150*(3), 531–538. doi:10.1111/j.1365-2249.2007.03522.x

129. Vissers, Y. M., Snel, J., Zuurendonk, P. F., Smit, B. A., Wichers, H. J., & Savelkoul, H. F. J. (2010). Differential effects of Lactobacillus acidophilus and Lactobacillus plantarum strains on cytokine induction in human peripheral blood mononuclear cells. *FEMS Immunology & Medical Microbiology*, *59*(1), 60–70. doi:10.1111/j.1574-695X.2010.00662.x

130. Angelakis, E., Armougom, F., Million, M., & Raoult, D. (2012). The relationship between gut microbiota and weight gain in humans. *Future Microbiology*, *7*(1), 91–109. doi:10.2217/fmb.11.142

131. Jain, P. K., McNaught, C. E., Anderson, A. D. G., MacFie, J., & Mitchell, C. J. (2004). Influence of synbiotic containing Lactobacillus acidophilus La5, Bifidobacterium lactis Bb 12, Streptococcus thermophilus, Lactobacillus bulgaricus and oligofructose on gut barrier function and sepsis in critically ill patients: a randomised controlled trial. *Clinical Nutrition*, *23*(4), 467–475. doi:10.1016/j.clnu.2003.12.002

132. Ahmed, M., Prasad, J., Gill, H., Stevenson, L., & Gopal, P. (2007). Impact of consumption of different levels of Bifidobacterium lactis HN019 on the intestinal microflora of elderly human subjects. *The journal of nutrition, health & aging*, *11*(1), 26–31.

133. Prasad, J., Sazawal, S., Dhingra, U., & Gopal, P. K. (2012). Detection of viable Bifidobacterium lactis HN019 (DR10™) in stools of children during a synbiotic dietary intervention trial. *International Dairy Journal*. doi:10.1016/j.idairyj.2012.12.001

134. Chiang, B. L., Sheih, Y. H., Wang, L. H., Liao, C. K., & Gill, H. S. (2000). Enhancing immunity by dietary consumption of a probiotic lactic acid bacterium (Bifidobacterium lactis HN019): optimization and definition of cellular immune responses. *European Journal of Clinical Nutrition*, *54*(11), 849–855. doi:10.1038/sj.ejcn.1601093

135. Shu, Q., & Gill, H. S. (2001). A dietary probiotic (Bifidobacterium lactis HN019) reduces the severity of Escherichia coli O157:H7 infection in mice. *Medical Microbiology and Immunology*, *189*(3), 147–152. doi:10.1007/s430-001-8021-9

136. Liu, C., Zhang, Z.-Y., Dong, K., & Guo, X.-K. (2010). Adhesion and immunomodulatory effects of Bifidobacterium lactis HN019 on intestinal epithelial cells INT-407. *World Journal of Gastroenterology*, *16*(18), 2283–2290. doi:10.3748/wjg.v16.i18.2283

137. Sazawal, S., Dhingra, U., Hiremath, G., Sarkar, A., Dhingra, P., Dutta, A., et al. (2010). Effects of Bifidobacterium lactis HN019 and Prebiotic Oligosaccharide Added to Milk on Iron Status, Anemia, and Growth Among Children 1 to 4 Years Old. *Journal of Pediatric Gastroenterology and Nutrition*, *51*(3), 1. doi:10.1097/MPG.0b013e3181d98e45

138. Gill, H. S., Rutherfurd, K. J., Cross, M. L., & Gopal, P. K. (2001). Enhancement of immunity in the elderly by dietary supplementation with the probiotic Bifidobacterium lactis HN019. *Am J Clin Nutr*, *74*(6), 833–839.

139. Gopal, P. K., Prasad, J., & Gill, H. S. (2003). Effects of the consumption of Bifidobacterium lactis HN019 (DR10 TM) and galacto-oligosaccharides on the microflora of the gastrointestinal tract in human subjects. *Nutrition Research*, *23*(10), 1313–1328. doi:10.1016/S0271-5317(03)00134-9

140. Liu, Z. H., Huang, M. J., Zhang, X. W., Wang, L., Huang, N. Q., Peng, H., et al. (2012). The effects of perioperative probiotic treatment on serum zonulin concentration and subsequent postoperative infectious complications after colorectal cancer surgery: a double-center and double-blind randomized clinical trial. *American Journal of Clinical Nutrition*, *97*(1), 117–126. doi:10.3945/ajcn.112.040949

141. Corthésy, B. (2007). Roundtrip ticket for secretory IgA: role in mucosal homeostasis? *J Immunol*, *178*(1), 27–32.

142. Sutherland, D. B., & Fagarasan, S. (2012). IgA synthesis: a form of functional immune adaptation extending beyond gut. *Current Opinion in Immunology*, *24*(3), 261–268. doi:10.1016/j.coi.2012.03.005

143. Slack, E., Balmer, M. L., Fritz, J. H., & Hapfelmeier, S. (2012). Functional flexibility of intestinal IgA - broadening the fine line. *Frontiers in immunology*, *3*, 100. doi:10.3389/fimmu.2012.00100

144. Brandtzaeg, P. (2011). The gut as communicator between environment and host: Immunological consequences. *European Journal of Pharmacology*, *668*(S1), S16–S32. doi:10.1016/j.ejphar.2011.07.006

145. Brenchley, J. M., & Douek, D. C. (2012). Microbial Translocation Across the GI Tract *. *Annual Review of Immunology*, *30*(1), 149–173. doi:10.1146/annurev-immunol-020711-075001

146. McFarland, L. V. (2010). Systematic review and meta-analysis of Saccharomyces boulardii in adult patients. *World Journal of Gastroenterology*, *16*(18), 2202–2222.

147. Billoo, A. G., Memon, M. A., Khaskheli, S. A., Murtaza, G., Iqbal, K., Saeed Shekhani, M., & Siddiqi, A. Q. (2006). Role of a probiotic (Saccharomyces boulardii) in management and prevention of diarrhoea. *World Journal of Gastroenterology*, *12*(28), 4557–4560.

148. Czerucka, D., Piche, T., & Rampal, P. (2007). Review article: yeast as probiotics -- Saccharomyces boulardii. *Alimentary Pharmacology & Therapeutics, 26*(6), 767–778. doi:10.1111/j.1365-2036.2007.03442.x

149. Buts, J.-P. (2009). Twenty-Five Years of Research on Saccharomyces boulardii Trophic Effects: Updates and Perspectives. *Digestive Diseases and Sciences, 54*(1), 15–18. doi:10.1007/s10620-008-0322-y

150. Kelesidis, T. T., & Pothoulakis, C. C. (2012). Efficacy and safety of the probiotic Saccharomyces boulardii for the prevention and therapy of gastrointestinal disorders. *Therapeutic Advances in Gastroenterology, 5*(2), 111–125. doi:10.1177/1756283X11428502

151. Earnest, C. P., Jordan, A. N., Safir, M., Weaver, E., & Church, T. S. (2005). Cholesterol-lowering effects of bovine serum immunoglobulin in participants with mild hypercholesterolemia. *Am J Clin Nutr, 81*(4), 792–798.

152. Pérez-Bosque, A., Amat, C., Polo, J., Campbell, J. M., Crenshaw, J., Russell, L., & Moretó, M. (2006). Spray-Dried Animal Plasma Prevents the Effects of Staphylococcus aureus Enterotoxin B on Intestinal Barrier Function in Weaned Rats. *J. Nutr., 136*(11), 2838–2843.

153. Klein, G. L., & Weaver, E. M. (2012). Improvement of chemotherapy induced colitis with serum-derived bovine immunoglobulin. *BCM Proceedings, 6*(Supp. 3), 26. doi:10.1186/1753-6561-6-S3-P

154. Asmuth, D. M., Ma, Z.-M., Albanese, A., Sandler, N. G., Devaraj, S., Knight, T. H., et al. (2013). Oral serum-derived bovine immunoglobulin improves duodenal immune reconstitution and absorption function in patients with HIV enteropathy. *AIDS (London, England), 27*(14), 2207–2217. doi:10.1097/QAD.0b013e328362e54c

155. Vrieze, A., Holleman, F., Zoetendal, E. G., de Vos, W. M., Hoekstra, J. B. L., & Nieuwdorp, M. (2010). The environment within: how gut microbiota may influence metabolism and body composition. *Diabetologia, 53*(4), 606–613. doi:10.1007/s00125-010-1662-7

156. Gevers, D., Pop, M., Schloss, P. D., & Huttenhower, C. (2012). Bioinformatics for the Human Microbiome Project. *PLoS Computational Biology, 8*(11), e1002779. doi:10.1371/journal.pcbi.1002779

157. Diamant, M., Blaak, E. E., & de Vos, W. M. (2011). Do nutrient-gut-microbiota interactions play a role in human obesity, insulin resistance and type 2 diabetes? *Obesity reviews : an official journal of the International Association for the Study of Obesity, 12*(4), 272–281. doi:10.1111/j.1467-789X.2010.00797.x

158. Tremaroli, V., & Bäckhed, F. (2012). Functional interactions between the gut microbiota and host metabolism. *Nature, 489*(7415), 242–249. doi:10.1038/nature11552

159. Gophna, U. (2012). The Guts of Dietary Habits. *Science, 334*(6052), 45–46. doi:10.1126/science.1213799

160. Wu, G. D., Chen, J., Hoffmann, C., Bittinger, K., Chen, Y. Y., Keilbaugh, S. A., et al. (2011). Linking Long-Term Dietary Patterns with Gut Microbial Enterotypes. *Science*, *334*(6052), 105–108. doi:10.1126/science.1208344

161. David, L. A., Maurice, C. F., Carmody, R. N., Gootenberg, D. B., Button, J. E., Wolfe, B. E., et al. (2013). Diet rapidly and reproducibly alters the human gut microbiome. *Nature*, –. doi:doi:10.1038/nature12820

162. Kau, A. L., Ahern, P. P., Griffin, N. W., Goodman, A. L., & Gordon, J. I. (2011). Human nutrition, the gut microbiome and the immune system. *Nature*, *474*(7351), 327–336. doi:10.1038/nature10213

163. Krajmalnik-Brown, R., Ilhan, Z.-E., Kang, D.-W., & DiBaise, J. K. (2012). Effects of gut microbes on nutrient absorption and energy regulation. *Nutrition in Clinical Practice*, *27*(2), 201–214. doi:10.1177/0884533611436116

164. De Filippo, C., Cavalieri, D., Di Paola, M., Ramazzotti, M., Poullet, J. B., Massart, S., et al. (2010). Impact of diet in shaping gut microbiota revealed by a comparative study in children from Europe and rural Africa. *Proceedings of the National Academy of Sciences of the United States of America*, *107*(33), 14691–14696. doi:10.1073/pnas.1005963107/-/DCSupplemental

165. Carrera-Bastos, P., Fontes-Villalba, M., O'Keefe, J. H., Lindeberg, S., & Cordain, L. (2011). The western diet and lifestyle and diseases of civilization. *Research Reports in Clinical Cardiology*, *2*, 15–35. doi:10.2147/RRCC.S16919

166. Xiao, S., Fei, N., Pang, X., Shen, J., & Wang, L. (2013). A gut microbiota-targeted dietary intervention for amelioration of chronic inflammation underlying metabolic syndrome. *FEMS microbiology ....* doi:10.1111/1574-6941.12228

167. Musso, G., Gambino, R., & Cassader, M. (2011). Interactions Between Gut Microbiota and Host Metabolism Predisposing to Obesity and Diabetes. *Annual Review of Medicine*, *62*(1), 361–380. doi:10.1146/annurev-med-012510-175505

168. Fung, Q. M., & Szilagyi, A. (2012). Carbohydrate Elimination or Adaptation Diet for Symptoms of Intestinal Discomfort in IBD: Rationales for "Gibsons' Conundrum." *International Journal of Inflammation*, *2012*(6), 1–19. doi:10.1111/j.1365-2036.2008.03911.x

169. Delzenne, N. M., & Cani, P. D. (2011). Interaction Between Obesity and the Gut Microbiota: Relevance in Nutrition. *Annual Review of Nutrition*, *31*(1), 15–31. doi:10.1146/annurev-nutr-072610-145146

170. HAMER, H. M., De Preter, V., Windey, K., & Verbeke, K. (2011). Functional analysis of colonic bacterial metabolism: relevant to health? *AJP: Gastrointestinal and Liver Physiology*, *302*(1), G1–G9. doi:10.1152/ajpgi.00048.2011

171. Kimura, I., Inoue, D., Maeda, T., Hara, T., Ichimura, A., Miyauchi, S., et al. (2011). Short-chain fatty acids and ketones directly regulate sympathetic nervous system via G protein-coupled receptor 41 (GPR41). *Proceedings of the National Academy of Sciences of the United States of America, 108*(19), 8030–8035. doi:10.1073/pnas.1016088108/-/DCSupplemental/pnas.201016088SI.pdf

172. Ulven, T. (2012). Short-chain free fatty acid receptors FFA2/GPR43 and FFA3/GPR41 as new potential therapeutic targets. *Frontiers in endocrinology, 3.* doi:10.3389/fendo.2012.00111/abstract

173. Samuel, B. S., Shaito, A., Motoike, T., Rey, F. E., Bäckhed, F., Manchester, J. K., et al. (2008). Effects of the gut microbiota on host adiposity are modulated by the short-chain fatty-acid binding G protein-coupled receptor, Gpr41. *PNAS, 105*(43), 16767–16772.

174. Schwiertz, A., Taras, D., Schäfer, K., Beijer, S., Bos, N. A., Donus, C., & Hardt, P. D. (2010). Microbiota and SCFA in lean and overweight healthy subjects. *Obesity, 18*(1), 190–195. doi:10.1038/oby.2009.167

175. Tiihonen, K., Ouwehand, A. C., & Rautonen, N. (2010). Effect of overweight on gastrointestinal microbiology and immunology: correlation with blood biomarkers. *British Journal of Nutrition, 103*(7), 1070–1078. doi:10.1017/S0007114509992807

176. Fava, F., Gitau, R., Griffin, B. A., Gibson, G. R., Tuohy, K. M., & Lovegrove, J. A. (2012). The type and quantity of dietary fat and carbohydrate alter faecal microbiome and short-chain fatty acid excretion in a metabolic syndrome ‘at-risk’ population. *International Journal of Obesity,* 1–8. doi:10.1038/ijo.2012.33

177. Al-Lahham, S. H., Peppelenbosch, M. P., Roelofsen, H., Vonk, R. J., & Venema, K. (2010). Biological effects of propionic acid in humans; metabolism, potential applications and underlying mechanisms. *Biochimica et Biophysica Acta (BBA) - Molecular and Cell Biology of Lipids, 1801*(11), 1175–1183. doi:10.1016/j.bbalip.2010.07.007

178. van Zanten, G. C., Knudsen, A., Röytiö, H., Forssten, S., Lawther, M., Blennow, A., et al. (2012). The Effect of Selected Synbiotics on Microbial Composition and Short-Chain Fatty Acid Production in a Model System of the Human Colon. *PLoS ONE, 7*(10), e47212. doi:10.1371/journal.pone.0047212.s003

179. Payne, A. N., Chassard, C., & Lacroix, C. (2012). Gut microbial adaptation to dietary consumption of fructose, artificial sweeteners and sugar alcohols: implications for host-microbe interactions contributing to obesity. *Obesity Reviews,* no–no. doi:10.1111/j.1467-789X.2012.01009.x

180. Panickar, K. S. (2013). Effects of dietary polyphenols on neuroregulatory factors and pathways that mediate food intake and energy regulation in obesity. *Molecular Nutrition & Food Research, 57*(1), 34–47. doi:10.1002/mnfr.201200431

181. Tuohy, K. M., Conterno, L., Gasperotti, M., & Viola, R. (2012). Up-regulating the Human Intestinal Microbiome Using Whole Plant Foods, Polyphenols, and/or Fiber. *Journal of Agricultural and Food Chemistry, 60*(36), 120521051833005. doi:10.1021/jf2053959

182. Geurts, L., Neyrinck, A. M., Delzenne, N. M., Knauf, C., & Cani, P. D. (2013). Gut microbiota controls adipose tissue expansion, gut barrier and glucose metabolism: novel insights into molecular targets and interventions using prebiotics. *Beneficial Microbes, 1*(-1), 1–15. doi:10.3920/BM2012.0065

183. Raman, M., Ahmed, I., Gillevet, P. M., Probert, C. S., Ratcliffe, N. M., Smith, S., et al. (2013). Fecal Microbiome and Volatile Organic Compound Metabolome in Obese Human Beings With Nonalcoholic Fatty Liver Disease. *YJCGH*, 1–11. doi:10.1016/j.cgh.2013.02.015

184. Alkhouri, N., Eng, K., Cikach, F., Patel, N., Yan, C., & Brindle, A. (2013). Breathprints of Childhood Obesity- Changes in Volatile Organic Compounds in Obese Children and Adolescents Compared to Healthy Controls. *Gastroenterology, 144.5*(S-30).

185. Nyangale, E. P., Mottram, D. S., & Gibson, G. R. (2012). Gut Microbial Activity, Implications for Health and Disease: The Potential Role of Metabolite Analysis. *Journal of Proteome Research*, 121101161847008. doi:10.1021/pr300637d

186. Jacobs, D. M., Gaudier, E., van Duynhoven, J., & Vaughan, E. E. (2009). Non-digestible food ingredients, colonic microbiota and the impact on gut health and immunity: a role for metabolomics. *Current Drug Metabolism, 10*(1), 41–54.

187. Maslowski, K. M., & Mackay, C. R. (2011). Diet, gut microbiota and immune responses. *Nature Publishing Group, 12*(1), 5–9. doi:10.1038/ni0111-5

188. Mai, V., McCrary, Q. M., Sinha, R., & Glei, M. (2009). Associations between dietary habits and body mass index with gut microbiota composition and fecal water genotoxicity: an observational study in African American and Caucasian American volunteers. *Nutrition Journal, 8*(1), 49. doi:10.1186/1475-2891-8-49

189. Gregersen, S., Samocha-Bonet, D., Heilbronn, L. K., & Campbell, L. V. (2012). Inflammatory and oxidative stress responses to high-carbohydrate and high-fat meals in healthy humans. *Journal of Nutrition and Metabolism, 2012.*

190. Turnbaugh, P. J., Ridaura, V. K., Faith, J. J., Rey, F. E., Knight, R., & Gordon, J. I. (2009). The effect of diet on the human gut microbiome: a metagenomic analysis in humanized gnotobiotic mice. *Science Translational Medicine, 1*(6), 6ra14. doi:10.1126/scitranslmed.3000322

191. Winter, S. E., Lopez, C. A., & Bäumler, A. J. (2013). The dynamics of gut-associated microbial communities during inflammation. *EMBO Reports, 14*(4), 319–327. doi:10.1038/embor.2013.27

192. O'sullivan, O., Coakley, M., Lakshminarayanan, B., Conde, S., Claesson, M. J., Cusack, S., et al. (2012). Alterations in intestinal microbiota of elderly Irish subjects post-antibiotic therapy. *Journal of Antimicrobial Chemotherapy*, *68*(1), 214–221. doi:10.1093/jac/dks348

193. Cardona, F., Andres-Lacueva, C., Tulipani, S., Tinahones, F. J., & Queipo-Ortuño, M. I. (2013). Benefits of polyphenols on gut microbiota and implications in human health. *The Journal of Nutritional Biochemistry*, *24*(8), 1415–1422. doi:10.1016/j.jnutbio.2013.05.001

194. Etxeberria, U., Fernández-Quintela, A., Milagro, F. I., Aguirre, L., Martínez, J. A., & Portillo, M. P. (2013). Impact of Polyphenols and Polyphenol-Rich Dietary Sources on Gut Microbiota Composition. *Journal of Agricultural and Food Chemistry*, 130927121135003. doi:10.1021/jf402506c

195. Clemente-Postigo, M., Queipo-Ortuno, M. I., Boto-Ordonez, M., Coin-Araguez, L., Roca-Rodriguez, M. D. M., Delgado-Lista, J., et al. (2013). Effect of acute and chronic red wine consumption on lipopolysaccharide concentrations. *American Journal of Clinical Nutrition*, *97*(5), 1053–1061. doi:10.3945/ajcn.112.051128

196. Kelly, C. J., Colgan, S. P., & Frank, D. N. (2012). Of microbes and meals: the health consequences of dietary endotoxemia. *Nutrition in Clinical Practice*, *27*(2), 215–225. doi:10.1177/0884533611434934

197. Van den Abbeele, P., Verstraete, W., Aidy, El, S., Geirnaert, A., & Van de Wiele, T. (2013). Prebiotics, faecal transplants and microbial network units to stimulate biodiversity of the human gut microbiome. *Microbial biotechnology*, *6*(4), 335–340. doi:10.1111/1751-7915.12049

198. Spreadbury, I. (2012). Comparison with ancestral diets suggests dense acellular carbohydrates promote an inflammatory microbiota, and may be the primary dietary cause of leptin resistance and obesity. *Diabetes, Metabolic Syndrome and Obesity: Targets and Therapy*, *5*, 175–189. doi:10.2147/DMSO.S33473

199. Possemiers, S., Bolca, S., Verstraete, W., & Heyerick, A. (2011). The intestinal microbiome: A separate organ inside the body with the metabolic potential to influence the bioactivity of botanicals. *Fitoterapia*, *82*(1), 53–66. doi:10.1016/j.fitote.2010.07.012

200. Joven, J., Micol, V., Segura-Carretero, A., Alonso-Villaverde, C., & Menéndez, J. A. (2013). Polyphenols and the modulation of gene expression pathways: can we eat our way out of the danger of chronic disease? *Critical Reviews in Food Science and Nutrition*, 130308121420004. doi:10.1080/10408398.2011.621772

201. Nunn, A. V., Guy, G. W., Brodie, J. S., & Bell, J. D. (2010). Inflammatory modulation of exercise salience: using hormesis to return to a healthy lifestyle. *Nutrition & Metabolism*, *7*(1), 87. doi:10.1186/1743-7075-7-87

202. Joven, J., Rull, A., Rodriguez-Gallego, E., Camps, J., Riera-Borrull, M., Hernández-Aguilera, A., et al. (2013). Multifunctional targets of dietary polyphenols in disease: A case for the chemokine network and energy metabolism. *Food and Chemical Toxicology, 51*, 267–279. doi:10.1016/j.fct.2012.10.004

203. Williams, D. J., Edwards, D., Hamernig, I., Le Jian, James, A. P., Johnson, S. K., & Tapsell, L. C. (2010). Vegetables containing phytochemicals with potential anti-obesity properties: A review. *FRIN, 52*(1), 1–11. doi:10.1016/j.foodres.2013.03.015

204. Rooks, M. G., & Garrett, W. S. (2011). Bacteria, food, and cancer. *F1000 biology reports, 3*, 12. doi:10.3410/B3-12

205. Kemperman, R. A., Gross, G., Mondot, S., Possemiers, S., Marzorati, M., Van de Wiele, T., et al. (2013). Impact of polyphenols from black tea and red wine/grape juice on a gut model microbiome. *Food Research International.* doi:10.1016/j.foodres.2013.01.034

206. van Dorsten, F. A., Peters, S., Gross, G., Gomez-Roldan, V., Klinkenberg, M., de Vos, R. C., et al. (2012). Gut Microbial Metabolism of Polyphenols from Black Tea and Red Wine/Grape Juice Is Source-Specific and Colon-Region Dependent. *Journal of Agricultural and Food Chemistry, 60*(45), 11331–11342. doi:10.1021/jf303165w

207. Carrasco-Pozo, C., Morales, P., & Gotteland, M. (2013). Polyphenols Protect the Epithelial Barrier Function of Caco-2 Cells Exposed to Indomethacin through the Modulation of Occludin and Zonula Occludens-1 Expression. *Journal of Agricultural and Food Chemistry*, 130523151421000. doi:10.1021/jf400150p

208. Hooper, L. V. (2011). You AhR What You Eat: Linking Diet and Immunity. *Cell, 147*(3), 489–491. doi:10.1016/j.cell.2011.10.004

209. Cahenzli, J., Balmer, M. L., & McCoy, K. D. (2013). Microbial-immune cross-talk and regulation of the immune system. *Immunology, 138*(1), 12–22. doi:10.1111/j.1365-2567.2012.03624.x

210. Kiss, E. A., Vonarbourg, C., Kopfmann, S., Hobeika, E., Finke, D., Esser, C., & Diefenbach, A. (2011). Natural aryl hydrocarbon receptor ligands control organogenesis of intestinal lymphoid follicles. *Science, 334*(6062), 1561–1565. doi:10.1126/science.1214914

211. Esser, C. (2012). Biology and function of the aryl hydrocarbon receptor: report of an international and interdisciplinary conference. (Vol. 86, pp. 1323–1329). Presented at the Archives of toxicology. doi:10.1007/s00204-012-0818-2

212. Pot, C. (2012). Aryl hydrocarbon receptor controls regulatory CD4+ T cell function. *Swiss Medical Weekly, 142*, w13592. doi:10.4414/smw.2012.13592

213. Rastmanesh, R. (2011). High polyphenol, low probiotic diet for weight loss because of intestinal microbiota interaction. *Chemico-Biological Interactions, 189*(1-2), 1–8. doi:10.1016/j.cbi.2010.10.002

214. Flint, H. J., Scott, K. P., Duncan, S. H., Louis, P., & Forano, E. (2012). Microbial degradation of complex carbohydrates in the gut. *Gut Microbes*, *3*(4), 289–306. doi:10.4161/gmic.19897

215. Cani, P. D., Neyrinck, A. M., Fava, F., Knauf, C., Burcelin, R. G., Tuohy, K. M., et al. (2007). Selective increases of bifidobacteria in gut microflora improve high-fat-diet-induced diabetes in mice through a mechanism associated with endotoxaemia. *Diabetologia*, *50*(11), 2374–2383. doi:10.1007/s00125-007-0791-0

216. Delzenne, N. M., Cani, P. D., & Neyrinck, A. M. (2007). Modulation of glucagon-like peptide 1 and energy metabolism by inulin and oligofructose: experimental data. *The Journal of Nutrition*, *137*(11 Suppl), 2547S–2551S.

217. Verhoef, S. P. M., Meyer, D., & Westerterp, K. R. (2011). Effects of oligofructose on appetite profile, glucagon-like peptide 1 and peptide YY3-36 concentrations and energy intake. *British Journal of Nutrition*, *106*(11), 1757–1762. doi:10.1017/S0007114511002194

218. Dehghan, P., Gargari, B. P., Jafar-Abadi, M. A., & Aliasgharzadeh, A. (2013). Inulin controls inflammation and metabolic endotoxemia in women with type 2 diabetes mellitus: a randomized-controlled clinical trial. *International Journal of Food Sciences and Nutrition*, 1–7. doi:10.3109/09637486.2013.836738

219. Dewulf, E. M., Cani, P. D., Claus, S. P., Fuentes, S., Puylaert, P. G. B., Neyrinck, A. M., et al. (2013). Insight into the prebiotic concept: lessons from an exploratory, double blind intervention study with inulin-type fructans in obese women. *Gut*, *62*(8), 1112–1121. doi:10.1136/gutjnl-2012-303304

220. Lecerf, J.-M., Dépeint, F., Clerc, E., Dugenet, Y., Niamba, C. N., Rhazi, L., et al. (2012). Xylo-oligosaccharide (XOS) in combination with inulin modulates both the intestinal environment and immune status in healthy subjects, while XOS alone only shows prebiotic properties. *British Journal of Nutrition*, *108*(10), 1847–1858. doi:10.1017/S0007114511007252

221. Bouhnik, Y., Flourié, B., D'Agay-Abensour, L., Pochart, P., Gramet, G., Durand, M., & Rambaud, J. C. (1997). Administration of transgalacto-oligosaccharides increases fecal bifidobacteria and modifies colonic fermentation metabolism in healthy humans. *The Journal of Nutrition*, *127*(3), 444–448.

222. Pourghassem Gargari, B., Dehghan, P., Aliasgharzadeh, A., & Asghari Jafar-abadi, M. (2013). Effects of High Performance Inulin Supplementation on Glycemic Control and Antioxidant Status in Women with Type 2 Diabetes. *Diabetes & Metabolism Journal*, *37*(2), 140. doi:10.4093/dmj.2013.37.2.140

223. Russo, F., Linsalata, M., Clemente, C., Chiloiro, M., Orlando, A., Marconi, E., et al. (2012). Inulin-enriched pasta improves intestinal permeability and modifies the circulating levels of zonulin and glucagon-like peptide 2 in healthy young volunteers. *Nutrition Research*, *32*(12), 940–946. doi:10.1016/j.nutres.2012.09.010

INDEX

11beta-hydroxysteroid dehydrogenase type 1 (11beta-HSD1), 53

Made in the USA
Lexington, KY
08 March 2015